Pharmacy and Medicine in Ancient Egypt

Proceedings of the conferences held in Cairo (2007) and Manchester (2008)

Edited by

Jenefer Cockitt
Rosalie David

BAR International Series 2141
2010

Published in 2016 by
BAR Publishing, Oxford

BAR International Series 2141

Pharmacy and Medicine in Ancient Egypt

ISBN 978 1 4073 0682 7

BAR Publishing is the trading name of British Archaeological Reports (Oxford) Ltd. British Archaeological Reports was first incorporated in 1974 to publish the BAR Series, International and British. In 1992 Hadrian Books Ltd became part of the BAR group. This volume was originally published by Archaeopress in conjunction with British Archaeological Reports (Oxford) Ltd / Hadrian Books Ltd, the Series principal publisher, in 2010. This present volume is published by BAR Publishing, 2016.

Printed in England

BAR
PUBLISHING

BAR titles are available from:

BAR Publishing
122 Banbury Rd, Oxford, OX2 7BP, UK
EMAIL info@barpublishing.com
PHONE +44 (0)1865 310431
FAX +44 (0)1865 316916
www.barpublishing.com

THESE PROCEEDINGS ARE DEDICATED TO THE MEMORY OF OUR DEAR FRIENDS AND ESTEEMED COLLEAGUES AT THE NATIONAL RESEARCH CENTRE, CAIRO:

PROFESSOR FAWZIA HELMY HUSSIEN, PHD
AND
DR ALI EL-SAWAF

PREFACE AND ACKNOWLEDGMENTS

This monograph comprises the *Proceedings of The Pharmacy and Medicine in Ancient Egypt Conferences*, jointly organised by The University of Manchester, Britain, and the National Research Centre, Cairo, Egypt, and held at The National Research Centre (March 19-21, 2007) and The University of Manchester (September 1-3, 2008).

The conferences and *Proceedings* are one aspect of a major research programme, *Pharmacy in Ancient Egypt* that has been funded by a Research Grant (2006-2009) from the Leverhulme Trust (UK). The conferences have provided an opportunity to present new research in this field, and these findings now form the basis of this publication.

The conferences were attended by delegates from Germany, Hungary, Portugal, Romania, Spain, South Africa, and the United States of America, as well as Egypt and Britain. The delegates ranged from senior scientists and scholars based at universities and museums, through to early career researchers and postgraduate students. Lectures and poster presentations included a wide range of topics within the conference subject area, and there was coverage of the research in the local, national and international media. The conferences were opened, in Cairo, by the President of the National Research Centre, Professor Dr Hany El-Nazer, and, in Manchester, by the President and Vice-Chancellor of the University of Manchester, Professor Alan Gilbert. The Manchester conference was attended by Professor Maisa Farid, the Cultural Counsellor and Director of the Cultural Centre and Educational Bureau of the Embassy of the Arab Republic of Egypt, London.

We should like to thank the following for their support and encouragement for this international collaboration:

The University of Manchester and the National Research Centre; The K. N. Hinckley Charitable Trust; The Leverhulme Trust; The British Academy; The British Council in Cairo; Mr J. H. Davidson.

The City of Manchester and the Lord Mayor of the City of Manchester, Councillor Mavis Smitheman, who hosted a Civic Reception at the Town Hall for conference delegates.

Dr N. Merriman, Director of the Manchester Museum, who hosted a Conference Reception at the Museum; Dr Ann Young, John Rylands University Library, Manchester, who facilitated visits to the Library's special collections for the delegates; Professor Essam Abdelrazek of the University of Alexandria, Egypt, for support in liaising between the University of Manchester and the Egyptian delegates who attended the Manchester conference.

We should like to thank Miss Kay Hinckley and Miss Ann Gibson who provided considerable help and support throughout the planning of the Manchester conference; and the staff and students of the KNH Centre for Biomedical Egyptology, University of Manchester, for their dedicated assistance throughout the conference.

The research undertaken for the *Pharmacy in Ancient Egypt* project has received considerable international support which we should like to acknowledge here:

The Agricultural Museum, Cairo; the British Museum, London; the Royal Botanic Gardens, Kew, Britain; Cairo University; the Chelsea Physic Garden, London; the Egyptian Museum, Cairo; Hall Analytical Laboratories, Manchester; the Petrie Museum of Egyptian Archaeology, University College London; and the South Sinai Environmental Agency (Conservation and Sustainable Use of Medicinal Plants in Arid and Semi-Arid Ecosystems in Egypt).

With regard to the *Proceedings*, the editors would like to express their gratitude to the publishers The Egypt Exploration Society, London, and *Ancient Egypt* magazine for support towards this publication and Ryan Metcalfe and Angela Thomas of the KNH Centre for Biomedical Egyptology, University of Manchester, for their help with the manuscript.

Finally, we should like to thank the delegates who participated in these conferences; it is their important research that has made this publication possible.

Jenefer Cockitt and Rosalie David

The KNH Centre for Biomedical Egyptology, The University of Manchester

May, 2010

CONTENTS

THE 'PHARMACY IN ANCIENT EGYPT PROJECT' AT THE KNH CENTRE FOR BIOMEDICAL EGYPTOLOGY

A.R. David

KNH Centre for Biomedical Egyptology, University of Manchester, UK

Abstract: *Over the past thirty years, the Manchester Egyptian Mummy Research Project at The University of Manchester (UK) has pioneered and developed a multidisciplinary scientific approach, using a range of diagnostic tools, in order to investigate and identify disease in ancient Egyptian mummies.*

The Pharmacy in Ancient Egypt Project has extended this combined historical and scientific methodology to investigate the potential therapeutic regimes used by the Egyptians, many of which are listed in the ancient medical papyri. Although previous research has been undertaken on these texts, and there have been specific botanical studies of ancient Egyptian plants, this project is innovative in that it adopts a multidisciplinary approach. Historical and scientific analytical methods are being used to study the literary accounts, investigate plant and inorganic remains from Egypt, and identify in the mummified tissue any traces of pharmaceutical intervention, in order to determine the accuracy and therapeutic efficacy of these treatments.

This three-year study, supported by a Research Grant from The Leverhulme Trust (UK), has unprecedented access to collections of modern and ancient plants in Britain and Egypt, as well as samples of mummified tissue held in the International Ancient Egyptian Mummy Tissue Bank at the University of Manchester. The Project also draws on the expertise of a wide range of scientists and scholars. In particular, it is supported by partnerships between the KNH Centre for Biomedical Egyptology and the National Research Centre in Cairo, and the South Sinai Environmental Agency (Conservation and Sustainable Use of Medicinal Plants in Arid and Semi-Arid Ecosystems in Egypt).

This paper outlines the Project's structure, major aspects of the research, and its potential to change our perception of ancient Egyptian pharmacy and its place in the world history of pharmacy and medicine.

Key words: Egyptology, mummies, palaeopathology, archaeobotany, pharmacy

Introduction

Academic interest in Egyptian mummies dates back to the Renaissance when antiquarian collectors began to bring them out of Egypt to form, together with other antiquities, the nuclei of growing Egyptology collections owned by museums, learned societies and wealthy individuals in Britain, Europe and, later, the United States of America. From the sixteenth century onwards, it became fashionable to 'unroll' (unwrap) mummies: some of these events were watched by invited audiences, and although most were frivolous occasions that preserved little of scientific value and destroyed important evidence, a few were carried out by serious investigators who published their results. Such accounts can still provide valuable information, and in some cases (Osburn 1825), they have been used as the basis for current studies (David and Tapp 1992).

Unrollings had been largely discontinued by the mid-nineteenth century, but a new approach to examining mummified remains emerged in the early twentieth century, exemplified by Dr Margaret Murray's pioneering work at the University of Manchester. In 1908, she undertook one of the earliest scientific investigations of Egyptian mummies when, with her interdisciplinary team of specialists in anatomy, chemical analysis and textile studies, she unwrapped, autopsied and subsequently investigated the mummies and goods from the Middle Kingdom (c.1900 BC) tomb of two brothers excavated at Deir Rifeh. The published results (Murray 1910) again formed the basis for later studies (David 2007).

In 1973, a new pioneering study was initiated at Manchester when the Manchester Egyptian Mummy Project was established to examine all the Egyptian mummified remains in the Manchester Museum; this was later extended to include mummies from other collections (David 1997). Since then, an interdisciplinary team of scientists, drawn from the university, associated teaching hospitals and other institutions, has pursued the Project's main aims: to establish and develop a methodology for examining mummified remains; and to use biomedical and scientific techniques to increase knowledge about disease, diet, lifestyle, medical treatment, and religious beliefs and practices in ancient Egypt (David 1979). Working together continuously since 1973, this has become the longest established team project in palaeopathology.

A major development of the Manchester Project's work was the establishment, in 2003, of a university specialisation in Biomedical Egyptology which would have access to state-of-the-art bioscience facilities and the world's major bio-repository of ancient Egyptian tissues; together, these would provide unparalleled resources for research and training young scientists in this new field. The KNH Centre for Biomedical Egyptology, opened in 2003 by HRH The Earl of Wessex, is situated in the University of Manchester's Faculty of Life Sciences. As the new location for the Manchester Mummy Project, it is a unique university facility where Egyptology is pursued from the standpoint of bioscience. The Centre's main focus is to promote an interdisciplinary approach that combines historical and scientific methodology to research disease, medical treatments, lifestyle and mummification techniques in ancient Egypt. Teaching and research focus particularly on the use and development of a range of diagnostic tools that include radiology, histology, immunology, analytical methods and molecular techniques.

The KNH Centre has access to considerable scientific resources: in addition to the bio-science, radiological and analytical facilities available in Europe's largest Faculty of Life Sciences and other university departments and teaching hospitals, the Centre has its own dedicated laboratories and collections of human and plant remains. It houses the Ancient Bio-Repository, a unique resource that contains the International Ancient Egyptian Mummy Tissue Bank (IAEMTB) and the Grafton Elliot Smith anatomical collection. The IAEMTB, which holds over 1,500 samples of tissue, bone and hair samples from Egyptian mummies housed in collections around the world, was initially established through funding provided by a research grant from The Leverhulme Trust, and provides a unique resource for ongoing research and teaching (Lambert-Zazulak 2000). The Manchester Museum, a university department with one of Britain's outstanding Egyptology collections, holds human and animal mummies and associated funerary artefacts which provide an important resource for the KNH Centre's research and teaching activities.

Until the mid-1900s, Manchester's palaeopathological studies focused on investigating individual mummies or specific groups of human remains, usually held in museums, but in 1995, the researchers were invited to participate in the first major epidemiological project on disease in Egypt to cover a 5,000 year time-span, tracing the pattern of a parasitic disease, schistosomiasis, from ancient to modern times (Contis and David 1996). Major achievements of the Schistosomiasis in Ancient Egypt Project include the innovative development and application of immunocytochemistry as a diagnostic tool to identify disease in mummies, and the first identification of parasite (schistosome) aDNA in mummified remains (Rutherford 1999).

The Pharmacy in Ancient Egypt Project

The innovative, multidisciplinary 'Manchester Methodology', that combines historical and scientific approaches and was developed for disease studies on mummies (David 2008a), was extended in 2005 to investigate ancient Egyptian pharmacy, and to confirm if, alongside an at least partially science-based medical system, the Egyptians also had plant-based treatments that were therapeutically viable. The support of a Research Grant (2006-2009) from The Leverhulme Trust has enabled this project to appoint a specialist team to undertake the research, facilitate exchange visits between partners in Britain and Egypt, and organise two conferences (Cairo, 2007 and Manchester, 2008) on the themes of pharmacy and medicine in ancient Egypt.

Previous Studies

The most important literary source of ancient Egyptian pharmaceutical ingredients and therapeutic regimes are the Egyptian Medical Papyri; in addition, ancient plant remains have been recovered from funerary and domestic contexts in Egypt. Previously, both these sources have been studied separately, resulting in translations of the medical papyri and botanical surveys of the ancient and contemporary plants in Egypt.

Overview of the Research Plan

The current project is innovative however because it combines historical and scientific methods to investigate and identify the plants and inorganic remains employed in ancient Egyptian pharmacy. This involves not only study of the ancient literary accounts, but also analyses of the archaeobotanical and contemporary plant remains.

A pilot scheme carried out at Manchester by J.M. Campbell provided the basis for some of this research. This study focused on more than 1,000 prescriptions contained in four Medical Papyri; 379 drug substances were analysed and formatted in the style of the British National Formulary, detailing their active ingredients and therapeutic efficacy. A comparison of the compounding and administration of these prescriptions with contemporary pharmacy demonstrated that over two-thirds of the identified substances used by the ancient Egyptians remained in use in the twentieth century AD.

The current research has extended this identification of plants used in ancient Egyptian pharmacy. It has also sought to locate their geographical places of origin and associated trade routes; determine any traces of these pharmaceutical treatments that might remain in mummified tissue; confirm or revise existing translations of the Medical Papyri; assess the accuracy and therapeutic efficacy of these treatments; and examine the hypothesis that the ancient Egyptians practised pharmacy long before the Greeks. In general, the project provides a unique opportunity to use scientific analytical methods to assess the validity of the literary evidence.

Scientific Support and Collaboration

The project involves an international, interdisciplinary group of scientists: researchers include Egyptologists, botanists, palaeobotanists, earth scientists, pharmacists, pathologists, molecular scientists and chemists. The study has benefited from unprecedented access to the International Ancient Egyptian Tissue Bank, collections of modern and ancient plants in Britain and Egypt, and analytical facilities. Apart from the host institution, the University of Manchester, support and collaboration have been provided by Hall Analytical Laboratories, Manchester (UK); Cairo University; the Egyptian Museum and the Agricultural Museum in Cairo; in London, the British Museum, the Petrie Museum of Egyptian Archaeology, and Chelsea Physic Garden; and the Royal Botanic Gardens, Kew. A particularly important collaboration, based on a formal partnership established in 2004 between Manchester and the National Research Centre, Cairo, enabled the two institutions to become joint hosts for the Cairo and Manchester conferences on ancient pharmacy. Co-operation with the Medicinal Plant Conservation Project in Sinai (El-Demerdash 2008) has facilitated comparative studies on ancient Egyptian and modern traditional pharmaceutical regimes.

Over the period of the Project, KNH researchers and colleagues in Egypt have benefited from exchanges that have greatly facilitated the work, enabling collections to be studied, sites of special relevance to be visited, and important links to be forged.

The project has also facilitated the establishment of a new research resource. A Palaeopharmacognosy Bank, located in the Ancient Bio-Repository in the KNH Centre, contains contemporary and herbarium plant material and digital records of plant specimens used in Egyptian medicine. This collection will preserve fragile evidence, make data internationally available, and provide a benchmark for future archaeobotanical study.

The Contribution of Ancient Egyptian Pharmacy

The accuracy of earlier translations of the pharmaceutical ingredients in the Medical Papyri has been tested (Campbell and David 2010). This is important because the translations of some 30% of these ingredients are disputed. Translators rely heavily on the context of a word in order to infer its meaning, and usually a word will occur in a variety of contexts in Egyptian texts. However, many of the words for plants and minerals found in the Medical Papyri do not appear elsewhere, and thus early translators were obliged to make educated guesses as to meaning, often seeking an ingredient in contemporary pharmacopoeia that had the same medicinal use and was best fitted to the description.

The current project has analysed the ingredients in the prescriptions, and checked if the plant ingredients (as identified in existing translations) grew or were traded in Egypt when the text was written, and if the named ingredients would have worked in the way the prescription indicated. If the translated name did not meet these criteria, then alternative identifications of plant names have been sought.

Since the papyri are specific enough (providing all the necessary information - ingredients, method of preparation and dosage) to allow reproducibility, it has been possible to reproduce the prescriptions, investigate their effectiveness, and compare them with modern remedies. This has confirmed that, although the Egyptians were usually ignorant of causes and focused on symptoms, a considerable proportion of their treatments had a therapeutic value on a par with drugs used in conventional medicine in the last fifty years. It has also been possible to assess the similarities and differences between modern traditional medicine and the therapies recorded in the papyri, through collaboration with the Medicinal Plant Conservation Project in Sinai. Established in St Katherine's Protectorate in 2002, this project is conserving local, globally significant species that have medicinal properties; there is considerable involvement of the local Bedouin population whose knowledge is vital in identifying plants that are medicinally useful. This rare combination of Egyptological and ethnographic studies is important in helping to identify the existence of any similarities and routes of transmission that might demonstrate a continuous pharmaceutical tradition from ancient to modern times.

Evidence provided by reassessing the papyri contradicts the widely held scholarly belief that ancient Egyptian treatments were mainly 'magical' or 'non-rational' (David 2004); although some drugs had only a placebo effect, and prayers and incantations played an important role, there is now well-attested evidence that 'rational' treatments were predominant (David 2008b). The recent studies also confirm that the Egyptians had a valid and effective pharmaceutical tradition that pre-dates the Greek system, usually accredited as the source of modern pharmacy, by over 1,500 years. However, whereas the Greeks have left a vast legacy of medical texts which can be readily translated, only twelve Egyptian medical papyri have been discovered to date, and these contain many doubtful translations.

The research has also demonstrated that, although there is no evidence that the Egyptians had a pharmacopoeia (Campbell 2007), the papyrus prescriptions fulfil the role of a formulary, with the plausible identification of ingredients from plant, animal and mineral sources.

Molecular Methods for Studying Ancient Pharmacy

The innovative application of DNA analysis in the field of ancient pharmaceutical research has the potential to provide a variety of useful data (Metcalfe 2010). Experiments are being pursued to determine which plants are most promising for DNA analysis, which, combined with evidence from pharmacognitive research and palaeobotany, may help to identify the plant ingredients found in remedies in the Medical Papyri, and possibly in mummified remains.

An experimental model has been prepared to study DNA degradation in charred plant remains and to determine the best extraction method to use on similar samples. This will provide the basis and guide for extraction of DNA from ancient remains.

Because there are often technical difficulties associated with ancient DNA analysis, and it is a process that involves the destruction of irreplaceable ancient samples, it was decided to first develop and carry out tests on models, so that the resultant data could be analysed and used to guide sample selection for future research.

Sourcing the Pharmaceutical Ingredients

The identification of the geographical sources of some of the ingredients used medicinally as internal or topical treatments has also been pursued (Seath 2008). Although Egypt itself provided many of the pharmaceutical ingredients, such as plants from its agricultural industry, animal products from husbandry and hunting, and mineral products from mining, smelting and building, other ingredients (for example, frankincense, cedar and coriander) undoubtedly originated in trade between Egypt and her neighbours in the Near East, North Africa, Nubia, and the southern Mediterranean.

Once again, an interdisciplinary approach has been adopted. An analytical investigation was undertaken of resins and unguents found in predynastic graves in Egypt, to attempt to relate them to their geographical sources and to examine evidence linking trade networks to Egypt at this period.

A sample cohort was selected from material provided by museums in Britain. Because this material is a finite and limited resource, it was essential to utilise analytical techniques that are minimally invasive. By including visible light microscopy, environmental scanning electron microscopy, and Fourier transform infrared spectroscopy, it has been possible to characterise and identify unguents such as mineral waxes and resins.

This investigation has demonstrated that these graves contained a wide range of organic materials, some of which occur much later as pharmaceutical ingredients in the Medical Papyri, and that, as early as the Fourth and Third millennia BC, there was already an active trade in these commodities between Egypt and the Near East.

Reporting the Results

This ongoing project has generated widespread interest in the local, national and international media (Pain 2007), and is already the subject of several academic publications. Members of the team have given lectures to academic and lay audiences, and the subject is now included in university graduate courses. It was also the focus of a joint annual workshop held at the National Research Centre, Cairo, for staff and students from both institutions.

The research and results have been reported at two conferences, jointly organised by the KNH Centre and the National Research Centre and supported by funding from The Leverhulme Trust, The British Academy and The British Council in Cairo. The first, 'Pharmacy in Ancient Egypt', was held at the National Research Centre (March 19-22, 2007), and the second, 'Pharmacy and Medicine in Ancient Egypt', was hosted by the University of Manchester (September 1-3, 2008). This current publication of the Proceedings includes a selection of papers presented at both conferences.

Conclusion

Although pharmacy was probably not pursued as an independent profession in ancient Egypt, there is now considerable evidence that, from early times, their practitioners had professional standards and protocols, and that some medicinal ingredients were imported into Egypt through active trade routes. Generally, the results to date indicate that this research has the potential to revolutionise our knowledge and understanding of ancient Egyptian pharmacy, and to make a contribution not only to the subject area of Egyptology but also to the wider history of medicine and pharmacy.

Acknowledgements

The KNH Centre would like to thank the many academic colleagues in Egypt and Britain for their help and support, and to acknowledge our gratitude for the substantial financial contribution made to this project by: The Leverhulme Trust, KNHCT, The British Academy, The British Council in Cairo, Hall Analytical Laboratories and Mr J.H. Davidson.

References

Campbell, J.M. (2007) Pharaohs and the first prescriptions. *The Pharmaceutical Journal* 279 (7483), pp. 735-737.

Campbell, J.M. and David, A.R. (2010) The Application of Archaeobotany, Phytogeography and Pharmacognosy to Confirm the Pharmacopoeia of Ancient Egypt, 1850-1200 BC, In Cockitt, J. and David, A.R. (eds.) *Proceedings of the 'Pharmacy and Medicine in Ancient Egypt' Conferences, Cairo (2007) and Manchester (2008).* BAR Publishing, pp. 20-29.

Contis, G. and David, A.R. (1996) The Epidemiology of Bilharzia in ancient Egypt: 5000 years of schistosomiasis. *Parasitology Today* 12 (7), pp. 253-255.

David, A.R. (1979) *The Manchester Museum Mummy Project: Multidisciplinary Research on Ancient Egyptian Mummified Remains.* Manchester Museum.

David, A.R. and Tapp, E. (eds.) (1992) *The Mummy's Tale. The Scientific and Medical Investigation of Natsef-Amun, Priest in the Temple of Karnak.* Michael O'Mara Books Limited.

David, A.R. (1997) Disease in Egyptian mummies: the contribution of new technologies. *The Lancet* 349, pp. 1760-1763.

David, A.R. (2004) Rationality versus irrationality in Egyptian medicine in the Pharaonic and Graeco-Roman Periods, in Horstmanhoff, H.F.J. and Stol, M. (eds.) *Magic and Rationality in Ancient Egyptian, Near Eastern and Graeco-Roman Medicine.* Brill.

David, R. (2007) *The Two Brothers. Death and the Afterlife in Middle Kingdom Egypt*. Rutherford Press Limited.

David, R. (ed.) (2008a) *Egyptian Mummies and Modern Science*. Cambridge University Press.

David, R. (2008b) The art of healing in ancient Egypt: a scientific appraisal. *The Lancet* 372, pp. 1802-1803.

El-Demerdash, M.A. (2008) The Conservation and Sustainable Use of Globally Significant Medicinal Plant Biodiversity in St. Katherine's Protectorate (Sinai, Egypt). *The Pharmacy and Medicine in Ancient Egypt Conference, Manchester (2008).* Abstract.

Lambert-Zazulak, P. (2000) The International Ancient Egyptian Mummy Tissue Bank at the Manchester Museum. *Antiquity* 74, pp. 44-48.

Metcalfe, R. (2010) Molecular Methods for the Study of Ancient Pharmacy, in Cockitt, J. and David, A.R. (eds.) *Proceedings of the 'Pharmacy and Medicine in Ancient Egypt' Conferences, Cairo (2007) and Manchester (2008)*. BAR Publishing, pp. 110-112.

Murray, M.A. (1910) *The Tomb of Two Brothers.* Sherratt and Hughes.

Osburn, W. (1828) *An Account of an Egyptian Mummy presented to the Museum of the Leeds Philosophical and Literary Society by the late John Blayds, Esq.* Leeds Philosophical and Literary Society.

Pain, S. (2007) The Pharaohs' Pharmacists. *New Scientist* 196, (2634), pp. 40-43.

Rutherford, P. (1999) Immunocytochemistry and the diagnosis of schistosomiasis; ancient and modern. *Parasitology Today* 15, (9), pp. 390-391.

Seath, J. (2008) Preliminary Study of Predynastic Period Unguents to Identify Medicinal Plant Origin and Identity. *The Pharmacy and Medicine in Ancient Egypt Conference, Manchester (2008).* Abstract.

COMPLEMENTARY MEDICINE IN ANCIENT AND MODERN EGYPT

R. Baligh

Mansoura University, Mansoura, Egypt

Abstract: *Ancient Egyptian Medicine depended on a number of factors. It has long been known that the ancient Egyptians were advanced in medicine and practised certain kinds of surgery such as skull surgery and setting bones. They were also famous for having the first specialists in a certain area of medicine such as ophthalmology. Dentistry was also practised as a branch of medicine. In addition to conventional medicine, the ancient Egyptians practised a number of complementary treatments such as herbal medicine, aromatherapy and had knowledge of essential oils and flower remedies. Natural treatments were employed, such as balanced diet and exercise, hydrotherapy, and some aspects of homeopathy, as were stress management techniques and body work techniques such as massage and reflexology. Classical writers had mentioned that the famous hospital in Memphis established by Imhotep included treatment with unconventional techniques such as colour therapy, music therapy, and aromatherapy. At the time, those therapies were strange enough to merit commenting about them and were clearly considered unusual. It also appears that the physicians prepared their own remedies, but there is reference in a text that a person who prepares the remedies, meaning a pharmacist, missed certain days of work. Ancient Egyptian medicine also included certain aspects of traditional treatments such as incantations and religious words. Nowadays in Egypt, many people are using Islamic or prophet Mohamed's treatments which depend on incantations of verses of the Quran while moving the hands over a person, using honey as a remedy and creating a vacuum over infected areas known as al-hagamah. Certain of these methods were used in ancient Egypt, such as the use of honey and religious incantations.*

Key words: Alternative, complementary, medicine, pharmacy, ancient Egypt, reflexology, aromatherapy, massage, homeopathy, diet, Islamic medicine.

Introduction

This paper will be touching on both medicine and pharmacy. The term complementary medicine is one which is preferable to alternative medicine, a more common term. The word alternative or complementary 'medicine' itself has given the syndicate of medical doctors and the Ministry of Health in Egypt the right to prevent many practitioners of complementary treatments from obtaining a licence to practise those kinds of 'medicine' without an official medical degree from one of the recognized or accredited faculties of medicine in universities. It is therefore best to refer to them as Complementary Treatments or Therapies while the medicines should be best referred to as Complementary Remedies. The term 'complementary' also refers to something completing another. The term complementary treatments or therapies includes but is not limited to the following: herbal medicine, aromatherapy, acupuncture, reike, jin chin jitsu, reflexology, massage, and meditation to name but a few.

Alternative or Complementary Medicine

Alternative or complementary medicine in present day Egypt known in Arabic as '*al-.tibb al-bad-il*' has become a subject for serious debate in recent years. This is part of a world-wide movement where people have started to realize that modern medicine has severe limitations and does not offer all it is supposed to offer in terms of reducing pain and suffering and offering fast relief from symptoms. To the contrary, it usually offers a lengthy process where relief and medical treatment for the masses is not all it should be. The higher classes usually go for private health care or seek treatment outside the country. Egypt was a pioneering nation in medicine and there was even a system of health care for workers as far back as the Old Kingdom and the age of pyramid building (ca. 2460 BC) (Hawass 2006, 167-8, 172-3). Other countries are now starting to embrace certain aspects of ancient Egyptian medicine while the Egyptians themselves remain largely ignorant of their fine medical heritage and seek other forms such as western medicine since they are very influenced and impressed by the advancement of the west.

Pharmacy

It is thought that the medical knowledge of the Egyptians started in the prehistoric era and went through trial and error before it was recorded in a number of papyri around the New Kingdom (Kahun, Edwin Smith, Ebers, Hearst, Berlin, Chester Beatty, London, Carlsberg (Stetter 1993, 29-34)). Other references include Junkers, Leiden and Westcar (Ghalioungui 1958, 16-17).

The Materia Medica of the ancient Egyptians included plant, animal and mineral remedies. They also used substances which are considered poisonous or harmful such as snake venom, poisonous plant extracts such as hemlock, aconite and opium, in addition to heavy metals such as lead and antimony, human or animal excrement and urine. There is reference on an ostracon from the 19th Dynasty from Deir el Medina in the British Museum, no. BM 5634, which mentions that a certain Paher Pedjef did not come on certain days. That would make this the first pharmacist known by name from ancient Egypt (Nunn 1996, 132). Herbalists were considered the earliest pharmacists in ancient Egypt (Gabra 1960, 13).

Magic

Magic is the ability to cause things to happen by the power of the spoken word, or through utilizing a certain cosmic energy. Both magic and religion depend on blind faith since you cannot see with your eyes how something comes to happen. In ancient Egypt, society was still going through the phase when magic, religion and medicine were all interrelated (Ghalioungui 1958, 11-12). The power of the written word and incantations can be seen through the system of the Horus cippi. These were stone stelae from the Late and Graeco-Roman periods which had raised reliefs of Harpocrates or Horus the Child holding snakes and scorpions. People who were stung by either kind were treated by drinking water which was poured over the shapes and words on the cippus, and then caught in a small crucible. Coffin Text no. 341 implies that the system of dissolving words in water then drinking the water was in practice. '*This spell should be spoken over seven sacred eyes in writing: to be washed in beer and natron and to be drunk by the man.*' (Faulkner 1973, 276; Ritner 2001, 325 - variation in translation). The Pyramid Texts nos. 273-274 have some cannibalistic references which indicate that eating enemies adds their intelligence to the one who devours (Faulkner 1969, 80-84).

Treatment for stings is one of the oldest forms of magic in ancient Egypt as we can see from Pyramid Texts nos.: 226-244, 276-299, 314, 375-399, 499-500, 501, 538, etc. (Faulkner 1969, 53-206; Halioua 2004, 158-9; Gayyar 1996, 72-3). The Ebers Medical papyrus has around 875-77 general prescriptions, 47 diagnoses and spells (Halioua 2004, 218-9), and 17 spells and two pieces of advice on giving birth which may be considered magical, while a diseased heart is said to be because of the evil breath and the actions of a lector priest (Nunn 1996, 30-4; 98-9). In Coffin Texts no. 81, the person is supposed to lick the prescription written on his hand, 'to be recited over eight chaos gods inscribed with yellow pigment and Nubian ochre on the hand of the man, to be rinsed off every day very early' (Faulkner 1973, 87). Traditional magic /medicine in the Egyptian countryside still depends on curing a person by writing the prescription using an ink made out of rose water and saffron, then dissolving the writing in water, and drinking it or bathing with it.

Other forms of magic in medicine included magical semi-circular ivory or bone wands associated with women and childbirth, fertility dolls, paper dolls which receive pin incisions and are burnt to save a patient from the evil eye, and knives which were brandished in a certain way to keep away evil. Egyptian kings are often shown with something in their hands resembling rods. In the present day, certain wands are sold over the Internet which are said to have the healing properties of the ancient Egyptian rods, although the rods were thought to be amuletic, rather than therapeutic.

Herbal Remedies

Herbal remedies are probably the widest known and were used by ancient and modern societies. The Egyptians used plants in treatment whether by brewing them and drinking their teas, eating them, or applying them locally-in addition to extracting aromatherapy extracts from them such as essential oils (Manniche 2006, 64-5; Manniche 1999, 7-9; 133-25). They also used all the different parts of the plant depending on the condition. In the Ebers papyrus there is a long list of different plants and their medical uses. Opium, called '*shepen*', was used as a remedy as was *Hashish* or *Cannabis sativa*, known as '*shemshemet*,' (Nunn 1996, 155-156), the lotus and the willow tree which were used to reduce pain (Nunn, 1996, 146). In fact, the use of the lotus so commonly appears, especially in tomb scenes, it has led to studies which proved that the lotus had a number of excellent health benefits, including increased virility (Manniche 1999, 97-100). Some spices with therapeutic effects were coriander, which was found in the tomb of Tutankhamun, cinnamon, and oregano. Fruits used by the ancient Egyptians in treatment included dates, figs, *doum* from special palm trees, grapes, olives and apples. Vegetables included onions, leeks, lettuce, celery and radishes. Seeds included lentils and lupins (Nunn 1996, 14-15).

Aromatherapy

This line of complementary medicine is based on the healing properties of certain aromas derived from different sources. The Egyptians used a variety of essential oils and aromatic fatty substances. Acacia oil was used to 'take the blood to the heart and spread it' according to Papyrus Berlin no. 3038 (Manniche 1999, 114). A warm piece of cloth with the oil is applied locally. Other examples include the use of basil, celery and daisies (Manniche 2006, 136; 82-3). Cumin was called '*tepnen*' and was used for several ailments (Manniche 2006, 102-4). Perfumed oils and fats were used often in festivals such as the Beautiful Feast of the Valley. The lotus flower had a special position and was depicted very often in funerary scenes. It appears to have had a role in rejuvenation. The lotus was also used a lot in treating ailments such as fever. The patient would be placed in a warm room to allow him to sweat heavily. His body would then be anointed with lotus oil and placed in a lukewarm bath (Manniche 1999, 121).

Reflexology

Certain tomb scenes tell us that the ancient Egyptians knew the art of reflexology. This therapy depends on pressing and coaxing certain zones in the soles of the feet, the palms of the hands, and the ears, which in turn affect the whole body including the internal organs. The tomb of Ankhmahor and Khentika from the 6th Dynasty in Saqqara has a scene with men applying a massage to the hands and feet of others with a certain therapeutic effect. The scene reads 'Make those sweet dear.' The man holding the foot says 'I shall work for thy praise.' In another scene, it reads 'Cause the giving of strength to these'. This shows that the ancient Egyptians believed that the massaging of the hands and feet had a therapeutic healing effect (Nunn 1996, 133).

Precious Stones

The ancient Egyptians knew the therapeutic effect of many gems. Lapis lazuli had a very good reputation and was called *tfrr* and *khesbed ma`*. It was known to purify the soul and keep the mind away from worldly troubles. It was brought from Asia and was used abundantly by the pharaohs, especially in the New Kingdom. Tuthmosis III received a gift of good lapis lazuli from Babylon (The New Guide to Remedies 2002, 163), and another from Assyria (Saleh 2006, 234) (*Urk.* IV, 668, 13 and 6). The famous boy king Tutankhamun also had several jewellery items with lapis lazuli.

Music Therapy

Certain Greek writers had reported that the Academy of Imhotep, attached to the famous temple of Ptah, was run by priest scientists, and used unorthodox methods of treatment such as music, colours, olfactory remedies, and herbs (Personal archive of Dr. Sayyid Karim 1985). Musical groups used to play for treatment in certain places such as the temple of Abydos. They were present in most medical centres for that reason (Youssef 1999, 31). Imhotep was the architect of the Step Pyramid Complex of King Zoser, Dynasty 3. He was worshipped as a god of medicine from around 2850 BC to 525 BC.

Colour Therapy

A study about colour symbolism in ancient Egypt touches on this issue. White was considered a colour indicating purity and clarity like the day (El-Rashiedy, 2004, 217) and was also associated with children and new beginnings. Present day Egyptians use colour in treatment by dressing a measles patient in red, covering him with a red blanket and leaving him in a red light. Jaundice patients are dressed in yellow in some parts of the countryside. The effect of colour on the psychological condition and energy is common knowledge, hence the use of black as a mourning colour, white as a wedding colour, and bright and vivid colours for festivals, for children and to improve a person's morality which is a kind of psychological treatment.

Directions and Energy Fields

People who use the pendulum today say that the ancient Egyptians knew about the flow of cosmic energy and designed and located their monuments according to these unseen energy paths. Certain objects in the Egyptian Museum in Cairo may have been used as pendulums in the past, such as JE 51045, a brown stone, and JE 40353, a grey one. They are in Room 34 in the Museum in Tahrir Square. The Egyptian engineer Ibrahim Karim has formulated a theory known as biogeometry which concentrates on this issue of energy fields. According to founder Dr Ibrahim Karim, 'biogeometry is a powerful science which shows how to use shapes, patterns, colours, sounds and motion to create specific energy effects. It clearly identifies core principles as well as providing a wide range of practical techniques.' (http://www.rexresearch.com/biogeom/biogeom.htm).

Pyramid Shape

Several modern day Egyptians believe in the medicinal properties of the pyramids. Some reproduce pyramidal shapes from substances such as wood or cardboard, and place water underneath them to become energized and then use the water in treatment (Schul 1983, 112). The people who use this technique today insist that the pyramid has to be made in the exact proportions of the Great Pyramid of Cheops or Khufu in Giza. The water needs to be placed in the centre of the hollow pyramid for at least a week before drinking it, bathing with it, or sprinkling the house with the positively energized water. Many people believe the pyramids were not just tombs and were not located haphazardly throughout Egypt. They think they had an important function to establish harmony and positive energy within a certain area.

Homeopathy

Homeopathy is a system of medical treatment or complementary therapy which was developed by the German physician/chemist Samuel Hahnemann around 1800 AD. It depends on treatment with natural substances which, if taken in very small quantities, cause the same symptoms as the medical condition they are to treat. The root of the word 'homeo' means similar and is based on the theory that 'like cures like' (Gemmell 1997, 3). Preparation of the homeopathic remedies depends on succussion and extraction of the very essence and energy of the substance, then diluting it repeatedly with the theory that the more diluted potencies are actually the more effective. The ancient Egyptians used poisonous substances in small concentrations, and human and animal excrement (Halioua 2004, 44; Gayyar 1996, 76).

Treatment with Urine

The use of urine as medicine is hardly a novelty in traditional societies. The ancient Egyptians included urine, mostly human, in prescriptions which were usually for external use. In one case mentioned in the Ramesseum papyrus 3A, 19-20, it advises that human urine be applied to the eyes (Nunn 1996, 149). In modern Egypt, Bedouin healers use the urine of small male camels to treat certain kinds of hepatitis. New controversial treatments practised in modern day Egypt include:

Bee Sting Treatment: This method depends on making live bees sting the area where there is joint or bone pain. Bee sting poison is also used in medicines sold in pharmacies.

Treatment with the back side of pigeons: Based on placing the back side of a pigeon on an infected area.

Less controversial methods include:

The Prophet's Medicine (Islamic Medicine): This system depends on a combination of methods such as the use of herbs and other natural substances such as honey, olive oil and the black seed. It also depends on reading certain verses of the holy Quran, treatment with hot pressure cups or '*hagamah*' which is performed on certain days of the Arabic month, and what is known as 'ironing' which is a treatment with fire. Fevers are treated with a combination of water and Quran verses. Due to the return to Islamic origins probably caused by the dire economic conditions, it is now used excessively in modern Egypt. Some aspects of it such as the use of honey in treatment, herbal remedies, treatment of fever with water and the recitation of certain words or verses, were also used in ancient Egypt.

Diet

The Egyptians knew the importance of proper diet. They believed that most ailments were caused by an excess of food and drink. Modern theories also place a lot of importance on diet. Egypt was a major agricultural nation and was known as the bread basket of the Roman Empire. The ideal form for beauty in ancient Egypt included a slim, well-formed body for both men and women. Most of our information about diet comes from either feasts for the dead, or offering scenes in tombs and temples. In Herodotus Book II:77, it mentions that the Egyptians ate bread and drank wine made of barley and certain kinds of fish that they ate raw, salted or dried. He mentioned that they ate quails, ducks and other kinds of birds and fish that they did not worship, as they worshipped a number of animals including fish (Nunn 1996, 19). The Egyptians also believed in clearing their bowels by getting frequent enemas up to three times a month (Kamal 1967, 114).

Cleanliness

Cleanliness and personal hygiene constitute the first step towards preventative medicine. In the so-called 'negative confession' scenes, the deceased person says in front of the gods that he did not do certain things such as 'wading in water.' This alone is proof of the understanding of the Egyptians that you must keep water clean (Kamal 1967, 339). The Egyptians used a combination of fat and sodium as coarse soap. Salt and fragrant spices were used as a mouth wash. Cleanliness to the Egyptians included shaving off bodily hair as it was considered unclean. A variety of perfumes and fragrances were used to improve body odour. Special very thin combs were used to get rid of lice in the hair. Bathrooms were known in richer houses. A traditional bathroom consisted of a hole in the ground with a foot rest on both sides. One of the earliest examples of such a bathroom comes from the palace of the pharaoh Amenhotep III in Malkata, Dynasty 18. This form of bathroom is still often used in the countryside and is called '*hammam baladi*' in Arabic. It is more hygienic than toilet seats which can transfer diseases easily.

Conclusion

The new millennium in Egypt was marked with a great interest in alternative or complementary therapies. The ancient medical knowledge of the Egyptians is now embraced by foreign nations while the Egyptians have embraced western medicine. The best situation would be one in which the most effective techniques of ancient Egyptian and other cultures are embraced and built upon. Western Medicine should be more flexible towards complementary practitioners since at the moment it is placing obstacles and almost disregarding any kind of medicine other than western medicine.

References

Faulkner, R.O. (1973) *The Ancient Egyptian Coffin Texts, vol. I: Spells 1-354*. Aris and Phillips Ltd.

Faulkner, R.O. (1969) *The Ancient Egyptian Pyramid Texts*. Clarendon Press.

Gayyar, J. and Ritter, L. (1996) *Medicine and mummification in the time of the pharaohs*. Second edition. Trans. into Arabic by Anton Zikri. Madbouli Bookstore.

Gemmell, D. (1997) *Everyday Homeopathy*, Second edition. Beaconsfield Publishers Ltd.

Ghalioungui, P. (1958) The *Medicine of the ancient Egyptians*. Dar el Maarif.

Hawass, Z. (2006) *Mountains of the pharaohs: the untold story of the pyramid builders*. The American University in Cairo Press.

Halioua, B. and Ziskind, B. (2004), *Le médicine au temps des pharaons*, 2002. Trans. by Kamal al-Sayyid. The Higher Council of Culture.

Kamal, H. (1967) *A Dictionary of Pharaonic Medicine*. The National Publication House.

Manniche, L. (1999) *Egyptian luxuries: fragrance, aromatherapy, and cosmetics in pharaonic times*. The American University in Cairo Press.

Manniche, L. (2006) *An Ancient Egyptian Herbal*. The American University in Cairo Press.

Nunn, J.F. (1996) *Ancient Egyptian Medicine*. British Museum Press.

El-Rashiedy, T.A.F.A. (2004) *Colour symbolism and their connotations in ancient Egyptian architecture and arts to the end of the New Kingdom (religious-archaeological study)*. Unpublished Masters Degree Thesis, Faculty of Archaeology, Cairo University.

Ritner, R.K. (2001) Magic: An Overview. In Redford, D.B. (ed.) *The Oxford Encyclopedia of Ancient Egypt*, Vol. 2. The American University in Cairo Press.

Saleh, A. al-A. (2006) *The Ancient Near East*, Vol. I. Anglo Egyptian Bookstore.

Schul, B. and Pettit, E. (1983) *The secret power of pyramids*, Trans. by Amin Salama. The Anglo-Egyptian Bookstore.

Stetter, C. (1993) *The Secret medicine of the pharaohs*. Quintessence Publishing.

Youssef, N.M. (1999) *Treatment with music*. Cairo.

HOW THE SUCCESS OF THE ANCIENT EGYPTIANS DEPENDED ON PLANTS

J. Bellinger

Independent Scholar

Abstract: *This paper considers the climate and seasons of Egypt and contemplates how the ancient Egyptians' effective management of the land allowed them to make a good living. The success of the Egyptian civilisation depended almost entirely upon the annual inundation of the Nile Valley down to the Delta from Neolithic times. The efficient use of this excess of water and the fertile alluvial soils brought with it were the key to their success. Brief consideration will be given to the nutrients that the alluvial soils provided which, with plentiful supplies of water, enabled the plants and trees to flourish. Some examples will be given of the plants that favour these ideal conditions and others that can survive drier areas and even brine affected areas in the Delta.*

The Middle East including Egypt is one of the most important areas of botanical diversity responsible for providing some of the world's major crops. The effect the water table can have on a plant's ability to take up water through the root system will be discussed. Most importantly, the medicinal herbs that were used to treat the wounds, diseases and infections common in ancient Egypt will be examined. Advice is given on the recognised methods of propagation and growing on before permanent planting out and general care. Finally, other applications such as use in cooking, cosmetics, perfumery and a few interesting anomalies will be highlighted.

Introduction

The success of the Egyptian civilisation from Neolithic times depended almost entirely upon the annual inundation of the Nile Valley down to the Delta and a few oases. They realised the potential of the fertile land bordering the Nile and learned how to manage the flooding which brought with it the fertile alluvial soils and allowed plants and trees to flourish. Indication that the flooding season had started could be observed by the beginning of July at Aswan and could take until September to reach an optimum level of 8m and 7m by the time it reached the environs of Cairo (Nunn 1997, 8). The height of the inundation varied from year to year, particularly high levels were experienced during the Middle Kingdom and resulted in ruined crops, loss of habitation and loss of life.

Heavy summer rains caused the Blue Nile to rise during May, June and July bringing with it vast quantities of silt from the Ethiopian highlands. Soils transported by water are gradually sifted with the heavier particles being deposited first and the lightest last, the finest silt being found in the delta areas of rivers. The silts consisted of mineral deposits washed from the volcanic rocks of the area. The White Nile and its tributaries were similarly affected by tropical rainstorms near its source around the borders of Uganda and Sudan. A region known as the Sudd, a little way south of Khartoum, and the confluence of the rivers which join the Nile was a vast area of low lying marshland by the river which from January to the end of March was intensively grazed by wild animals and domesticated cattle at a density of 1,000 animals per square kilometre. By the beginning of April when the rainy season began, the grazing animals would have left to find grasses and other vegetation elsewhere. The land of the Sudd would be stripped bare of grazing but the ground could have an appreciable distribution of animal waste, which had been left behind. This area became extensively flooded by the fast flowing river at its highest level in June, July and August. It is quite likely that the decaying animal waste was washed away by the river, most of it being carried downstream and possibly some of it deposited on the land in the Nile Valley. This dark brown or black sediment was probably this colour due to mineral deposits being combined with organic matter which remained on the lands as the flooding subsided, creating enriched soils which enabled crops to flourish with no need for fertilisers. The flood water brought down by the fast flowing Nile covered the cultivated lands in the Nile valley, sometimes to an excessive level.

In order to manage the flood waters from the Nile as the river began to rise the labourers built dykes and dams to hold the excess for later and distribute it along channels to the cultivated land after the waters had subsided. The fields were divided into small squared off areas by means of mud walls a few inches high. In between the squares a small channel was created to convey water to the plants. Each square could be watered separately by removing a mud wall blocking the channel and then breaking an opening in the mud enclosure of the square to be watered. When one square had been sufficiently watered the opening was closed and a break in the wall of the next square was created in order to water another area, the same procedure being repeated for successive squares (Murray 1931, 63). The water channels were also blocked and opened where irrigation was required; in this way one field could be watered selectively according to the need of the crop.

The soil in the Nile Valley is mainly composed of sand, which soon dries out. The water percolates between the grains of sand and silt layer drawn down by gravity until it reaches the permanently saturated area known as the water table. As the water drains through it, it wets the humus in the soil and leaves a film on each grain.

Shallow surface roots of plants are able to absorb water and nutrients from these particles, which is essential for their growth. Many of the crops grown alongside the Nile needed to be irrigated frequently so that they would flourish. The problem with light sandy soil is that the water soon dissolves the essential nutrients. Fortunately, the flooding of the Nile Valley revitalised the banks every year. The sort of plants needing regular watering included the following: *Lactuca sativa* (Cos lettuce), *Allium cepa* (onions), *Allium porrum* (leeks), *Apium graveolens* (celery), *Citrullus Lanatus* (syn c.vulgaris) (water melons), *Hordeum vulgare* (barley), *Triticum dicoccum* (Emmer wheat) and *Trigonella foenum-graecum* (fenugreek) for animal fodder and human consumption.

There are several plants and trees that are not dependent on regular supplies of water provided by irrigation, some can survive desert conditions for months or even years in the desert or dry rocky soils. Examples include: *Punica granatum* (pomegranate), *Ficus carica* (common fig), *Myrtus* (myrtle), *Mandragora officinarum* (mandrake), *Ceratonia siliqua* (carob), *Phoenix dactylifera* (date palm) and *Tamarix aphylla* (syn T.articulata) (tamarisk). These have very deep roots that can seek out water at low levels. The plants and trees that grew near the Nile depended upon water to survive during the summer when the river was at its lowest level. Generally speaking, the water table would be at the same level as the river, and the soil within a short distance of it would be at the same level.

Beyond the narrow fertile strip of land alongside the river, plants had to seek out water at greater depths and developed tap roots which penetrated the compacted soil. In rocky dry soils it is known that grape vine roots can reach up to a depth of ten metres and tamarisk to a much greater depth than that. Plants that have adapted to desert climates have developed mechanisms which help them to conserve what little water there is in the soil or in the atmosphere during dew fall. For example, Aloe vera has thick, fleshy leaves which have a high water content and reduce water loss through transpiration down to a bare minimum because of a waxy epidermis. The *Capparis spinosa* (caper) has hard, fleshy leaves and stems which are greyish green, and have a dense covering of fine downy hairs which restrict water loss. It is often found growing by sea shores and can withstand salt spray. The *Phoenix dactylifera* (date palm) is very adaptable, often growing beside the Nile. It is not affected by the hot, dry summers. Conversely, they will withstand flooding for several months without detriment and can also be irrigated with brine affected water.

The climate in the Nile Valley and the Delta being next to the desert is very hot and dry and mid-day temperatures sometimes reach 40°C during May to September. The cultivated land became parched, affected by drying southerly winds, and due to the low level of the Nile, irrigation of growing crops at this time would have been impractical due to lack of water and when the land became inundated no cultivations could take place.

In the period between November and February it was important to provide shelter for young delicate plants as the temperature sometimes dips below freezing point. In the early spring strong cold winds can delay growth and some trees may suffer damage to leaves and branches. Later on in the spring there is a hot wind known as the "Khamsin" which usually lasts for fifty days. The heat is debilitating and can damage the flowers even of indigenous species resulting in poor crops later on. These winds also cause dust storms which would have made it almost impossible for the garden labourers to work. It is easy to see why many of the temple gardens had walls high enough to provide shelter for the plants and humans.

Several medical papyri have been discovered from ancient Egypt and research to date has identified that the ancient Egyptians were one of the first known civilisations to use herbs for the treatment of diseases, infections and wounds. The lowly peasants worked long hours particularly if they laboured on the land, life expectancy was about thirty years. Serious injuries were quite common, diseases and infections were rife and the privileged were not immune either. Parasitic infestations were common, especially as water was often contaminated; the medical papyri document many plants that were specified to deal with different types of worm. The roots of *Punica granatum* (pomegranate) were ground to a pulp in water and drunk for the elimination of tapeworm and roundworm. *Teucrium polium* (mountain germander/cat thyme, hulwort) was also used for the same purpose, using a decoction of the dried plant. Cannabis sativa (hemp) was used as a plant for making rope fibres, for inflammatory conditions and also as a laxative and as a sedative. Research into the papyri so far seems to suggest they were not aware of its use as a narcotic (Nunn 1997, 156).

Medicinally Useful Plants from Ancient Egypt

Allium cepa (onion): This was used in ancient Egypt to add flavour to cooked food just as it is today. The juice extract from the bulb is antibiotic and helpful in reducing the effects of colds, ejecting phlegm for coughs and encouraging discharge of urine (diuretic). It is also capable of lowering blood pressure, encouraging clotting and reducing blood sugar levels. In Pharaonic times, perhaps because of its antibiotic properties, the onion was used in the mummification process (Manniche 1989, 75).

Allium sativum (garlic): Used to clear bacterial infections.

Aloe vera: It is known that the Copts prescribed Aloe for digestive problems and external inflammations (Manniche 1989, 78). It is interesting to note that it is used for the same disorders today and to treat skin problems, such as eczema, burns and scalds.

Capparis spinosa (caper): So far not identified in the papyri, but used as a folk medicine in the Mediterranean area for liver and chest diseases, sciatica and gastric pain (Batanouny 2006, 11). The immature flower buds are pickled in vinegar and add a piquant flavour to meats and salads.

Coriandrum sativum (coriander): The seeds have a sharp spicy flavour appreciated as an ingredient in curries, pickles and for seasoning meats. Oil is extracted from the seeds which are used medicinally and for perfumes (the leaves contain the same oil). Coriander is also used in cooking for flavour. Pliny said that when coriander is combined with honey or raisins it healed spreading sores, diseased testes, burns, carbuncles and sore ears.

Hordeum (barley): Grown frequently in Egypt and Israel for bread-making, it is also used in recipes for laxatives, expelling intestinal parasites and poultices for burns and fractures.

Lawsonia inermis (henna): In ancient Egypt, henna was used as a dye for hair and cloth and for painting nails. The dried leaves of the plant are powdered and small amounts of water added to make a paste which produces an orange/red dye which these days is mainly used as a hair dye though it does have some medicinal value. The identification of this plant in the medical papyri is not certain, but if the translation does prove to be correct it was used as a remedy for hair loss in ancient Egypt (Manniche 1989, 120). Today, it is used medicinally for skin diseases (including leprosy), wounds, ulcers and herpes.

Myrtus communis (myrtle): Used by the Ancient Egyptians for its medicinal properties, assuming it has been correctly identified in medical papyrus texts. If this is the case then Myrtle leaves are used as ingredients in poultices applied externally for swellings (The Hearst Papyrus 37), pains (The Ebers Papyrus 129), stiffness of limbs (The Ebers Papyrus 672) and removing mucus from the left or right chest (The Berlin Papyrus 142). It is also a treatment for urinary disorders using ground leaves in fermented plant juice applied externally. Interestingly today the medical herb is used for urinary infections, dry coughs, bronchial congestion and sinusitis. The oil is still an ingredient in perfumes and used to add flavour when cooking pork, lamb and poultry.

Nymphaea lotus and N. caerulea (White and Blue Lotus): These were combined with other herbs and used to treat the liver, constipation and to cool a high temperature.

Papaver rhoeas (field or corn poppy): All parts of the plant are toxic, except for the seeds that can be used for culinary purposes. The dark brown seeds are added to breads, pastries and meat dishes and to cooked foods for a decorative effect. Medicinally, it is used as a sedative for coughs and digestive problems.

Papaver somniferum (opium poppy): An effective painkiller, the seeds were sprinkled on bread and added to meat dishes. The seeds are safe to use as they are alkaloid free.

Ricinus communis (castor-oil plant): Used as a purgative, but also often used for anointing of body and as lamp oil.

Trigonella foenum-graecum (fenugreek): Used to induce childbirth and to encourage weight gain after illness. The seeds have a high protein content and in Egypt today are used as a remedy for painful menstruation. The seeds were added to stews and bread to add spice and the leaves added to salads and for cattle fodder.

Ziziphus spina-christi (Christ Thorn): The timber of the tree was used for carpentry in ancient Egypt as the wood is very durable, and in some cases, it was used for coffins. As a herbal medicine, the leaves of the Christ Thorn were used to treat constipation. Also, the fruit was sometimes used to make zizyphus bread.

Medicinal Plant Propagation

Many of the medicinal herbs could be propagated from seed directly sown where required to grow. After the flooding had subsided in November winter sowing could begin; very little preparation would be needed because of the fine, silty soil. Probably, the seed was sown thinly in rows and later when the seedlings had emerged thinned out with a hoe, so that the young plants had sufficient space to grow. It has always been common practice to sow the seeds of cereal crops by sowing broadcast as thinly as possible over the whole field. The following herbs can be sown directly: *Coriandrum* (Coriander), *Capparis* (caper), *Carthamnus* (safflower), *Centaurea* (cornflower). *Capparis spinosa* (caper) seeds have to be sown direct as soon as the seeds are ripe; otherwise if the seeds are left too long they become dormant and have to be soaked in warm water for twelve hours and refrigerated for three months (Batanouny 2006, 9). *Acacia nilotica* (Nile acacia) can be reproduced from seeds, but needs mechanical scarification, which penetrates the hard seed coat allowing the seeds to absorb moisture and germinate. Alternatively, the seeds could be soaked in boiling water and left for twelve hours. Today, it is the normal practice to soak the seeds in dilute acid solution to penetrate the seed coat (Ismail 2006, 53-4).

Division: Some herbs like *Origanum syriacum* (marjoram) can be reproduced by lifting large clumps of plants and dividing them into small sections; it is better to use the younger growth around the outside and discard the growth in the centre which is old and weak. The divisions can be planted in their permanent positions and soon become established and ready for cropping again (Hammouda 2006, 71).

Layering: For example, *Myrtus communis* (myrtle) – plant stocks of the shrub can be increased by layering. For this purpose, small young branches are chosen which are growing horizontally near the ground. The branches are lowered until they touch the ground and a long slanting cut is made so that half the stem is cut through. The branch is then pegged down just before the cut in the stem and a mound of soil is earthed up to cover this area. In a few months time the stem will have developed its own root system and can be cut free from the parent plant. The young shrubs can be planted out retaining as much soil as possible into their permanent positions and watered until well established to prevent the roots from drying out.

From Offsets: Aloe vera stocks can be increased from offsets - these are small plantlets that grow from the base of mature specimens. The plants can be lifted once the offsets have made sufficient root growth so that they do not die when separated from the parent plants. The young offsets can be planted in a nursery bed until sufficiently large enough to place in more permanent positions.

From Softwood Cuttings: *Lawsonia inermis* (henna), *Myrtus communis* (myrtle) and *Punica granatum* (pomegranate) can be propagated from softwood cuttings, ideally take the cuttings from mature plants that have young strong growth. Trim the cuttings with a sharp knife and cut to a length of about 10cm taking care to cut just below a leaf joint. Remove most of the leaves except for two or three leaves near the growing tip. Loosely fill 9cm pots to the brim with a compost mixture composed of 50% gritty sand and 50% of peat or peat substitute. Having treated the cuttings with a solution of rooting hormone, insert the stems of four or five cuttings around the inside edge of the pot and lightly firm. Water thoroughly and place in a mist propagator with bottom heat of 23 - 26°C and 21°C at leaf level. Leave until they become well rooted and gradually acclimatised, removing the young plants from the pots and placing them in individual pots; later, plant out when large enough into their permanent positions.

From Semi-hardwood Cuttings: Cuttings can be obtained from woody, broad-leaved, evergreen species during summer using the current year's growth that has partially matured or hardened, for example, *Olea europaea* (olive) and *Thymus spicata* (wild thyme). Take cuttings 7.5 – 15 cms in length making a clean cut just below the leaf joints or nodes and remove the lower leaves close to the stem leaving 2 to 3 leaves at the tip. If the leaves are very large it is advisable to reduce the leaf area, possibly by 50%. Ideally, this type of cutting should be rooted in a mist propagator with bottom heat having been treated with hormones or growth regulators.

Summary

The importance of the annual inundation and the plant species this event supported can be easily recognised. Management of their unique environment provided the ancient Egyptians with the means to cultivate a large range of plants, including those of medicinal value. Consideration of plant propagation methods used today highlights that many of these were available to the ancient Egyptians and may have been used to grow plants for a variety of purposes, including their use in pharmaceutical remedies.

References

Batanouny, K. H. (2005) (Ed) *Encyclopaedia of Wild Medicinal Plants in Egypt, Vol 1.* Project of Conservations and Sustainable Use of Medicinal Plants and Arid and Semi-Arid Ecosystems in Egypt.

Bircher, W.H. (1960) *Gardens of the Hesperides: A book on old and new plants for Egypt and similar climes.* Anglo Egyptian Bookshop.

Bown, D. (1995) *RHS Encyclopaedia of Herbs and Their Uses.* Dorling Kindersley Ltd.

Hartmann, H.T. and Kester, D.E. (1959) *Plant Propagation: Principles and Practice.* Prentice-Hall, Inc.

Hepper, F.N. (1990) *Pharaoh's Flowers: Botanical Treasures of Tutankhamun.* Stationery Office Books.

Hepper, F.N. (1993) *Baker Encyclopaedia of Bible Plants: Flowers and Trees, Fruits and Vegetables,* Ecology, Baker Publishing Group.

Holmes, M., Maxwell, G. and Scoones, T. (2004) *Nile.* BBC Books, BBC Worldwide Ltd.

Manniche, L. (1999). *An Ancient Egyptian Herbal.* British Museum Press.

Murray, M.A., (1931) *The Splendour That Was Egypt.* Sidgwick and Jackson.

Nunn, J.F. (1997) *Ancient Egyptian Medicine.* British Museum Press.

Walker, W. (1979) *All the Plants of the Bible.* Doubleday and Company Inc.

Withers, P. (1909) *Egypt of Yesterday and Today.* Grant Richards.

DO THE FORMULATIONS OF ANCIENT EGYPTIAN PRESCRIPTIONS STAND UP TO PHARMACEUTICAL SCRUTINY?

J.M. Campbell[1], J.R. Campbell[2] and A.R. David[1]

[1] **KNH Centre for Biomedical Egyptology, The University of Manchester, UK.**
[2] **Member of the Royal Pharmaceutical Society of Great Britain**

Abstract: *Amongst the problems in assessing ancient Egyptian remedies from a pharmaceutical standpoint is the reliance on textual information from the medical papyri, for unlike other technologies and practices in ancient Egypt, there is no ancient formulated remedy to analyse. Evaluation is therefore based on placing the ingredients in a known order and structure compliant with defined pharmaceutical formulations. A critical assessment of 1000 ancient Egyptian prescriptions confirms that the majority of remedies, by virtue of their ingredients and preparation, comply with the classical formulations detailed in the British Pharmaceutical Codex of 1973. They are less likely to comply with 21st century formulations.*

Key words: Ancient Egypt, drug formulations, archaeobotany, medical texts

Introduction

Much of what is known of pharmacy in ancient Egypt is based on the textual evidence of the medical papyri, in particular the Kahun (Griffiths 1898; Quirke 2002), Ebers (Ebbell 1937; Ghalioungui 1987), Edwin Smith (Breasted 1930) and Chester Beatty (Jonckheere 1947), which between them contain some 1000 prescriptions representing 50% of the known prescriptions from pharaonic Egypt. Scholars (Jonkheere 1947; 1955; 1958, Dawson 1967; Ghalioungui 1980; Nunn 1992; 1996; Manniche 1999) have variously described medicine and the materia medica of the ancient Egyptians but none have considered the pharmaceutical merit of the formulations.

The remedies are generally written in a formulaic style detailing the various ingredients, the method of preparation and on occasion, the measurements to be used. Moreover, the instructions describe the dosage and frequency of administration. The formulation has to be such that the drugs are presented in a form which allows the remedy to be administered and transported to the site of action without destruction of the active principle.

Our aim was to evaluate the textual evidence, consider the remedy, its component drugs, method of preparation and compare it to modern pharmaceutical protocols relevant at a time when drugs were regularly made in the dispensary. Accordingly the British Pharmaceutical Codex (1973) and the British Pharmacopoeia (1973) were used as the basis of comparison. Many of the formulations prevalent during the 1970s are available today but are manufactured at source.

Consequently, the formulations defined as creams, draughts, enemata, extracts, eye lotions, drops, ointments, infusions or inhalations are no longer made in the pharmacy but, as with liniments, linctuses, lotions, mixtures, mouth washes, ointments, pessaries, pills, powders, solutions, suppositories and tablets, are provided prepared and packaged, often in single dose format.

Other formulations such as pastes, paints, poultices or electuaries - common only 50 years ago in western medicine and pharmacy - have passed into pharmaceutical antiquity but nevertheless serve as a valid comparison for the remedies of ancient Egypt.

The efficacy and safety of any medicinal product depends upon the purity and stability of the active ingredients and their physical form, the method of preparation and presentation to the patient. Additionally, there must be no adverse interaction between any of the selected ingredients and the formulation has to be able to withstand the obstacles of the body to reach its site of physical or physiological action (Wilkinson 2001).

Furthermore, just as the ingredients in a contemporary formulation by virtue of their ingredients (oil, paste, liquid, powder) give an indication of the consistency and character of the finished preparation so the constituents in ancient Egyptian remedies by and large afford the same information. Substances that were oils 4000 years ago remain so today, similarly honey will be little changed in character and the description powder affords an immediate assessment regarding character, behaviour and nature of the formulation.

In much the same respect, the sourcing of raw materials would have been little different; for example, frankincense trees must be cut to permit the flow of tears, colocynth fruit and castor oil seeds are still picked, as are pomegranates, and seed oil is still the source of many medicaments. There is some uncertainty regarding some of the drugs, particularly the plants (Germer 1998; Campbell 2007; Campbell and David 2007) but the various options have been taken into account. Indeed the formulation has an influence on the identity of the drug.

Formulations

Creams are viscous emulsions of semisolid consistency and are either oil in water type mixtures (aqueous creams) or water in oil type (oily creams). Contemporary ingredients include waxes, soaps, fats, beeswax and water based products, with the ingredients generally being melted. There are only two creams in the Ebers papyrus, one for the anus - remedy 161 (Ebbell 1937, 44) - and the second - remedy 637 (Ebbell 1937, 95) - to soften all limbs, but each deployed a natural disperse phase analogous with the definition as they used animal fat from goose or ass and oil from seeds or beeswax. The liquids were water or weak alcohol and each was used topically and efficaciously.

Draughts are liquid preparations for oral administration formulated in single dose volumes of 50ml. Popular until the late 20th century, they are seldom used now other than in herbal or traditional medicine. Draughts are variously described in the Ebers for the belly (e.g. remedy 6 (Ebell 1937, 30)), as a laxative, to stop diarrhoea as an anthelminthic, or for a cough. Draughts are also identified in the Chester Beatty papyrus (remedy 14 (Jonckheere 1947, 25)) where they are taken orally as an anal demulcent. They are always instructed to be left during the night in dew. The water would have extracted the alkaloids whilst other constituents would have been extracted in alcohol, typically beer but occasionally wine. In every case the liquid medium was appropriate for an aqueous or non-aqueous extraction.

Enemata are aqueous or oily solutions or suspensions for rectal administration. Any substance, solid or oil, contained in them should be dissolved or uniformly dispersed. They are given for their analgesic, anthelminthic, anti-inflammatory, nutritive, purgative or sedative effects. All should be warmed to body temperature before administration. Ancient Egyptian use of enemata is explicitly described in all the papyri studied, reflecting very similar indications as those where enemata are prescribed today. Commonly used as demulcent preparations (e.g. (Ebbell 1937, 43), they also served as laxatives and sedatives:

> *'For the anus*
> *Water of ammi, Water of smsm, (cannabis??)*
> *Bread , Oil of mrḫ.t, Lotus flowers, Acacia flowers*
> *Mix the ingredients, Inject into anus for 4 days'*

(remedy 14 (Jonckheere 1947, 25))

The medium was either water or beer (rarely wine) and the active ingredient was demulcent carob (*Ceratona siliqua*), acacia mucilage (*Acacia sp*), or an unspecified oil usually carrying an antiseptic or bacteriocide as in Ebers 143 (Ebbell 1937, 43):

> *'Balanites oil, Water of ḏ3rt (Carob), Oil, Honey 5ro*
> *Injected into the hinder part'*

Enemata intended as a stimulant laxative carried irritants such as pine oil or turpentine. These remained in use until 50 years ago. The enema in Ebers case 265 (Ebbell 1937, 61), indicated for a bladder complaint, may indicate that schistosomiasis was clinically so advanced that it resulted in rectal irritation:

> *'To expel heat in the bladder. Suffers from edbw in the urine. Northern salt 0.5 ro, mlwj 5ro, Balanites oil, Honey, Sweet beer. Injected into the anus.'*

The use of balanites oil, recently recognised for its anthelminthic property to schistosomiasis (Whitefield 1996), is significant as it suggests the ancient physicians may have recognised the associated rectal symptoms of the disease.

Liquid extracts are concentrated products containing the active principles of crude drugs prepared by maceration with solvents followed by concentration. There is no evidence that the ancient Egyptians practised distillation, but extracts are concentrated drugs and Ebers 217 instructs that 31*ro* of liquid should be reduced in volume until 10*ro* are left (Ebbell 1937, 56). Whilst not as efficient as today's extractions or as quantitatively reliable, the procedure was utilised and indicates measurement at a fine level.

Eye drops are sterile aqueous solutions or suspensions for instillation into the eye. They are prepared by dissolving the medicament in an aqueous vehicle, then filtering to clarify it. The ophthalmic section in the Ebers papyrus details examples of eye drops which are to be 'instilled' into the eye (remedy 340 (Ebbell 1937, 68)) using the hollow quill of a bird. Whilst non-conforming, it is explicit. Eye lotions without medicament employed fresh milk, particularly from a woman who had just borne a male child, e.g. Ebers 415 (Ebbell 1937, 75). Eye drops with a drug component were typically delivered in carob water as in Ebers case 360 (Ebbell 1937, 70). The ancient remedies show no concept of sterility, but neither did contemporary western medicine until the 19th century AD.

Suitable bases for contemporary eye ointments are liquid paraffin, wool fat and yellow soft paraffin, mixed and filtered whilst hot. Harder paraffins are advised for tropical climates. Again, the Ebers ophthalmic section details formulations which comply with the definition bar sterility. Some are the very antithesis of sterility, as they use animal dung.

Infusions are dilute solutions containing readily soluble constituents of crude drugs. They are prepared by macerating the drug for a short period in cold or boiling water, or by diluting one volume of a concentrated infusion in ten volumes of water.

Infusions are liable to fungal and bacterial growth, and their short life seems to have been recognised in ancient Egypt because in every case, after infusing overnight, the remedy was used immediately (e.g. remedy 50 (Ebbell

1937, 34)). Only those infused in alcohol or with high sugar concentration, as in Ebers case 137 (Ebbell 1937, 42), could have been used for longer.

Inhalations are liquid preparations containing volatile ingredients which when vaporised are brought into contact with the lining of the respiratory tract. Some ingredients are volatile at room temperature and can be inhaled from a pad, others must be added to hot water and the vapour inhaled. Whilst there is no example of a liquid inhalation in ancient Egypt there is a clear reference in Ebers case 326 (Ebbell 1937, 67) to an inhalation of fumes from a fire to treat a cough:

> *'To expel cough. Orpiment ?, Bitumen, s'm, Fat. Heat seven stones on a fire. Place ingredients on hot stone. Place perforated vessel on top. Place reed in vessel. Inhale smoke through reed. Afterwards eat fat or oil.'*

Similarly, Dioscorides described the heating of orpiment, an arsenic-containing mineral (Gunther 1934). A further formulation (Ebers case 763 (Ebbell 1937, 105)) instructs that gum be inserted into the nostril as an inhalant somewhat reminiscent of Penetrol™, from the mid 20th century AD.

Cough linctuses are viscous liquid preparations usually containing sucrose and medicinal substances and possessing demulcent, expectorant or sedative properties, usually used for the relief of a cough and administered in doses of small volume. Whilst Ebers case 322 (Ebbell 1937) is compliant with the demulcent properties, it is not known to be sedative, but the ingredients remain in efficacious use today in clinical and herbal medicine:

> *'To expel cough*
> *Berry juice Figs 4ro, Sebesten 4ro, Raisin 4ro, Cumin 0.5ro, acacia 1ro, Ink powder 0.5ro, njwjw 1ro, Senna ?? 4ro, Sweet beer.*
> *Leave overnight in dew. Take for four days.'*

Liniments are liquid or semi liquid, usually oil-based preparations which are intended for external application and may contain substances possessing analgesic, rubefacient, soothing or stimulating properties. These were commonly described in ancient Egyptian remedies, the ingredients always being used topically and never ingested. Many of the ingredients and drug components remain in clinical use today. Liniments are typically applied with a bandage, e.g. Ebers 610 (Ebbell 1937, 92).

Mixtures are liquid preparations for oral administration consisting of one or more medicaments suspended in an aqueous or non-aqueous vehicle. Insoluble substances which do not diffuse evenly are finely powdered and mixed with a suitable suspending agent such as acacia or carob. The majority of ancient Egyptian mixtures utilise a wide variety of ingredients, and are comprised of an active principle, some flavouring, and a vehicle in which it is swallowed, usually water, beer or wine. Occasionally it is to be eaten, and sometimes infused overnight to extract the active ingredient. Ebers case 298 (Ebbell 1937, 64) instructs the fruits to be mixed, acting as a bulk laxative, whilst cumin acts as a carminative. The mixture uses beer as the vehicle and acacia as a stabiliser to keep it in even suspension.

Ointments are semi-solid preparations consisting of a medicament or mixture of medicaments, dissolved or dispersed in a suitable, often anhydrous, base. They are used as emollients, as protective preparations of the skin, or as a means for the local application of medicaments. They may contain vegetable oils or wool fat (lanolin), together with inert bases such as paraffin. A mildly antiseptic or astringent powder may be added. The proportion of paraffins, oils, fats and waxes may be varied in ointments intended for tropical or subtropical climates. Ointments may be diluted or strengthened as required.

Ancient Egyptian remedies are often described as ointments, but not all are compliant with the definition. Most are used to bring the active ingredient in close proximity with the wound, others to exclude air and bacteria, yet others to be soothing and comforting. Ebers case 620 (Ebbell 1937, 93) for an infected toe complies with the definition, being detailed in preparation and application, and having antibacterial properties:

> *'For an ill toe - Yellow ochre, Natron, Sory, Red ochre*
> *ḫnnw from the courtyard, Flax seed, Starch*
> *Marrow, Grease, Honey*
> *Warmed and ground.'*

Pessaries are solid bodies for vaginal administration, containing medicaments which are usually intended to act locally, prepared by moulding or by compression. Oil is used as a basis and all are characterised by having a maximum disintegration time of 1 hour.

The Kahun and Ebers papyri each instructs the use of pessaries to cure vaginal problems, the preparations bringing the principal ingredients into close proximity with the mucous membranes as in Ebers case 829 (Ebbell 1937, 112). In Ebers case 805 (Ebbell 1937, 109) a pessary containing juniper is used to induce birth. Juniper is a uterine stimulant specifically prohibited today in pregnancy.

Poultices are thick pasty preparations usually intended to be used extemporaneously for application to the skin with the objective of reducing inflammation and allaying pain. They are usually applied warm. The ancient poultices are varied yet compliant. Ebers case 246 (Ebbell 1937, 58-59) cites the use of statue clay, which is directly comparable with kaolin poultices that were popular up to the mid 20th century AD. Ebers case 536 (Ebbell 1937, 85) describes a warm mixture of a heat retaining substance (zizyphus bread) applied to soothe aching limbs or bring infection to a head, as in Edwin Smith case 41.

Suppositories are solid bodies, cone shaped for rectal administration. They are prepared by incorporating the requisite quantity of finely powdered medicament in the melted base, and pouring the mixture into previously lubricated moulds. Where threobroma was specified in the BPC 1973, it can be replaced by any other suitable base such as palm kernel oil or other suitable hydrogenated vegetable oil, provided that the melting point of the suppositories is not more than the body temperature (37°C). If suppositories are intended for use in tropical or subtropical countries, the melting point of the base may be raised by the addition of white beeswax. There is a standard disintegration time of 30-60 minutes. Ancient Egyptian formulations follow this protocol, as in Ebers case 141 (Ebbell 1937, 43). As an alternative to oil, the ancient recipe used carob, which rehydrates with body fluids, to hold the antimicrobial salt and frankincense in place. The Chester Beatty papyrus, devoted entirely to colorectal problems, cites only one suppository (remedy 6 (Jonckheere 1947)).

Non-conforming Remedies

There are numerous recipes within the papyri which, whilst of therapeutic benefit, do not conform to the formulations used today. These vary in composition and use. Crocodile dung is mentioned in both the Kahun (remedy 31) and the Ebers papyri where it is eaten (remedy 334) or where it is put in the eye (remedy 379). Animal dung remained in British formularies until Hans Sloane published his London Pharmacopoeia in the 17th century.

Other nonconforming remedies would now be regarded as nutraceuticals, as their role is nutritional. Examples include Ebers remedy 352 (Ebbell 1937), where consuming ox liver is advised to improve night blindness, and remedy 748 (Ebbell 1937) where celery is chewed with beer to strengthen the gums.

The most outlandish and nonconforming are the animal based prescriptions, such as Ebers remedies 425, which uses lizard's blood, and 429 (Ebbell 1937) where gall of bird is inserted into the eye.

Other formulations such as fumigations or douches are no longer in vogue. Douches were popular in Victorian England for obstetric and gynaecological conditions, and are cited in the Ebers Papyrus (Ebbell 1937) to contract the womb (remedy 822), to stop bleeding (remedy 827), to cool the womb (remedy 820) and for a vaginal discharge (remedy 815) (Campbell 2007, 160-162).

Discussion and Conclusion

The pattern of the formulae is consistent throughout and remarkable in its similarity to the formulae of 20th century medicines. The most potent ingredient is cited first and the lesser important cited next, the vehicle being cited last.

The mix of ingredients in the prescriptions of ancient Egypt also follows a similar format. The vast majority of prescriptions include the active ingredient, ancillary drugs which may alleviate some of the severe side effects of the therapeutic drug (such as flavourings to disguise a bitter or unpleasant taste) and a vehicle to carry the ingredients in even distribution and permit measurement of a suitable volume.

Our analysis has shown that of the 1000 ancient remedies, 70% are complaint with the protocols for formulation described in the BPC of 1973. The advent of parenteral administration makes them less comparable today but we can with confidence conclude that the formulations in ancient Egypt stand up to pharmaceutical scrutiny.

Acknowledgements

The authors would like to thank the Leverhulme Trust who funded this research.

References

Breasted, J.H. (1930). *The Edwin Smith Surgical Papyrus*. Vol. 1. University of Chicago Press.

B.P. (1973). *British Pharmacopoeia*. Her Majesty's Stationery Office.

BPC (1973) *The British Pharmaceutical Codex*. The Pharmaceutical Press.

Campbell, J.M. and David, A.R. (2005). Some Aspects of the Practice of Pharmacy in Ancient Egypt 1850B.C. to 1300B.C. *Journal of Biological Research* LXXX, pp. 331-334.

Campbell, J.M. (2007). Unpublished PhD. *An assessment of the pharmaceutical and therapeutic merit of remedies within the Kahun, Edwin Smith, Ebers and Chester Beatty ancient Egyptian medical papyri*. The University of Manchester.

Campbell, J.M. and David, A.R. (2007). The application of archaeobotany and pharmacognosy to reassess the translation of *šnj-t3* and *d3rt* in the medical papyri. In Griffin, K. (ed.) *Current Research in Egyptology 2007: Proceedings of the Eighth Annual Conference*, pp. 15-24.

Dawson, W.R. (1967). The Egyptian medical papyri. In Brothwell, D. and Sanderson, A.T. (eds.) *Diseases in antiquity*. Charles, C. Thomas.

Ebbell, B. (1937). *The Papyrus Ebers*. Oxford University Press.

Germer, R. (1998). The Plant Remains found by Petrie at Lahun and some remarks on the problems of identifying Egyptian plant names. In Quirke, S. (ed.) *Lahun Studies*. SIA Publishing.

Ghalioungui, P. (1980). Medicine in Ancient Egypt. In Harris, J.E. and Wente, E.F. (eds.) *An X-ray Atlas of the Royal Mummies*. University of Chicago Press.

Ghalioungui, P. (1987). *The Ebers Papyrus: A new English translation, commentaries and glossaries.* Academy of Scientific Research and Technology.

Griffith, F.Ll. (1893). A Medical Papyrus from Egypt. *British Medical Journal.* 3rd June, pp. 1172-1175.

Griffith, F.Ll. (1898). *The Petrie Papyri: Hieratic Papyri from Kahun and Gurob.* Bernard Quaritch.

Gunther, R.T. (1934). *The Greek Herbal of Dioscorides.* Oxford University Press.

Jonckheere, F. (1944). *Une maladie Égyptienne. L'hématurie parasitaire.* Fondation Égyptologique Reine Élisabeth.

Jonckheere, F. (1947). *Le Papyrus médical Chester Beatty.* Fondation Égyptologique Reine Élisabeth.

Jonckheere, F. (1955). Le 'préparateur de remèdes' dans l'organisation de la pharmacie Égyptienne. In Firchow, O. ed., *Äegyptologische Studien.* Deutsche Akademie de Wissenschaften zu Berlin 29, pp. 160-161.

Jonckheere, F. (1958). *Les Médecins de l'Égypte Pharaonique: essai de prosographie.* Fondation Égyptologique Reine Élisabeth

Manniche, L. (1999). *An Ancient Egyptian Herbal.* British Museum Press.

Nunn, J.F. (1992) The Medical Skills of the Ancient Egyptians. *Journal of Egyptian Archaeology,* 78, pp. 317-318.

Nunn, J.F. (1996) *Ancient Egyptian Medicine.* London: British Museum Press.

Quirke, S. (2002). *Manuscript for Health of Mother and Child. The Kahun Medical Papyrus or Gynaecological Papyrus.* University College London (Unpublished transcript by kind permission of the author).

Whitefield, P.J. (1996). Novel anthelminthic compounds and molluscicides from medicinal plants. *Transactions of the Royal Society of Tropical Medicine and Hygiene* 90, p. 596.

Wilkinson, G.R. (2001). Pharmacokinetics: The Dynamics of Drug Absorption, Distribution, and Elimination. In Hardman, J.G. and Limbard, L.E. (eds.) *A. Gilman. Goodman and Gilman's: The Pharmacological Basis of Therapeutics.* 10th International Edition. McGraw-Hill.

THE APPLICATION OF ARCHAEOBOTANY, PHYTOGEOGRAPHY AND PHARMACOGNOSY TO CONFIRM THE PHARMACOPOEIA OF ANCIENT EGYPT 1850 -1200 BC

J.M. Campbell and A.R. David

KNH Centre for Biomedical Egyptology, The University of Manchester, UK

Abstract: *This paper aims to confirm the materia medica and pharmacopoeia of ancient Egypt and to demonstrate that it was used appropriately and therapeutically. We intend to prove that the Egyptians were practising a credible and reproducible form of pharmacy as early as the 19th century BC, 1800 years before Galen, the acknowledged 'father of medicine'.*

The prescriptions in the medical papyri, which provide the literary research source, are noted for their uncertainty in interpretation and translation of drugs. Consequently, although much has been published, the materia medica of ancient Egypt is questionable and the efficacy of prescriptions uncertain.

Verification of the drug substances was sought in archaeobotanical and phytogeographical evidence, and to determine the availability, dynastic prevalence and predominance at the time of the papyri. Attestation was sought in contemporary pharmacognosy of the plants and their clinical application, to measure the medicinal uses in ancient Egypt. Efficacy was established by comparing the ancient remedies against modern pharmaceutical protocols including drug source, extraction, pharmacognosy, phytochemistry, pharmacology, formulation, preparation, dosing regime, administration and therapeutic activity.

Most drug sources have been verified, some 25% were determined to be of improbable use, alternative drugs being proposed. Significantly, 50% of the drug sources used by the ancient Egyptians remain in use today, albeit that many are now synthesised. The first scientific estimate of pharmaceutical merit demonstrates 64% of remedies in the medical papyri have therapeutic value in physiological or physical action, 3% are toxic, 1.5% sub-therapeutic, 20% undetermined and the remainder with no known therapeutic activity.

It is concluded that the application of archaeobotany and pharmacognosy may assist the identification of plants once available to ancient Egyptian medicine and consequently, to endorse the ancient texts.

Key words: Ancient Egypt, pharmacopoeia, papyri, archaeobotany, phytogeography.

Introduction

Much of what we know of medicine in ancient Egypt is recorded in twelve medical papyri, four of which provide the literary research source for this investigation: Kahun (Quirke 2002), Ebers (Ebbell 1937), Edwin Smith (Breasted 1930) and Chester Beatty (Jonckheere 1947). There is a general consensus on their origin, provenance and the medical conditions described in them, but uncertainty remains on the translation and identity of the drug substances cited. This uncertainty creates doubt about the entire materia medica used in ancient Egypt and consequently, about the pharmaceutical merit of the remedies described and the formulary /pharmacopoeia used in Pharaonic Egypt.

Scholars of the medical papyri have consistently endeavoured to reconcile a given translation with a particular plant, animal or mineral, rarely finding independent attestation for the unique vocabulary (Dawson 1925-1934, Manniche 1999, Nunn 1996). Botanic evidence was limited to the scholarly work of Loret (1887; 1892) and Schweinfurth (1883 1884)

Only in the last 40 years have botanists comprehensively investigated the flora of ancient Egypt (Tackholme 1941-1974, Boulos 1999-2005, Germer 1985); consequently, comprehensive herbaria exist, but still translations are less than reliable.

The purpose of this research was to undertake a scientific study of the ancient Egyptian remedies, to evaluate their pharmaceutical and therapeutic merit employing comparative analytical and historical methods.

Methods and Protocols

The translations of plants and minerals proposed by different scholars were compared (Aufrere 1986-1987; Breasted 1930; Charpentier 1981; Ebbell 1937; Dawson 1925-1934; The Grundriss (1954-73); Germer 1985; Ghaliounghui 1987; Loret 1898; Jonckheere 1947; Manniche 1999; Nunn 1996; Quirke 2002) and this showed considerable variance.

Scholars generally, but not always, agreed on the translation of trees used, but there was less agreement on cereals and grasses, even less on vegetables, shrubs, and minerals, and little agreement on herbs. Occasionally, the translators agree on the plant, but disagree on the part used. Moreover, plants of the same family and genus may have markedly different medicinal properties, but bear the same common name. This said, within the last 100 years, translations have been proposed for some 90 flora and 35 minerals (albeit opinion varies) but a further 130 drugs remain unidentified (Campbell 2007, 100-112). This disparity called for an additional means of identifying the plants used in the ancient Egyptian prescriptions.

It was essential to identify the species if we were to evaluate the remedy. Attestation to the translation was therefore sought in archaeobotanical evidence, pharmacognosy, phytochemistry, phytogeography and the prevalence and predominance of flora at the time of the papyri (1850 to 1200 BC) to confirm genus and species of plants hitherto described by common name. To accomplish this, c.800 archaeobotanical remains within the British, Petrie and Cairo Museums and the Royal Botanic Gardens, Kew (Campbell 2007, 341-362) were evaluated, supplemented with a review and evaluation of botanical evidence from published archaeobotanical reports and data sources (Vartavan and Amoris 1997), to record dynastic prevalence and predominance.

Dynastic Prevalence and Dominance Results

The results showed the biodiversity of medicinal flora increased as the dynasties advanced (Campbell 2007, 119-125). Plants and minerals cited in the Kahun (Quirke 2002) and Edwin Smith (Breasted 1930) papyri had an onset appearance from the Old Kingdom or earlier whilst the Chester Beatty papyrus (Jonckheere 1947) cites plants some of which have an onset appearance from the Middle Kingdom. It is significant that some of the flora cited in the Ebers papyrus, an early New Kingdom text, were not evident until the Graeco-Roman Period. Indeed, most of the flora of uncertain translation are not prevalent until this time, after which there are abundant archaeobotanical remains. Amongst these are aniseed (*Pimpinella anisum*), cinnamon (*Cinnamonium zeylanicum)*, opium poppy (*Papaver somniferum*), thyme (*Thymus vulgaris*), fennel (*Ferrula gummosa*) and others. This late onset appearance renders their inclusion in the medical papryi uncertain, but does not preclude their import through trade routes, confirming Germer's view (1998, 84).

The plants commonly used in pharmaceutical preparations that were undisputed in translation were also everyday food sources: dates, figs, Egyptian sycamore fruit, barley, wheat, beer and wine. In addition, a number of archaeobotanical remains of known medicinal value were observed in museum collections, which are not known to be identified in the medical papyri:- *Alium sativum*, *Calatropis procera*, *Carthamus tinctorus*, *Hyphaenea thebaica*, *Lathyrus sativum*, *Medima argun*, *Origanum marjorana* (Campbell 2007, 126-128). We propose that these might be candidates for some of the unknown translations. Consideration should be given to a plant having a different name when used in a medical application. Work is ongoing in this area.

Dynastic prevalence and dominance also showed the emergence of new species as the dynasties advanced, e.g. there is no evidence of *Acacia arabica* until the New Kingdom, but *Acacia nilotica* is dominant from the Predynastic Period. Similarly *Balanites aegyptica*, indigenous to Egypt's Nile Valley, has an early onset appearance yet *Balanites roxburghii*, indigenous to India, is not recorded in Egypt until the 3rd Intermediate Period (Table 1). *Tamarix nilotica* has an early onset appearance whilst *Tamarix aphylla* is not only less dominant, but is not evidenced until the Middle Kingdom. There is no archaeobotanical evidence of *Salix fragilis,* a natural source of salicin which is similar to aspirin. However, *Salix subserrata*, although yielding less salicin, has an onset from the New Kingdom and is a dominant tree species.

Pharmaceutical Merit of Prescriptions

Archaeobotany alone was insufficient to confirm the drug translation. Additional evidence was sought by evaluating the pharmaceutical merit of each prescription on the premise that the pharmacognosy of a species could be used to support the identification of the plant or query the accuracy of a translation when evaluated against the medical indication for which it was cited. The objective was to identify which medicinal species available in ancient Egypt have a pharmacological action in contemporary species, and to compare the medicinal application in ancient Egypt with contemporary use. Measurement was also of vital importance and present in 25% of the prescriptions examined (Campbell and David 2005); the work of Pommerening (2003; 2005) has significant bearing on this evaluation.

When the varying list of plants proposed by all the translators is taken as *de facto*, 70% of the plants proposed were used in medicine and pharmacy within the last 100 years (Campbell, Campbell and David 2005). When however, botanic evidence is examined along with the pharmaceutical merit of prescriptions, a different picture emerges - this reduces to 60%, suggesting the presence of a plant does not necessarily indicate appropriate clinical use.

Archaeobotany Results

Archaeobotany demonstrated that the range of medicinal plants available to the ancient physicians was wide and there is evidence of acacia (*Acacia nilotica* and other species), onion (*Allium sp*), celery (*Apium graveolens*), date (*Pheonix dactylifera*), dill (*Anethum graveolens*), flax (*Linum usitassimum*), frankincense (*Boswellia sp*), juniper (Juniperus sp), pomegranate (*Punica granatum*), *Zizyphus spina christi* and others, but there is no evidence of aniseed, cinnamon, cannabis, opium, senna or valerian until long after the papyri were written (Campbell 2007, 122-123).

Whilst the genus of a species might not be in dispute, the species often was. *Acacia nilotica* has always been considered the species indicated in ancient Egyptian remedies, but whilst the acacia is widespread, the species often has a specific phyteogeography. *Acacia tortilis* and *albida* are species predominant in Sinai and evident in archaeological remains from the Predynastic Period. The demulcent, stabilising and antiseptic properties of its resin equal that of *Acacia nilotica* and would have equal efficacy in ancient prescriptions. In another example,

Artemesia was assumed to be wormwood (*Artemesia absynthimum*), used in early 20th century medicine in England (BPC 1911) and the most predominant artemesia species in phytogeography and archaeobotany from the Archaic Period until the Graeco-Roman Period. *Artemisia inculta* is also evident, and whilst having none of the sophorific properties of *absynthimum,* it does have clinical application in menstrual regulation for which *'s 'm* is used in Kahun case 13. It also has application for colds and as an anthelminthic as in Ebers case 122 and 56.

Pharmaceutical Merit Results

Therapeutic merit was determined on the basis that the correct drug was prepared and formulated to be appropriately administered, transported to the site of action where it would have therapeutic effect. The drug had therefore to be appropriate for the symptom cited. The drugs used in ancient Egypt were considered according to therapeutic group and evaluated as having therapeutic, sub therapeutic or toxic effect (Campbell 2007, 170-183).

As an example, *ỉms.t* is proposed as dill (*Anethum graveloens*). Dill has been found in a predynastic grave at Heirakonpolis (Friedman 2003). The seeds, identified by Fahmy (2003), were contained in a basket amongst other plants of known medicinal property, in the crook of an arm of a predynastic female burial. Furthermore, the plant has a natural phytogeography in Egypt in the areas of the Fayoum, Delta and Nile valley (Boulos 2000). The pharmacognosy of Dill is carminative and aromatic whilst *ims.t* had no equivalent properties. The prescriptions using *ims.t* include its use for a headache (Ebers case 249) and a shoulder poultice (Ebers case 650); there are no equivalent properties and consequently, there is no pharmaceutical evidence to support dill being *ims.t* (Campbell 2007, 153).

Similarly, valerian (*Valeriana officinalis*) is proposed by Ghalioungui (1987) to be *š3š3*. The phytochemistry together with the analysis of prescriptions demonstrates that *š3š3* was used for the bowels in Ebers case 38, as a demulcent for haematuria in Ebers case 239, and topically for the skin in Ebers case 382; valerian has none of these clinical properties. It was also prescribed for the stomach 'gastric obstacle' in Ebers case 193 and valerian is bitter, hitherto used as a digestive and carminative. Valerian depresses the central nervous system, and is psychologically sedative, whilst *š3š3* had no similar application. The many and varied uses of š3š3 are incompatible with the pharmacognosy of valerian and we therefore preclude *š3š3* from being valerian (Campbell 2007, 145). The uses in the ancient prescriptions are compatible with the clinical application of mountain nard cited in Dioscorides 1.8.

Pharmacognosy proved to be a useful tool in supporting one view above another, but it is not definitive. For example, when determining if *b3k* is *Balanites aegyptica* or *Moringer aptera,* Ebbell (1937) proposes *Balanites* for *b3k* whilst the Grundriss, Ghalioungui, Germer, Charpentier and Loret propose Moringer, clearly representing the majority. Balanite oil is an anthelminthic specific to schistosomiasis consistent with *b3k,* which was used to control haematuria, a symptom of schistosomiasis (Ebers 143, Chester Beatty 27/29). Balanite oil is a lubricant laxative and an emollient as was *b3k.* However, balanite oil is anti-diabetic, but *b3k* had no similar use in ancient remedies other than the symptomatic cure to remove excess urine in Ebers case 265. Moringer is also a lubricant laxative and an emollient as was *b3k*, but unlike balanites has no known medicinal properties as an anthelminthic nor does it have any known anti-diabetic or urinary properties.

The archaeobotany confirms that *Balanites aegyptica* is indigenous to Egypt, and is evident from the Predynastic Period, whilst Moringer became apparent from the Middle Kingdom (Table 1). *Balanites aegyptica* was more readily available for pharmaceutical use. *b3k* has comparable medicinal application in ancient remedies compatible with the known pharmacognosy of *Balanites aegyptica* and it therefore favours *b3k* being Balanites, not Moringer. It is also significant that there is greater archaeobotanical evidence of *Balanites aegyptica* in tomb assemblages than of Moringer, yet each is a robust fruit (Table 1).

Other Aspects of Pharmaceutical Merit

Pharmaceutical merit was considered not only for the principal drug, but for all aspects of the prescription and structure, from its formulation and preparation to its administration. The prescription formulation demonstrated a pattern comprising the principal drug, often accompanied by a secondary drug to alleviate the effects of the main drug, a flavouring to make it palatable, or an ingredient to make it soothing. The ancient Egyptian formulations fell into the categories defined in the British Pharmaceutical Codex as creams, enemata, extracts, infusions, pessaries, poultices and other formulations well documented pharmaceutically (Campbell and David 2010).

Other than the 48 cases of the Edwin Smith Surgical Papyrus (Breasted 1930) the evidence is in favour of the ancient Egyptians having treated the symptom and not the disease, a practice often evident today until a diagnosis has been made. Routes of administration are well documented (Nunn 1996), but to have pharmaceutical merit, the route of administration must carry the drug to the site of action, overcoming any of the natural obstacles in the body, e.g. the acid of the stomach or motility of the rectum. The majority of prescriptions complied with this requirement, employing oral, topical, vaginal, rectal nasal and aural routes of which oral administration was the most popular, much as it is today.

In Support of Translations

Using the technique of comparative pharmacy based on a critical assessment of archaeobotany and pharmacognosy, we were able to support the translations and clinical application for the species detailed in Table 2. There is no evidence, and indeed there is often contrary evidence, to support the proposals for the species in Table 3, when the clinical application in ancient prescriptions is taken into account. Others species such as chaste tree, fava bean, garlic and grass pea remain uncertain in use and identity, yet there is ample archaeological evidence of their presence at an early stage. Where there is conflicting opinion the application of archaeobotany and pharmacognosy has been useful in supporting one translation over another.

There remain over 100 remedies with drugs of unknown identity and whilst the application of pharmacognosy and phytogeography are useful in limiting the possible options, we concur with Quirk (2005) that 'Some of the transliteration will forever remain unknown'.

Conclusion

Most drug sources have been verified, with some 25% being determined to be of improbable use, with alternative drugs being proposed. Significantly, 50% of the drug sources used by the ancient Egyptians remain in use today, although many are now synthesised. The first scientific estimate of pharmaceutical merit demonstrates 64% of remedies in the medical papyri have therapeutic value in physiological or physical action, 3% are toxic, 1.5% sub-therapeutic, 20% undetermined and the remainder have no known therapeutic activity.

We concluded that the application of archaeobotany and pharmacognosy may assist the identification of plants once available to ancient Egyptian medicine and consequently, may endorse the ancient texts. The aim was to confirm the pharmacopoeia of ancient Egypt and to demonstrate that it was used appropriately and therapeutically, demonstrating that the Egyptians were practising a credible and reproducible form of pharmacy as early as the 19th century BC, 1800 years before Galen, the acknowledged 'father of pharmacy'. Our technique usefully identifies which plants can be dismissed in the ancient Egyptian texts, but it is less useful in determining the identity of the 130 unknown plants and to date, has only served to shortlist the possible contenders for identification.

Acknowledgements

The authors would like to thank The Leverhulme Trust who funded this research.

References

Aufrere, S. (1986). Études de Lexicologie et d'Histoire Naturelle VII-XVII. Remarques au sujet des vegetaux interdits dans le Temple d' Isis a Philae. *Bulletin de l' Institut Français d' Archéologie Orientale* 86, pp. 2-31

Aufrere, S. (1987). Études de Lexicologie et d'Histoire Naturelle XVIII-XXVI. *Bulletin de l' Institut Francais d' Archéologie Orientale* 87, pp. 21-44.

Boulos, L. (1999). *Flora of Egypt*, Vol. 1 (*Azollaceae – Oxalidaceae*). Al Hadara Publishing.

Boulos, L. (2000). *Flora of Egypt*, Vol. 2 (*Geraniiaceae- Boraginaceae*). Al Hadara Publishing.

Boulos, L. (2002). *Flora of Egypt*, Vol. 3 (*Verbenaceae – Compsitae*). Al Hadara Publishing.

Boulos, L. (2005). *Flora of Egypt*, Vol. 4 (*Alismataceae-Orchidaceae*). Al Hadara Publishing.

Breasted, J.H. (1930). *The Edwin Smith Surgical Papyrus*. Volume 1. University of Chicago Press.

B.P.C. (1911). *The British Pharmaceutical Codex*. London: The Pharmaceutical Press: http://www.bpc1911/species.html 2006

Campbell, J.M. and David, A.R. (2005). Some Aspects of the Practice of Pharmacy in Ancient Egypt 1850 B.C. to 1300B.C. In Massa, E.R. (ed.), Proceedings: V World Congress on Mummy Studies, *Journal of Biological Research* Vol. LXXX, N.1, pp. 331-334.

Campbell, J.M. and David, A.R. (2010) Do the Formulations of Ancient Egyptian Prescriptions Stand Up to Pharmaceutical Scrutiny?, In Cockitt, J. and David, A.R. (eds.) *Proceedings of the 'Pharmacy and Medicine in Ancient Egypt' Conferences, Cairo (2007) and Manchester (2008).* BAR Publishing, pp. 15-19.

Campbell, J.M., Campbell, J.R. and David, A.R. (2005). An insight into the Practice of Pharmacy in Ancient Egypt'. *Pharmaceutical Historian* 35 (4), pp. 62-68.

Campbell, J.M. (2007). *An assessment of the pharmaceutical and therapeutic merit of remedies within the Kahun, Edwin Smith, Ebers and Chester Beatty ancient Egyptian medical papyri.* Unpublished PhD. The University of Manchester.

Charpentier, G. (1981). *Recueil de Matériaux Épigraphiques Relatifs à la Botanique de l'Égypte Antique.* Trismégiste.

Dawson, W.R. (1925). Studies in Ancient Materia Medica. *American Druggist* 73, pp. 22-24.

Dawson, W.R. (1926). The Plant called 'Hairs of the earth'. *Journal of Egyptian Archaeology* 12, pp. 240-241.
154.
Dawson, W.R. (1932). Studies in the Egyptian Medical Texts I. *Journal of Egyptian Archaeology* 18, pp. 150-

Dawson, W.R. (1933). Studies in the Egyptian Medical Texts II. *Journal of Egyptian Archaeology* 19, pp. 133-137.

Dawson, W.R. (1934). Studies in the Egyptian Medical Texts III. *Journal of Egyptian Archaeology* 20, pp. 41-46.

Dawson, W.R. (1935). Studies in the Egyptian Medical Texts V. *Journal of Egyptian Archaeology* 21, pp. 37-38.

Ebbell, B. (1937). *The Papyrus Ebers*. Oxford University Press.

Evans, W.C. (2002). *Trease and Evans Pharmacognosy*. W.B. Saunders.

Fahmy, A. (2003). A Fragrant Mixture: Botanicals from the Basket in B333. In Friedman, R. (ed.) *Nekhen News* 15, pp. 20.

Friedman, R. (2003). A Basket of Delights: The 2003 Excavations at HK43. In Friedman, R. (ed.) *Nekhen News* 15, pp. 18-19.

Germer, R. (1979). *Untersuchungen uber Arzneimittelpflanzen im Alten Ägypten*. Unpublished PhD Thesis. University of Hamburg.

Germer, R. (1985). *Flora des Pharaonischen Ägypten*. Philipp von Zabern.

Germer, R. (1998). The Plant Remains found by Petrie at Lahun and some remarks on the problems of identifying Egyptian plant names, in S. Quirke (ed.), *Lahun Studies*. SIA Publishing.

Ghalioungui, P. (1987). *The Ebers Papyrus: A new English translation, commentaries and glossaries*. Academy of Scientific Research and Technology.

Grapow, H. (1954). *Anatomie und Physilogie*. Grundriss der Medizin der Alten Ägypten 1. Akademie Verlag.

Grapow, H. (1955). *Von den medizinischen Texten*. Grundriss der Medizin der Alten Ägypten 2. Akademie Verlag.

Grapow, H. (1956). *Kranker, Krankheiten und Arzt*. Grundriss der Medizin der Alten Ägypten 3. Akademie Verlag.

Grapow, H. (1958) *Die medizinischen Texte in Heiroglyphischer Umschreibung Autographiert*. Grundriss der Medizin der Alten Ägypten 5. Akademie Verlag.

Griffith, F.Ll. (1898). *The Petrie Papyri: Hieratic Papyri from Kahun and Gurob*. Bernard Quaritch

Hardman, J.G., Limbard, L.E., Gilman, A. (2001). *Goodman and Gilman's: The Pharmacological Basis of Therapeutics*. 10th International Edition. McGraw-Hill.

Harris, J.R. (1971). Medicine. In Harris, J. (ed), *The Legacy of Egypt*. 2nd edition. The Clarendon Press.

Jonckheere, F. (1944). *Une maladie Égyptienne. L'hématurie parasitaire*. Fondation Égyptologique Reine Élisabeth.

Jonckheere, F. (1947) *Le Papyrus médical Chester Beatty*. Fondation Égyptologique Reine Élisabeth.

Manniche, L. (1999). *An Ancient Egyptian Herbal*. British Museum Press.

Loret, V. (1887). *La Flore pharaonique d'après les documents hiéroglyphiques et les spécimens découverts dans les tombes*. 1st edition. Ernest Leroux.

Loret, V. (1892). *La Flore pharaonique d'après les documents hiéroglyphiques et les spécimens découverts dans les tombes*. 2nd edition. Ernest Leroux.

Martindale. (1958). *The Extra Pharmacopoeia*. 24th Edition. The Pharmaceutical Press.

Newberry, P. (1890). An examination of the botanical remains from excavations. In Petrie, W.M.F. (ed) *Kahun, Gurob and Hawara*. Kegan, Trench, Trübner and Co., pp. 46-50.

Nunn, J.F. (1992) The Medical Skills of the Ancient Egyptians. *Journal of Egyptian Archaeology* 78, pp. 317-318.

Nunn, J.F. (1996) *Ancient Egyptian Medicine*. British Museum Press.

Pommerening, T. (2003) Altägyptische Rezepturen Metrologisch neu interpretiert. *Berichte zur Wissenshaftsgeschichte* 26, pp. 1-16.

Pommerenering, T. (2005). Pommerening, T. (2005). Die Altägyptische Hohlmaße. *Studien zur Altägyptische Kultur* 10. Buske Verlag, pp. 239-261.

Quirke, S. (ed) (1998) *Lahun Studies*. SIA Publishing.

Quirke, S. (2002) *Manuscript for Health of Mother and Child. The Kahun Medical Papyrus or Gynaecological Papyrus*. University College London: (Unpublished transcript by kind permission of the author).

Täckholm, V. and Täckholm, G. (1941). *Flora of Egypt I*. Fouad University. Bulletin of the Faculty of Science, Vol 17. Cairo University Press.

Täckholm, V. and Drar, M. (1950). *Flora of Egypt II*. Fouad University. Bulletin of the Faculty of Science 28. Cairo University Press.

Schweinfurth, G. (1883a). Neue Beitrage zur Flora des alten Äegyptens. *Berichte der deutschen botanischen Gesellschaft* 1, pp. 544-546.

Schweinfurth, G. (1883b) La Flore de l'ancienne Égypte. *Revue Scientifique* 32, pp. 72-77.

Schweinfurth, G. (1884) Further Discoveries in the Flora of Ancient Egypt. *Nature* 29, pp. 312-315.

Vartavan de, C. and Amoros, V.A. (1997). *Codex of Ancient Egyptian Plant Remains.* Triade Exploration Ltd.

Von Deines, H., Grapow, H. and Westendorf, W. (1958). *Ubersetzung der medizinischen Texte.* Grundriss der Medizin der Alten Ägypten 4 (1). Akademie-Verlag.

Von Deines, H., Grapow, H. and Westendorf, W. (1958). *Erlauterungen.* Grundriss der Medizin der Alten Ägypten 4 (2). Akademie-Verlag.

Von Deines, H. and Grapow, H. (1959). *Wörterbuch der ägyptischen Drogennamen.* Grundriss der Medizin der Alten Ägypten 6. Akademie-Verlag.

Von Deines, H. and Westendorf, W. (1961). *Wörterbuch der medizinischen Texte.* Grundriss der Medizin der Alten Ägypten 7. Akademie-Verlag.

Von Deines, H., Grapow, H. and Westendorf, W. (1973). *Erganzungen, Drogenquanten, Sachgruppen, Nachtrage, Bibliographe, Generalregister.* Grundriss der Medizin der Alten Ägypten 9. Akademie- Verlag.

Westendorf, W. (1962) *Grammatik de medizinshen Texte.* Grundriss der Medizin der alten Ägypten 8. Akademie Verlag.

Common Name	Scientific Name	PD/ AP	OK	FIP	MK	2IP	NK	3IP	LP	GR
Acacia	*Acacia nilotica*	14	9		3		25			
	Acacia seyal									[illegible]
	Acacia arabica						2			[illegible]
	Acacia tortilis	1								
	Acacia albida	1	1				2			[illegible]
	Acacia species	10	4		18		15		6	[illegible]3
Balanite	*Balanites aegyptica*	3	2	1	5		5	2	1	[illegible]
	Balanites roxburghii							2	1	[illegible]
Chaste Tree	*Vitex agnus castus*									
Cedar	*Cedrus libani*	2		1		1	5	2		[illegible]
	Cedrus trew	4	1	3	3		3			[illegible]
Cinnamon	*Cinnanomum zeylanicum*									
Carob	*Ceratonia siliqua*				2		1			[illegible]
Date	*Phoenix dactylifera*	13	4		10		46		8	[illegible]8
Fig	*Ficus carica*	3			2		3		3	
Juniper	Juniperus drupacea						1			
	Juniperus oxycydedrus	3			5		5		2	[illegible]
	Juniperus phoenicea		1				4			[illegible]
Moringer	*Moringer aptera*				1					
Pomegranate	*Punica granatum*				1	2	7		1	[illegible]
Sebesten	*Cordia myxa*				2				2	[illegible]
	Cordia sinensis		1				1			
Sycamore fig	*Ficus sycomorus*	15	4	2	11	2	21	5	3	[illegible]
Tamarisk	*Tamarix nilotica*	1	2			1	1			[illegible]
	Tamarix aphylla				1			1		[illegible]
	Tamarix sp	27	2	3	6		14	2	4	[illegible]4
Willow	*Salix fragilis*									
	Salix subserrata						3	4		[illegible]
	Salix sp.	1	1				1	1		[illegible]
Zizyphus	*Zizyphus spina christi*	10	4	1	4		17	2		[illegible]

Table 1: The onset appearance and dynastic prevalence of trees cited within the medical papyri evidenced in archaeobotanical remains, detailing the number of archaeological finds in each dynasty.

Common name and classification	Uses BPC/ Martindale	Ancient Egyptian uses
Artemisia absinthium *Artemisia.* ***inculta***	Menstruation, Flu, Colds, Bitter, Appetite stimulant, Anthelminthic	**'s 'm** Menstruation K 13 ; Cough E122; Lung infection E190; Anthelminthic E56
Acacia nilotica, *arabica tortilis, albida*	Demulcent – Throat, Diarrhoea Cough and Gen. stabiliser	***šnd·t*** Demulcent colic E29; anus E161; ES V; chest E187; laxative E30; enema CB41
Aloe vera	Burns, skin, skin growth, antidiabetic, immunostimulant	***h·t-'w3*** E259 cool head; E378 sight; E424 grain eye E419 catarrh; E420 catarrh; E392 infection
Ammi majus and *visnaga.*	Anti-(inflammatory, allergic, tumour); gastric protection, vasodilator	***mjmj, mm*** CB16 Anus- anti-inflam. E175 Cystitis- anti-inflam; E215/203 Heart- vasodilator; CB17 Enema anus; E818 Cool womb
Balanite saegyptica	Not in BPC; recent research oil molluscide for Schistosomiasis. TM chest complaints/ Aqueous extract oral antidiabetic	**b3k/ išd** E41/42 Laxative-lubricant; E214 , E309 , E327 Chest/cardia-expectorant; CB 27 /29 Anus-molluscide? E143 Anus molluscide?; E265/4 Excess urine-antidiabetic?;E258 Head E687 Muscles; E32 Enema
Hordeum distichon, vulgare, hexastichum	Nutritive, carminative, demulcent , fibre, Hordenine is adrenalinic	***It*** E37 laxative - E37; adrenalinic -E240, E100 , K; demulcent belly- E133 –Demulcent skin -E497, E579 demulcent bladder E630
Bryonica dioica/ alba	Anti-tumour, purgative, irritant vasodilator, allay cough and pleurisy	***ḫ3šj·t*** laxative- E19 and 39; E122 mouth infection; heart/chest - E191/ E194/ E209; E247 and 249 head illness; rubefacient -E 610/ E614/ E649 and 657/ E666 and 86 / E693 limb stiffness
Ceratonia siliqua	Anti-diarrhoeal ,Anti-emetic, Mucilage, Demulcent	***ḏ3rt*** demulcent:- CB24, CB7,30,8,16, CB21, CB18, E8, E159, E135 antidiarrhoeal :- E44,47,48; colic :- E301
Apium graveolens	Rheumatism, arthritis, diuretic.	***m3t.t*** E145 haemorroids; E226 haematuria: diuretic; E634 stiffness; E655 rubefacient; E364 temple, E748 gums; E292 appetite stimulant; E701 tongue;E555 mouth ulcers
Citrullus colocynthis	Cathartic	***snj-t3*** Purgative E301; E132; E9 E193; E320. Cough- E331 Skin E577 Impotence E663
Coriandrum sativum Use uncertain	Carminative	***š3w*** E145 Haemorrhoids; E661 Soften erection E628 Muscles; E239 Haematuria/belly : carminative E652 Muscles
Cucumis sativus Cucurbita maxima	Carminative, diuretic, Mild laxative	***šsp·t*** E219/220 indigestion,E631for left side
Cordia Myxa tree	Nutritious Laxative	***išd*** E6,17,36,39,46,79,87,88,89,97,122, 126,137,152,186, 198,210, 219,229, 233,274,279, 284,297,300,321,327,477,480,593,631,637,754, 777,703,747, 805,177,577, 678: mild laxative / nutritive uses
Cuminum cyminum Cuminum nigrum	Carminative dose 300-600mg 0.06-2.0ml for diarrhoea, dyspepsia and as diophoretic	***tpnn*** E176, E285, E144, CB 12, E164, CB37 carminative; E254 head E700 tongue, E234 haematuria ,E766 ear-uncertain role, E89 purulency E742 mouth ulcers
Phoenix dactylifera	Highly nutritious. No formal medicinal uses are cited,	*bnr* [*bnrit*] **wdw of dates**:E189 antispasmodic; E100 purulency **Date wine**:E11 dejections, E441 skin lotion E442 scalp **Dates:** E19 belly, E423 eye, E284 urine **Powdered dates**: E103 purulency, E309 cough,E314 Cough
Ficus carica	Bulk Laxative, Demulcent Nutritive, antioxidant. poultice (BPC1911)	***d3b*** E202 stomach, E137, E97 E298 , E6, E186 laxative. E322, E328 cough, E226 haematuria
Linum usitatissimum	Poultice: inflammation, constipation Cough, urinary mucous, skin	**i3r/ *mhj* The seed**: E197: for the belly; E775: baldness E495: burns, E 110 for fever. **Dressings** ES 1-28 for wounds Lint: ES 1-48 wounds
Boswellia carteri	Fumigating powders Rubefacient, Antiseptic	***sntr*** Fumigation: K20, K1 womb; antiseptic : E 765, E742, E731 E338 ; rubefacient E638; control urine E 284
Vitis vinifera .	laxative, emetic, haemorrhage, urinary complaint,hypertension, HDC skin rashes. Oral inflammation or eyes.	***i3rr't*** E172, E186 laxative; E223 haematuria E631 muscle relaxant also grape wine
Gall nut	Used as astringents and styptics	**'3gj·t** E594 for a nest of blood-[possible styptic]
Hyoscyamus Muticus	Urinary and smooth muscle Anti-spasmodic and anticloinergic.	***pšd*** E 98 in a laxative- antispasmodic, E66 roundworm-antispasmodic E204 malaria- [possibly angina] E671 limbs
Juniperus Oxycedrus Juniperus phoenice	Colic,Flatulence carminative Antibacterial properties Antiseptic Uterine stimulant	***w'n*** E585/31/137 laxative; E140/164 antibacterial; E 184 epilepsy; E254/257 head; E631/675 muscles; E480 Jaundice Kahun onset labour? E805 0nset labour
Lactuca sativa Wild lettuce: fresh flowering herb	sedative , hypnotic irritable cough rheumatic pain, whooping cough hyperactivity anxiety necrosis insomnia. 'non addictive opium'	E 64: roundworm –pain?E608, 670 :stiff knee limbs -antirheumatic Possibly *'f3* see melilot
Fraxinous Ornus	Mild laxative flatulence griping, laxative for infants	***w 'h*** E132, E178, E43 belly and anus; E224, E230, E49 haematuria E261 remove urine retention

Melilotus officinalis	headache, neuralgia, palpitation, insomnia, veins, period pain, bruising, rheumatism, boils and	*'f3* E 64: roundworm –pain? E608 :stiff knee-antirheumatic E 670: stiff limbs- antirheumatic
Sinapsis alba/nigra	Emetic and externally as skin irritant, warming, poultice	***sh.t*** E191 for the heart, E209 for epilepsy ?, E757 Bandaged
Moringer aptera	No recorded medicinal use.	***ndm*** E80 for tapeworm
Myrtus communis	No use in formal medicine. Bown 1995:316 herbal application warming, Liver, bladder	***ht-ds*** E200 cardia,E249 The head, E672 the limbs, E175 bladder, E110 fever, E580 exudation, E472 for hair to grow
Olea Europea	Nutrient, demulcent laxative,limits gastric secretion; enema , emollient	Could be any of oils in Chester Beatty or Ebers papyri
Allium cepa	.Antithrombitic, Hypolipidaemic Hypoglycaemic, Hypotensive diaphoretic, expectorant, Antibiotic	***hdw*** E192 Lung E331 asthma E724 'blood eating' E519 wound antiseptic, K28 pregnancy test
Pistacia lentiscus *Pistacia terebinthus*	P. *lentiscus* dental caries P. *terebinthus* astringent and restorative	***'rw*** E99 to clear purulency, E127 for purulency, E225 for haematuria Consistant with P. *terebinthus*
Papaver *Rhoeas-*	somniferum extensive application as opium	***spn*** Ebers 782: stop baby crying Opium improbable but red poppy possibility. E441 and446 for scalp
Punica granatum	Tapeworms, Nausea ,vomiting, anti diarrhoea anti dysentery anti diarrhoea	***inhmn*** E50 to kill round worm, E63 to kill roundworm[possibly tapeworm]
Ricnus communis	Mild purgative,Colic in children Skin, Bed sores,Conjuctiva	***dgm**; k3k3* E123 skin, E438 scalp; E601 spots,CB 160, CB18 anus, E25 laxative
Carthamus tinctorius	bitter, circulation, heart, uterus, reducing fevers, inflammation, relieving pain, lowering cholesterol.. Externally for rheumatism bruising, sprains skin inflammation, wounds or paralysed joints	E295 rheumatism in sacral region, E296 Rheumatism in neck E759 Paralysis on one side
Ficus sycomorus	No formal use recorded	***nht* : tree** To heal wounds: E582 for the skin E491 for burns, E749 gum ulcers As a carminative: E202 E154 ; E18 laxative; E623 for the fingers E632 for the muscles,E570 skin purulency E478 for jaundice
Tamarix nilotica *tamarix aphylla*	used for sore throats in herbal pharmacopoeia.	***i3'm,im3isr / isr*** E764 for the hearing, E483 for burns, E473 to make hair grow. E535 promote new flesh
Oleo terebinth or other sp. of pinus	s antimicrobial, anti-ulcer, cardiovascular active surfactant Used as an enema, cathartic, rubefacient, antiseptic. arbortifacient	***sft*** E 679 for the limbs: rubefacient,E246 for all infection, E492 for burns: antiseptic, E519, E617: antiseptic E75, E76, E 77 anthelminthic
Triticum aestivum, durum dicoccum- emmer,	Dusting powders, Skin emollient Enemata, Demulcent, Drying	*Db·t* CB 33, CB34, CB29 : enemata. E275, E276, E278 E100 urinary demulcent, E587 demulcentE652, E679 muscle-? E90 fever:
Salix alba, Salix subserrata	Analgesic, anti-inflammatory	*tr.t* E766 to treat an ear –antiseptic: anti-inflammatory E294 : appetite stimulant
Zizyphus lotus Zizyphus spina Christi	Demulcent and nutritive. Throat and bronchial admin. Conjuctivitis, ulcers, carbuncles, boils. Purgative, colic **Herbal medicine**:Dysentery, diarrhoea, influenza, cold, boils	*nbs* E226 haematuria-demulcent,E631 treat the left side-pulmon'y E663 impotence:?? E766 the ear :astringent E481 jaundice: E213 the cardia: gastric demulcent E230, E272 haematuria, E582 for skin exudation: astringent

Table 2: Species for which archaeobotanical and pharmacognosy evidence supports their use in ancient remedies. Source material: A summary of drug monographs (Campbell 2007, 374-395)

Common name and classification	**Uses BPC**	**Ancient Egyptian uses deemed improbable**
Pimpinella anisum	Carminative, mildly expectorant	*inst* E219,230,237 Heart E633, 632 Muscles E234,226 Haematuria E267 Urinary
Melissa officinalis	Carminative, Diaphoretic Stimulant, skin Digestive stimulant	*snn* E368, E412 E379, E414
Myrica cerifera	Astringent, Fevers, head cold influenza catarrh diarrhoea colitis heavy menstruation	*p3'r.t* E257 headache salve
Cannabis sativa	Anticonvulsnant Analgesic Sedation Antifungal Antimicrobial, Anti inflammatory Narcotic Hypnotic	*smšmt* CB for the anus suppository? .
Cinnanomum zeylanicum	Germicide, carminative. astringent. anti- diarrhoeal	*tj-šps* E140 cool anus- anti-diarrhoeal E677 stiffness E553 gum ulcers –antiseptic E259 cool head – astringent E686 muscles E811 malabrathon???
Anethum graveolens	Relieve flatulence- ,Carmative Aromatic	*ims.t* E 650 Shoulder poultice, E249 Headache
Commiphora molmol	Mildly expectorant, diaphoretic, diuretic, mouth washes.	***'ntjw*** E140 anus suppository E145 anus tampon Cb10 anus bandaged E 258 head bandaged E392 the eye E466 skin bandaged E614 ankle E95 fever E529 a wound
Crocus sativas	anticancer anti arthritic antihypertensive powerful antioxidant	***śnwtt*** E295 for rheumatism E296 Rheumatism in neck E759 for paralysis down one side
Thymus vulgaris	Antiseptic, carminative cough linctuses whooping cough antispasmodic Externally:- Rubifacient counter irritant, deoderant	***innk*** E249 head,E20, E99 laxative; E194 , 191 cardia E69 to stop pain caused by tapeworm is therapeutic
Valeriana officinalis	sedative and psychotic carminative	***š3š3*** E38 E193 bowels, E239 E233 E266 E382 E593 topical: demulcent?

Table 3: Species for which there is no archaeobotanical or pharmacognosy evidence to support their use in ancient remedies. Source material: A summary of drug monographs (Campbell 2007, 374-395)

A REASSESSMENT OF WARREN DAWSON'S '*STUDIES IN ANCIENT EGYPTIAN MEDICAL TEXTS*' 1926-1934, IN THE LIGHT OF ARCHAEOBOTANICAL AND PHARMACOLOGICAL EVIDENCE

J.M. Campbell[1], E. El Saeed[2] and A.R. David[1]

[1] **KNH Centre for Biomedical Egyptology, The University of Manchester, UK**
[2] **The Faculty of Arts, The University of Alexandria, Egypt**

Abstract: *Warren R. Dawson, a distinguished Egyptologist, studied the original hieratic text of the medical papyri and published prolifically in the early 20th century, remaining an authority long after his death. Unlike subsequent scholars, he had neither the benefit of an Egyptian botanical Herbal nor the translations of Ebbell, Jonckheere or Charpentier. His work was original, diligently referenced and analysed, yet much uncertainty still characterises the materia medica of ancient Egypt and more so the pharmacopoeia. We have used forensic and comparative pharmaceutical techniques to reassess Dawson's proposals.*

We conclude that, although Dawson's technique has sustainable validity, the combined application of phytogeography, archaeobotany and pharmacognosy are useful in identification of drugs cited in the medical papyri. Consequently, we propose that ḏ3rt is Ceratona siliqua, šnj-t3 is Citrulus colocynthis, 'f3 is Melilotis officinalis, m3tt is Apium graveolens, and mm is Ammi visnaga / majus, There is however no pharmacological evidence to suggest that thwj is any variety of pea, or that šnj-t3 is Trigonella foenum graecum or that ḏ3rt is Citrulus colocynthis. There is insufficient evidence to support or refute h3syt as Bryonia diöica.

Key words: Ancient Egypt, drug identification, archaeobotany, medical texts

Introduction

The scholarly work of Warren Dawson (1926; 1932; 1934a; 1934b; 1935) is prominent for its analysis of drug translations, the difficulties still being encountered today. Dawson proposed each word from a literal translation, coupled with plants of a known morphology, characteristics of the literal description and the medicinal use. Amongst his studies in ancient Egyptian medical terms, Dawson examined five words known to be plants, proposing species of known clinical application.

Our objective was to ratify Dawson's work and our methods combined the forensic techniques of phytochemistry, archaeobotany and pharmacognosy with philology. Verification of the proposed plants was sought in archaeobotanical evidence to determine availability, dynastic prevalence and predominance at the time of the papyri. Attestation was sought in contemporary pharmacognosy of plants and their clinical application. Efficacy was evaluated by comparing the ancient remedies against late 20th century pharmaceutical protocols.

The Drugs *šnj-t3* and *ḏ3rt*

Dawson (1926, 240-241) described a vegetable drug, *šnj-t3*, occurring frequently in the Ebers papyrus, whose literal translation was '*hairs of the earth*'. Observing the seeds were used accompanied by honey or sweet beer throughout the remedies, he deduced they were bitter. The drug was primarily used as a purgative and for various stomach and intestinal disorders and consequently, Dawson commented:-

> '*we have accordingly to find a plant which fits in with the foregoing data and of which the appearance lends justification to the ancient name*'.

This rational approach was beset by uncertainty recognised by Dawson and he said of *šnj-t3*:-

> '*I have been able to find no other plant which so completely satisfies the requirements of the case and I think we may, with great probability, provisionally at least, equate hairs of the earth with fenugreek*'..

Some ten years later, Ebbell (1937) concluded the transliteration *šnj-t3* was of 'colocynth', also satisfying the parameters, but unlike fenugreek, it is an aggressive purgative. Some years earlier than Ebbell, Dawson had also considered the word *ḏ3rt*, and deduced it to be colocynth (Dawson (1934b, 41-44). His analysis was based on *ḏ3rt* being sourced from the oasis, versatile, and its sap, pulp, fruit, meal, powder, shoots, buds and fibre all found in medicinal use. It was cited for internal and external application and whilst predominantly used for gastro intestinal problems, was also used topically. Opinion still varies today (Campbell 2007, 100-102; Campbell and David 2007, 16).

Literary Evidence of *šnj-t3* and *ḏ3rt*

In examining the literary evidence, the word šnj-t3 occurs for the first time in the Ebers papyrus. It is translated as colocynth by Ebbell (1937, 31), fenugreek by Dawson, *Cyperus esculentis* by Gardiner (2001), Charpentier (1981, 682) and Germer (1979), whilst Ghalioungui (1987, 274), deems it unknown. The word *ḏ3rt* occurs on the perfumery door at Edfu denoting the determinative of a tree. This caused Charpentier to favour carob and not colocynth, a shrub. Ebers cases 10 and 212 cite both *šnj-t3* and *ḏ3rt*. The clinical significance is that each of these species is widely different in pharmaceutical activity and clinical application.

Archaeobotanical and Phytogeographical Evidence

Each species has an early appearance in Egypt. There is archaeobotanical evidence of colocynth from the Predynastic Period and throughout the dynasties (Campbell and David 2007, 16-24). A Badarian whole fruit specimen, complete with seeds, is housed at Kew (Figure 1).

Colocynth's phytogeography is extensive throughout the Nile Valley, the Mediterranean, Eastern Desert, southern Sinai, Western Desert and south to the mountainous region of Gebel Elba. The plant is characterised by its rough leaves, procumbent growth and hairy stems (Boulos 2000, 140), befitting the literal description 'hairs of the earth' (Figure 2).

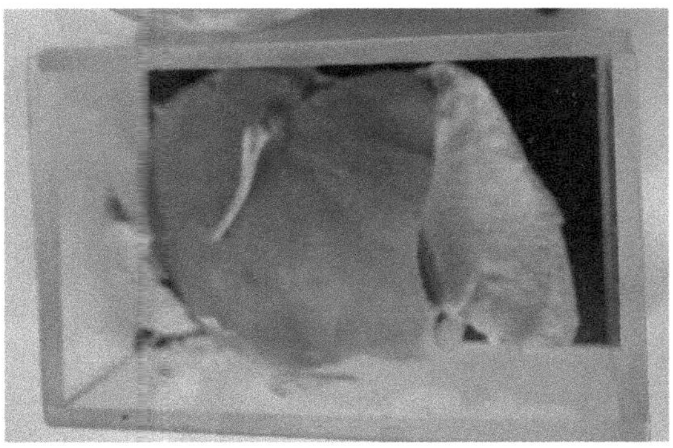

Figure 1: Fruit of *Citrullus colocynthis*, Badarian Specimen RBGK Kew Cat 40700 Image J.R. Campbell with permission Economic Botany Unit

The onset appearance of carob (*Ceratonia siliqua*) is later than colocynth, first evidenced in the Middle Kingdom tomb remains at Hawara (Newberry 1890, 46-50), and the wood was separately identified by Lucas (1948, 440). Pods were found at Deir el Medinah (de Vartavan and Amoros 1997, 70).

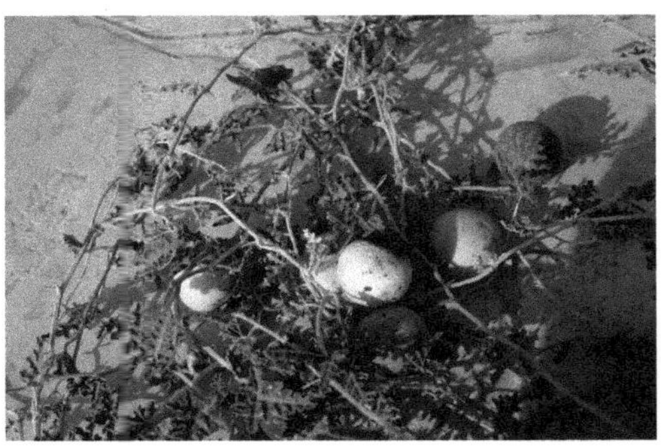

Figure 2: Citrullus colocynthis plant growing wild in the Sinai desert plain at the Medicinal Plant Project St Katherine. Image JR Campbell.

It is depicted amongst the trees in the botanical garden of Tuthmosis III at Karnak and also in the tomb of his official, Ineni (Aufrere 2005, 10). Predominance however is in the Graeco-Roman Period, when it became endemic (Campbell 2007, 119), its growth confined to the phytogeographical regions of the Fayoum, the northern Nile Delta and southern Sinai (Boulos 2000, 361).

Other plants variously proposed as *šnj-t3* or *ḏ3rt* :- Fenugreek

Dawson proposed that *šnj-t3* was fenugreek (*Trigonella foenum graecum*), a herb of southern Mediterranean origin. Archaeobotanical evidence was found by Newberry in Tutankahmun's collection (de Vartavan et al. 1997, 258) and Granger (1996) identified remains in Amenhotep's tomb. Its growth today is confined to the Mediterranean coast line of Egypt and it is improbable that it was ever grown further south than this phytogeographical region, remaining a rare plant in pharaonic times (Boulos personal communication 2006).

Rush nuts

Germer proposed *šnj-t3* as *Cyperus esculentis* of which rush nuts are its swollen tubers. The plant is indigenous to Egypt and evident in archaeobotanical remains from the Predynastic Period (Figure 3). Archaeological evidence indicates that the plant was widely available in the Nile Delta and its marshes and tributaries and it remains so today. Archaeobotanical evidence alone cannot be used to attest to the translation of these plants other than to indicate that each species was available at the time of the papyri and morphological examination of each indicates a robust, transportable fruit capable of trading. However, when the pharmacognosy of each plant was examined distinct patterns emerged.

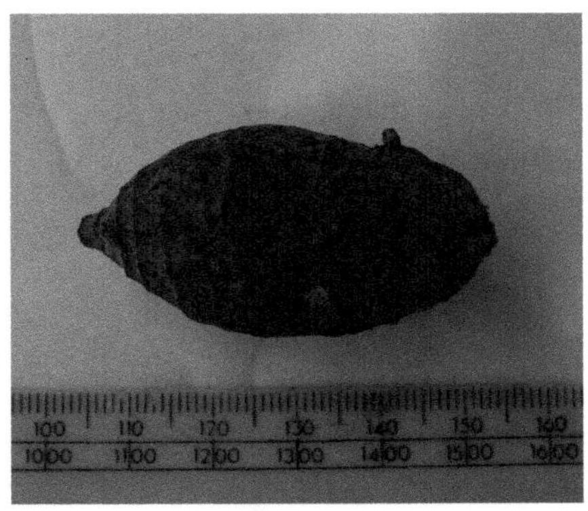

Figure 3: *Cyperus esculentis* tuber Royal Botanic gardens Kew cat. 26582. Image JR Campbell with permission RBGK

Pharmacognosy of Species Proposed as *šnj-t3* and *ḏ3rt*

The carob pod yields a mucilaginous gel, used clinically for centuries. Pharmaceutically, the pods are harvested in autumn, pressed, powdered and stored. Carob is used pharmaceutically as an anti-diarrhoeal agent, anti-emetic, thickening mucilage and demulcent for both skin and alimentary canal. It remains in clinical use today, marketed as Cheshire Gum (Martindale 1977, 921).

Colocynth is the very antithesis of carob. It is a ground covering shrub bearing small round fruits about the size of an apple and is melon-like in appearance (Figure 2). The drug is the dried pulp of the rind containing not more than 5% seed and 2% rind. The seed contained within the pod yields oil with pharmaceutical properties (Martindale 1958, 98). It is harvested in Egypt between July and October and grows spontaneously after water inundation, indicating the seed bed is long established. The pulp contains an alkaloid alpha eleterine and citrullol, once used as a potent purgative causing gross abdominal pain. Excess use or dose causes rectal bleeding.

Fenugreek has no formal clinical use but herbal medicine acknowledges its very mild laxative property (Bown 2002, 393). It also stimulates lactation, promotes healing and has some anti-diabetic properties.

A blind study of transposing *šnj*-t3 and *d̲3rt* against the known clinical uses shows that carob when fresh causes diarrhoea, when dry is anti-diarrhoeal, it is a digestive, carminative and demulcent as was *d̲3rt*. Colocynth is an aggressive purgative, causes griping as did *šnj-t3*. Colocynth is bitter and was always accompanied in recent pharmaceutical use by sweeteners as was *šnj-t3* - the ancient remedies used honey or sweet beer (Campbell et al. 2007, 18).

Typically of a potent purgative today, *šnj-t3* was usually prescribed in a single dose and was always accompanied by a carminative or antispasmodic herb, much as colocynth is always accompanied by a carminative or anti-griping agent such as hyoscine.

The efficacy of the ancient Egyptian remedies also has a significant bearing on the accuracy of the translation. Analysis of the prescriptions shows them to be pharmaceutically efficacious if *šnj-t3* is colocynth and *d3rt* is carob. The reverse does not apply.

Within the Ebers medical papyrus, 25 ancient Egyptian remedies employed colocynth efficaciously, 2 are deemed non-therapeutic, one for a cough, and two were toxic. Some 127 remedies deploy carob, each appropriate for the pharmacology (Campbell et al. 2007, 20-21). Moreover, 80% of those remedies comply with early 20th century pharmaceutical protocols of drug source, preparation, formulation, route of administration and above all, dosing regime. There was awareness of the appropriate extraction medium and selective solubility in water or alcohol.

In Ebers 10 and 212, colocynth acts as the purgative and carob the demulcent. The laxative properties of fresh carob are cited but it is an extremely mild laxative. Carob is often specified powdered and mixed with water. This rehydrates to form a demulcent lubricant, its demulcent properties affecting the skin, intestine and respiratory system. These demulcent properties are most evident in cases for the anus, a role that could not be substituted by colocynth. Neither can the clinical uses of fenugreek be substituted for either colocynth or carob pod.

The pharmacological evidence is overwhelmingly in support of *šnj-t3* fruit being colocynth and *d̲3rt* being carob.

Other drugs: *m3tt; thwj; h̲3sj·t.* ; *'f3; mjm*

The application of archaeobotany and pharmacognosy were used to reassess Dawson's other proposals:-

***m3tt* mandrake or celery?**

Dawson (1933) proposed *m3tt* as mandrake (*Mandragona officinarium*) but our analysis would indicate that it is *Apium graveolens,* wild celery (Figure 4).

Literary evidence of *m3tt*

The word *m3tt* occurs for the first time in Loret (1892) proposed as *Crocus hortensus* but subsequently revised by him to celery, after a study of the Coptic equivalent for the word. It is also proposed as celery by six scholars (Ebbell, Ghalioungui, Jonckheere, Germer, Manniche and Charpentier. Manniche also thinks consideration should be given to the plant being mountain parsley (1999, 82). Nunn is uncertain as to the translation (Campbell 2007, 104).

Dawson (1933) concluded:

> '*we are looking for a plant of magical worth which resembles the testicles of a man*' referring to Budge who described mandrake '*after the flower hath died away there remains on the top two little balls which are like the testicles of a man*'.

One of the Arabic names for mandrake is 'devil's testicles' and another 'male mandrake'. Dawson further supported Budge's view that *m3tt* was mandrake in that two varieties are cited in the papyri, one from the north (*Mandragona autumnalis*) and one from the Delta (*Mandragona officinarium*).

Celery also satisfies the phytogeoegaphy and literary description. Wild celery, *Apium graveloens*, grows in the Delta or other marshy places. It is a bulbous, partially grooved fleshy root from which arises a solid grooved stem. A hardier sub species grows in the hill country of Sinai. When young, the plant is short and leafy, resembling parsley (*Apium petrosolum*).

Archaeobotanical evidence is not prolific but the onset appearance of celery is Early Dynastic found at Tell Ibrahim in the Nile Delta (Thanheiser 1997) and it is next cited in the New Kingdom Tutankhamen assemblage (Newberry 1927). The plant is indigenous to Egypt, with growth confined to the phytogeographical regions of the Mediterranean, the desert east of the Nile Delta and southern Sinai (Boulos 2000).

Mandrake, however, is prolific in its artistic representations but the only archaeobotanical evidence is in the 18th Dynasty remains of Tutankhamen (Newberry 1927; Germer 1989, 89-95; de Vartavan et al. 1997, 168). Mountain parsley (*Apium petrosolum*) is not indigenous to Egypt and there is no archaeobotanical evidence of the species at this time. The pharmacognosy of each of these proposed plants demonstrates distinct patterns.

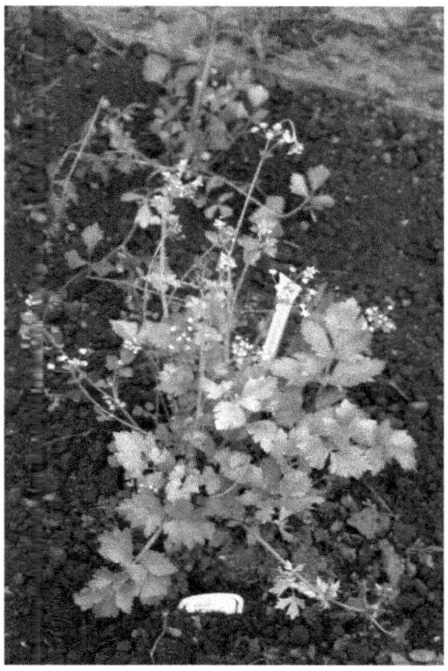

Figure 4: Wild celery (*Apium graveolens*) growing at the University of Manchester Botanic Garden, from seed provided by the Chelsea Physic Garden, London.

A blind study (Campbell 2007, 150) of transposing *m3tt* against the clinical uses in ancient prescriptions, shows that *Apium graveolens* is diuretic, as was *m3tt*, and has anti-rheumatic properties - *m3tt* was used to relieve back pain in Ebers case 634.

Parsley (*Apium petrosolum*), also having the diuretic properties of *m3tt*, is without anti-rheumatic characteristics. Furthermore, *m3tt* had none of the soporific, narcotic or poisonous properties of mandrake.

The pharmaceutical properties of the dried ripe fruit are renowned; as an anti-rheumatic, celery was an official monograph in the BPC until 1949 and is now revived in the British Herbal Pharmacopoeia. Acclaimed as a diuretic, it was used for haematuria in Ebers case 226 and was similarly advised by Dioscorides.

The pharmacological evidence is in support of *m3tt* being *Apium graveolens*, wild celery.

thwj peas?

Dawson proposed peas for *thwj*. Cited by Ghalioungui, it is in the generic form. The onset appearance of *Pissum* or *Lathyrus* species is from the Middle Kingdom (Vartavan et al. 1997 208) and the plant was used from the earliest times (Newberry 1890), but an evaluation of its phytochemistry and any medical use or application is inconsistent with the use of *thwj*.

An analysis of prescriptions shows that *thwj* was taken internally to control haematuria or for the stomach or the heart (Campbell 2007, 141). It was used topically for a burn or to dry a wound, for lameness or stiff joints. Pissum (pea) species have no such use. Consequently, there is no pharmacological evidence to suggest that *thwj* is any species of pea.

h̲3sj·t. bryony ?

Dawson proposed, with some reservation, that *h̲3sj·t.* was white bryony.

Archaeobotanical evidence is sparse, the pollen found at Naqada in a Predynastic grave remaining the only evidence of the plant (Vartavan et al 1997, 54). Neither is the species endemic to Egypt, its origin being the Levant and the southern Mediterranean; however, such close proximity does not exclude transportation.

The phytochemistry, with the analysis of ancient prescriptions, demonstrates *h̲3sj·t* was cited post epilepsy, and also for rheumatism, the liver, burns, blisters, pain in the joints, whilst bryony has no known clinical or herbal application in these areas. Bryony is however purgative and *h̲3sj·t* had laxative properties (Table 1). It was also used for the heart, and whilst bryony has no cardiac application, it has been used in contemporary herbal medicine to sedate a cough (Campbell 2007, 143). Consideration must be given that, if *h̲3sj·t* is bryony it might have been prescribed to cause blisters and burns and not cure them, a technique adopted until the late 19th century.

The limited archaeobotanical evidence, coupled with the phytogeography and pharmacognosy of bryony, suggests there is insufficient evidence to either reject or support *h̲3sj·t* as its translation, although the bias is against the translation.

'f3 melilot or lettuce?

Dawson proposed *'f3* as melilot (concurred by Grundriss, Ghalioungui, Charpentier and Nunn) whilst Ebbell and Loret proposed lettuce. It remains unknown to Germer. It is cited for roundworm (Ebers case 64) and for stiff knees (Ebers 608 and 670).

Lettuce is depicted artistically from early dynasties and there is archeobotanical evidence from the 3rd Intermediate Period. Lettuce, once wild but now cultivated, has a wide phytogeography throughout Egypt. Its symbolism is also well recorded (Aufrere 2005)

Melilot is evidenced from the Old Kingdom and from Kha's tomb in the New Kingdom. Melilot, also endemic to Egypt, grows wild in the Mediterranean region and the Dakhla Oasis where it is known as a weed of cultivation.

The phytochemistry, together with the analysis of prescriptions, demonstrates that lettuce sap is mildly narcotic and is used for insomnia, neurosis, whooping cough and hyperactivity (Martindale 1958, 1375) whilst *'f3* had no similar application in ancient remedies. However, lettuce is used for rheumatic pain and *'f3* was for stiff knees. But whereas *'f3* was for roundworm, lettuce has no anthelminthic properties. Melilot is used externally for bruising, rheumatism and swollen joints as was *'f3*. Melilot is taken internally for period pains; *'f3* was used for the pain of roundworm, a similar smooth muscle (Campbell 2007, 387). The pharmacognosy supports Dawson's analysis of melilot for *'f3* but our most recent work would indicate that the *Melilotis albus*, *sulcatis* or *elegans* should be considered possible species, each with similar clinical properties to *officinalis*.

mjmj ammi or emmer?

Ammi is proposed by Ebbell and Dawson for *mjmj* but suggested by Manniche and Ghalioungui as emmer, a variety of wheat. *mjmj* is a plant whose seeds are used for menstruation, as an anti inflammatory, demulcent, anti-asthmatic and cardio vasodilator. The species ammi is described as of age old cultivation in North Africa but is not evidenced until the New Kingdom (de Vartavan et al.; Thanheiser 1997, 38) and this has yet to be ratified. Emmer wheat is prolific from Neolithic times.

The pharmacological properties of ammi and wheat are markedly different. The phytochemistry, together with the analysis of prescriptions, demonstrates that wheat has properties as a dusting powder and a skin emollient; *mjmj* had no parallel application other than Ebers cases 109, 129, 330 where it is also combined with wheat in the same recipe. Wheat, however, has demulcent properties when applied as an enema and *mjmj* was given for a swollen belly.

Ammi visnaga and *majus* are anti-inflammatory, pulmonary and cardiac vasodilators specific for asthma, and have some properties for gastric protection, as did *mjmj*. Against the proposal that ammi is *mjmj* are the Chester Beatty prescriptions for the anus but ammi has no recorded colo-rectal properties. In each of these cases, *mjmj* water is defined.

Ammi is anti-allergic and has anti-tumour properties but there is no comparable use in ancient remedies. The evidence is compellingly in support of Dawson's proposal that *mjmj* is ammi but it is not conclusive.

Conclusions

Supported by evidence in archaeobotany and pharmacognosy, we propose that *d3rt* is *Ceratona siliqua*, *šnj-t3* is *Citrulus colocynthis*, *'f3* is *Melilotis officinalis*, *m3tt* is *Apium graveolens*, and *mjmj* is *Ammi visnaga/ majus*.

There is however, no pharmacological evidence to suggest that *thwj* is any variety of pea, or that *šnj-t3* is *Trigonella foenum graecum*, that *d3rt* is *Citrulus colocynthis* or that *h3syt* is *Bryonia dioica*.

Warren R. Dawson, unlike subsequent scholars, had neither the benefit of an Egyptian botanical Herbal nor the translations of subsequent scholars. His work was original, exquisitely referenced and analysed. We have used forensic botany and comparative pharmacy techniques to reassess Dawson's proposals and conclude that, although Dawson's technique has sustainable validity, the combined application of phytogeography, archaeobotany and pharmacognosy are useful in identification of drugs cited in the medical papyri. We think they are tools he would have found useful.

Notes

The consideration of *d3rt* and *šnj-t3* was first published by Campbell and David (2007).

Acknowledgments

The Leverhulme Trust who funded this research
Dr John Campbell MRPharmS, for pharmaceutical advice
Prof. Mohamed El Demerdash, The Medicinal Plant Project, St Catherine Sinai.
Prof. Hasne Hosni, The Vivi Tackholme Herbarium, The University of Cairo.
Dr Mark Nesbitt, The Royal Botanic Gardens Kew, Economic Botany Collection.
Prof Loutfy Boulos, Emeritus Prof of Botany, The University of Alexandria

References

Aufrere, S. (2005). *Plants, gardens and horticulture in their relationship to Egyptian culture and cosmology.* Clusius Lecture, Leiden University. http://www.clusiusstitching.nl/aufrere.html [Accessed 23/10/2006]

Boulos, L. (2000). *Flora of Egypt.* Volume 2 (geraniiaceae-boraginaceae). Al Hadara Publishing.

Boulos, L. (2006) *Personal Communication,* Cairo.

Bown, D. (2002). *The Royal Horticultural Society New Encyclopedia of herbs and their uses.* Dorling Kindersley Limited.

Breasted, J.H. (1930). *The Edwin Smith Surgical Papyrus.* Volume 1. University of Chicago Press.

B.P.C. (1949). *The British Pharmaceutical Codex.* The Pharmaceutical Press.

B.P.C. (1973). *The British Pharmaceutical Codex.* The Pharmaceutical Press.

Campbell, J.M. and David, A.R. (2005). Some Aspects of the Practice of Pharmacy in Ancient Egypt 1850B.C. to 1300B.C. In Massa, E.R. (ed.), V Proceedings: World Congress on Mummy Studies, *Journal of Biological Research* Vol. LXXX, N.1, pp. 331-334.

Campbell, J.M. (2007). Unpublished PhD. *An assessment of the pharmaceutical and therapeutic merit of remedies within the Kahun, Edwin Smith, Ebers and Chester Beatty ancient Egyptian medical papyri.* The University of Manchester: John Rylands University Library.

Campbell, J.M. and David, A.R. (2007). The Application of Archaeobotany and Pharmacognosy to Reassess the Translation of *šnj-t3* and *d3rt* in the Medical Papyri. *Current Research in Egyptology*. Oxbow Publications, pp. 15-24.

Charpentier, G. (1981). *Recueil de Matériaux Épigraphiques Relatifs à la Botanique de l'Égypte Antique.* Trismégiste.

Dawson, W.R. (1926). The Plant called 'Hairs of the earth'. *Journal of Egyptian Archaeology* 12, pp. 240-241.

Dawson, W.R. (1932). Studies in the Egyptian Medical Texts I. *Journal of Egyptian Archaeology* 18, pp. 150-154.

Dawson, W.R. (1933). Studies in the Egyptian Medical Texts II. *Journal of Egyptian Archaeology* 19, pp. 133-137.

Dawson, W.R. (1934a). Studies in the Egyptian Medical Texts III. *Journal of Egyptian Archaeology* 20, pp. 41-46.

Dawson, W.R. (1934b). Studies in the Egyptian Medical Texts IV. *Journal of Egyptian Archaeology* 20, pp. 185-188.

Dawson, W.R. (1935). Studies in the Egyptian Medical Texts V. *Journal of Egyptian Archaeology* 21, pp. 37-38.

Ebbell, B. (1937). *The Papyrus Ebers.* Oxford University Press.

Gardiner, A. (2001). *Egyptian Grammar: Being an introduction to the study of hieroglyphs.* 3rd edition revised. Griffith Institute.

Germer, R. (1979). *Untersuchungen uber Arzneimittelpflanzen im Alten Ägypten*. Unpublished PhD Thesis. University of Hamburg.

Germer, R. (1985). *Flora des Pharaonischen Ägypten.* Philipp von Zabern.

Germer, R (1989). Die Blütenhalskragen aus RT54. In Helk, H (ed) *Miscellanea Aegyptologica* 75. Archäologische Institut der Universität Hamburg, pp. 89-95.

Ghalioungui, P. (1987). *The Ebers Papyrus: A new English translation, commentaries and glossaries.* Academy of Scientific Research and Technology.

Granger, S., Tyson Smith, S. and Elder Smith, D. (1996). Report on Botanical samples TT294. In Strudwick, N. (ed). *The tombs of Amenhotep, Khnummose and Amenmose at Thebes.* Griffith Institute.

Grapow, H. (1955). *Von den Medizinischen Texten. Grundriss der Medizin der alten Ägypter* II. Akademie Verlag.

Griffith, F.Ll. (1893). A Medical Papyrus from Egypt. *British Medical Journal* 3rd June, pp. 1172-1175.

Jonckheere, F. (1947). *Le Papyrus médical Chester Beatty.* Fondation Égyptologique Reine Élisabeth.

Loret, V. (1892). *La Flore pharaonique, d'après les documents hiéroglyphiques et les spécimens découverts dans les tombes.* 2nd edition. Ernest Leroux.

Lucas, A. (1948). *Ancient Egyptian Materials and Industries*. 3rd edition. Edward Arnold and Co.

Manniche, L. (1999). *An Ancient Egyptian Herbal.* British Museum Press.

Martindale, W. (1958, 1977) *The Extra Pharmacopoeia* 27th Edition. The Pharmaceutical Press.

Newberry, P. (1927) Report on the floral wreaths found in the coffin of Tutankhamun. In Carter, H. (ed) *The tomb of Tutankhamun.* Cassel and Co.

Newberry, P. (1890). An examination of the botanical remains from excavations. In Petrie, W.M.F. (ed) *Kahun, Gurob and Hawara.* Kegan, Trench, Trübner and Co., pp. 46-50.

Nunn, J.F. (1996) *Ancient Egyptian Medicine.* British Museum Press.

Quirke, S. (2002). *Manuscript for Health of Mother and Child. The Kahun Medical Papyrus or Gynaecological Papyrus.* University College London: (Unpublished transcript by kind permission of the author).

Thanheiser, U. (1997). Local production versus import of cereals during the Predynastic Period in the Nile Delta. In Kryzaniak, L. (ed) *Interregional Contacts in the Later History of Northeastern Africa.* Poznan Archaeological Museum.

Vartavan de, C. and Amoros, V.A. (1997). *Codex of Ancient Egyptian Plant Remains.* Triade Exploration Ltd.

Prescriptions	Principal drug	Secondary drug(s)	Flavouring /other	Administration & formulation	Efficacy
Ebers 109, 129, 330,. For infection used topically	Ammi (*mjmj*) amongst others	Milk balanites Wheat Honey Myrtle	Honey beer or wine/ date wine, sweet	Topically and bandaged	Therapeutic physiol.
Ebers 121,125,173, 174.For infection	Hyoscyamous	honey Ammi (*mjmj*)	water	taken	Indeterminate Therapeutic physiol
Ebers 199, 204 For the heart	Ammi (*mjmj*)	Dates honey	Oil	Non conforming	Therapeutic physiol
Ebers 319, 323 for a cough	Ammi (*mjmj*)	Honey or beer	Honey or beer	taken	Therapeutic physiol and physical
Ebers 239 For haematuria	Ammi (*mjmj*)	Coriander Honey Unknown ingredients		mixture	Therapeutic physiol carminative
Ebers 383,572,582 eye treatments	Ammi (*mjmj*)	Fly's dirt Sycomore frt Zizyphus frt Willow frt	Viscous fluid	Eye paste non conforming	Unknown activity or pathogen
Ebers 739 Secure tooth	Ammi (*mjmj*)	Yellow ochre Honey		Paste	antiseptic none therapeutic
Ebers 818 Cool womb	Ammi (*mjmj*)	Rush nut	oil	Douche	Indeterminate
CB 13, 16 anus worms	Ammi water (*mjmj*)	Bread cake Lotus flowers Acacia flowers dates, carob honey	*smsm* water Oil of *mrẖ.t*	Enema or infusion	Unknown activity other than demulcent
Ebers 247,249,255,299 for the head	*ẖ3sj·t* bryony	Coriander. Dill, Thyme. Myrtle. juniper	grease	Topical preparation	Indeterminate
Ebers 39, for the belly (laxative)	*ẖ3sj·t* bryony	Figs, Raisin, Sycamore fruit, Yellow ochre, Frankincense.	Milk, Water	Internal, oral laxative	Therapeutic physiol, bulk laxative
Ebers 164 for the anus	*ẖ3sj·t* bryony	Natron , myrrh Juniper, Frankincense *ḏ3rt,* Cumin, Honey		Suppository	Antibacterial Astringent Demulcent Therapeutic physical
Ebers 191,194 For the heart	*ẖ3sj·t* bryony	mustard seed		Oral	Sub therapeutic physiol
Ebers 263,271,284 Urine	*ẖ3sj·t* bryony	Reed, Dates, Honey, juniper, Frankincense Rush nut, Yellow ochre, Porridge	Water	Infusion	Sub therapeutic physiol diuretic Or Non therapeutic
Ebers 610,614,649,655,657, 682,686,693 knee, ankle joints or muscles	*ẖ3sj·t* bryony	Honey celery seed, juniper Frankincense Wax	Oil grease	Topical	Therapeutic physiol
Ebers 111, 112 Skin disease	*m3tt* celery	Cumin, Wax, Dirt from courtyard, Milk of a woman, myrrh	Oil Balanites oil	Topical ointment	Therapeutic physical
Ebers 145 rectal prolapse	*m3tt* celery	Myrrh, Frankincense Rush nut, Coriander, Salt	Oil	Rectal Tampon	Anti-inflammatory Antiseptic Therapeutic physical
Ebers 228,229,233,283 Haematuria or urinary	*m3tt* celery	Figs, Yellow ochre, Honey	Sweet beer Water	Infusion	Non therapeutic or Indeterminate
Ebers 333 Blood, eyes	*m3tt* celery	Frankincense		Non- conforming	Indeterminate
Ebers 488,502 burns	*m3tt* celery	Pine tar Turpentine		Topical lotion/ointment	Therapeutic physical Therapeutic physiol
Ebers 335 asthma/cough	*m3tt* celery not dominant	Fresh bread Colocynth *pht* of an ass, juniper Cumin Figs Grapes	Wine *ḏśrt*-beer	Infusion	Therapeutic physical as laxative but non therapeutic for asthma /cough
Ebers 364 head	*m3tt* celery	Celery	Water	Lotion Cooling, Anti – infl'tory	Non therapeutic

Ebers 634,655,677,682 Stiffness, joints, rheumatics	*m3tt* celery	Frankincense Juniperus Coriander seed Hippopotamus fat	Beer/oil Hippo fat *ḏśrt* beer	Ointment	Antirheumatic Emollient Rubefacient Therapeutic:physiol Therapeutic:physical
Ebers 701,748 tongue, mouth, gums	*m3tt* celery	Rush nut Pine tar Yellow ochre Copper refuse Honey		Mouth wash	Antiseptic Anaesthetic, Sub- Therapeutic:physiol Therapeutic:physical

Table 1: The clinical applications of *m3tt; ẖ3sj.t;* and *mjmj.*

A GRAIN OF TRUTH? DETERMINING THE DIET OF THE ANCIENT EGYPTIANS

J.A. Cockitt

KNH Centre for Biomedical Egyptology, The University of Manchester, UK

Abstract: *Ancient Egypt provides us with a wealth of surviving evidence detailing the food sources available to the population. Despite this, do we really have a good understanding of the Egyptians' diet, and the implications of this for their nutritional state? The tomb and temple scenes preserved in the archaeological record appear to portray an idyllic life where food is plentiful and everyone - young and old, rich and poor - is healthy.*

This paper seeks to analyse the sources of dietary data currently available in an attempt to examine whether this is an accurate portrayal. Attention will also be paid to the factors that may have influenced the choice of food, or its availability. Careful scrutiny reveals that there still much to be learned about the importance of different food stuffs in ancient Egyptian society and the evolution of their diet over time.

Key words: Diet, grain, nutrition, food availability.

Introduction

Much of the dietary work conducted to date on the ancient Egyptian population has focussed on the domestication of cattle and the shift from a hunter-gatherer population to a more modern agricultural society. Comparatively little research has been undertaken on the pharaonic period. This is probably largely due to the significant number of reliefs, texts and models that have survived from the beginning of the dynastic period through to the end of Roman occupation in Egypt. The representation of food offerings in temples and tombs are some of the most iconic and easily identifiable images from ancient Egypt. They have served to provide scholars with an idea of what crops could be grown and which animals could survive in that environment, either naturally or with human intervention. They have also revealed which foods were considered suitable offerings to the gods, the pharaoh himself and the deceased. In addition, tomb scenes have recorded methods of growing and harvesting crops, hunting, fishing and hand rearing animals.

Information has also been preserved about the onwards processing of some food stuffs, such as the production of wine, bread and beer; the latter two forming the staples of the Egyptian diet. The importance of bread and beer to the ancient Egyptians is attested by the number of scenes, texts, models and archaeological remains associated with these industries. Adding a further dimension to our understanding of the importance of food in ancient Egyptian society are the scenes and texts that show the role of eating and drinking in festivals and banquets. It is obvious that food played an integral role in the development of a sophisticated society in Egypt, being entwined in religion, social status, entertainment, trade and politics.

Despite the wealth of surviving evidence, what is immediately obvious is the bias present in the majority of reliefs and texts. Most belong to the upper and middle classes and tend to show a stylised, idealised view of life. The main sources of information relating to the diet of the lower classes are from sources such as the ration texts and settlements such as Deir el Medina and Amarna. As stated above, the staples of the ancient Egyptian diet were bread and beer. The lower classes who worked on royal projects, on the land or in the army for example, were given rations that comprised largely of quantities of bread and beer, or the grain to make their own. According to Kemp (1989, 125) a basic wage would have consisted of ten loaves and a measure of beer, which was variable. The size of the ration awarded to workers would increase with their rank, usually in multiples of the basic ration. This diet would also have been supplemented with food that could be grown or caught e.g. fruit, vegetables, fish etc., and luxuries that were distributed during festivals, such as meat and wine. Additionally, any grain received as part of a ration that was not consumed could, in theory, be exchanged for other food stuffs (Nunn 1996, 20).

The main protein source for the ancient Egyptian population in general appears to have been fish, which were easily available from the Nile. Meat consumption seems to have been variable, with goat, sheep, fowl and pig being eaten at least in small quantities. The type(s) of meat eaten was, most probably, a reflection of several factors including social status, local prohibitions on certain foods, the environmental conditions and trade connections of a particular region. Classical authors have recorded a significant number of dietary prohibitions in evidence in ancient Egypt. The majority of these involve animals that are associated with particular gods, most frequently Osiris and Seth. These prohibitions appear to be quite restricted in their application, being linked to specific regions, periods or groups of people, and hence not part of the 'usual' Egyptian diet (Darby 1977).

Despite Herodotus' attestation that the ancient Egyptian has a plentiful daily supply of beef (Herodotus 2, 37), it is unlikely to have formed a major component of any ancient Egyptian diet. The only possible exceptions to this are the temple priests who were permitted to consume the food offerings made to the gods each day (David 1992, 75). This would have comprised a considerable proportion of beef, which was considered a luxury item.

Although this serves as an adequate overview of the diet of the ancient Egyptians and the social stratification evident in the historical record, there is a growing amount of evidence that suggests further work is needed in this area and the general idea of "one size fits all" is no longer tenable.

Nutrition

There are well-known nutritional implications for populations consuming a largely cereal based diet. As evidenced by modern West African societies, populations which rely on these types of diet are extremely susceptible to protein deficiency. Cereals contain much less protein than do meat or fish, and are deficient in particular amino acids; for example, wheat is low in lysine. In the most extreme cases, protein calorie malnutrition can result in the nutrition deficiency diseases kwashiorkor and marasmus and eventually death. Less severe examples involve growth retardation, developmental disabilities and a weakened immune system in individuals - these are still evidenced in Egypt today (WHO, 2005).

This aspect of the ancient Egyptian diet is not well understood; osteological research into stature has been conducted by many scholars (e.g. Zakrzewski 2003), but this has only generally been related to diet. Populations heavily reliant on cereals can avoid or reduce the effects of protein malnutrition with the consumption of legumes and fish, where meat is not available. Fish should have been readily available to the ancient Egyptians, and beans could have been easily grown with irrigation. Interestingly though, both of these food stuffs were subject to prohibitions during the pharaonic period (Darby 1977). Zakrzewski's work in 2003 on stature showed variation between different periods suggesting the availability of protein over time was variable.

Cereal based diets can provide further problems for populations due to the fact that they contain insufficient critical micronutrients, especially iron. Fruits, vegetables and legumes produce most of the micronutrients required daily, but unfortunately legumes and other plant proteins are known to inhibit the bioavailability of dietary iron (Larsen 2000, 26). There is therefore considerable potential for an ancient population like Egypt that does not consume much meat to have suffered from iron deficiency anaemia. This may have been exacerbated in individuals suffering from schistosomiasis which is also known to have caused hemorrhaging (Cheever cited in Rutherford 2008, 102). Skeletal material from ancient Egypt has revealed that a significant number of individuals showed evidence of cribra orbitalia and/or porotic hyperostosis, manifestations of chronic anaemia. Unfortunately, it is not possible to rule out other causes of anaemia for the bony changes, such as malaria.

The skeletal evidence from Egypt, in combination with modern nutritional studies, does not hold with the stereotypical vision of ancient Egyptian life. Studies of the ration texts do not endorse this view either. Miller (1991) produced calorific calculations of the daily rations allocated to various workers. Whilst those present in the Middle Kingdom fort of Uronarti were allocated 2136 kcal per day in bread, labourers in Abydos received only 1709 kcal per day. As Miller (1991, 259) points out this is below the maintenance level of rations determined for refugee camps, although not as low as the starvation threshold of 1300 kcal/day. It is anticipated that labourers working near settlements would have been able to supplement their rations, but this does not take into consideration the potential for one ration to have supported several family members. Workers in isolated areas would have had to rely entirely on the ration they were given. It is obvious from the ration texts that there was a great deal of variability in the diet of different levels of society; even within social levels there was a great deal of stratification.

Famine and Food Availability

The cereal-based diet favoured by the ancient Egyptians was one heavily dependant upon a good harvest and adequate distribution of food. As a significant percentage of the population was reliant on the food rations received in return for work on royal projects, it was important that promises were fulfilled, both for the workers' continued health and the continuation of royal authority. The first recorded strike in history dates to the reign of Ramses III (c.1184-1153 BC). The workers at Deir el Medina went on strike when their rations were not received (David 1996, 73). Productivity and supply can be affected by many factors including climatic or environmental change, disease, trade, war and political efficiency to name but a few. Although the specifics are different, this situation is the same today as it was in ancient times.

The most significant threat to the production of crops in Egypt is again the same as it is today – water availability. The fluctuations of the annual Nile inundations, and the impact this variation had on food productivity in the country has been well documented. Up until the building of the 1st Aswan dam, Egypt's harvest was at the mercy of the East African monsoons which are responsible for bringing water to the East African Rift Valley and controlled the amount of water brought in the inundation. Hassan (2007) cites numerous historical records of widespread famine in Egypt, due to both very low and very high flood levels, between 930 and 1500 AD. Although there is a growing amount of evidence about the climate of ancient Egypt during the pharaonic period, there has yet to be an attempt to apply this data to diet and food availability. The civilisation is noted for its long-term policy of grain storage and the central control of grain distribution, yet it seems unlikely that they could have stored enough grain to survive several years of low crop yield.

The storage of surplus grain in the country dates back at least to the Badarian Period (c. 4400-4000 BC). This feature of the society was an important factor in its success. It provided a buffer against short-term fluctuations in food availability, made long-term provision for seed cultivation and was a source of considerable wealth. There may also have been another unexpected positive aspect to this – a potential antibiotic effect caused by the consumption of stored grain. The work of Bassett et al. (1980) suggested that grain stored over a considerable period or in non-ideal conditions may become contaminated with the bacteria *Streptomycetes*. These bacteria are a source of tetracycline, an antibiotic, and so consumption may inadvertently have a positive effect upon the health of an individual. They found that 30% of the bone samples from an X-group cemetery near Wadi Halfa, Nubia produced a pattern of fluorescence identical to modern tetracycline-labelled bone when examined under a fluorescence microscope (Bassett et al. 1980, 1532). This raises the possibility that other regions of Egypt may show similar patterns.

There is, however, a negative side to the consumption of stored grain; cereals can potentially become contaminated with fungi and their metabolites - mycotoxins. These develop when storage conditions are not ideal, particularly where the humidity level is too high. The most well known of the mycotoxins are aflatoxins; the infestation of maize with the aflatoxin, *Claviceps,* is known to cause ergotism which is held responsible for high human mortality rates in the Medieval Period (Bhat and Miller 1991). Ergotism is known to affect the central nervous system, causing symptoms such as hallucinations, delusions and convulsions. Similar effects are encountered with aspergillotoxicosis, poisoning caused by *Aspergillus fumigatus* which affects cereals crops including wheat (Stathakopoulos 2004, 106). The latter remains active at high temperatures, so it could potentially have affected crops in Egypt.

There has been little research into the possibility that these may have caused problems in ancient Egypt, but famine periods may have necessitated the consumption of grain that would in ordinary circumstances have been discarded. Mycotoxins can also affect animals, so increased mortality rates in cattle may also have been experienced. There is however a suggestion that Egypt may have suffered from this problem. Stathakopoulos (2004, 104, 258) records an account of an epidemic in Alexandria in 507 AD that is consistent with ergotism type symptoms.

Dietary Stable Isotopes

Probably the most significant modern research conducted into the ancient Egyptian diet is the work on stable isotopes, which provide information about the bulk diet of individuals. Given sufficient sample numbers, this technique can also provide data about the diet of specific groups, social classes, populations, periods and areas of habitation. The studies conducted to date, although fairly small in number, have identified the potential for further research.

As discussed above the ancient Egyptian diet was largely comprised of bread and beer, with fruit and vegetables and very little meat. This is borne out by the available stable isotope data, which is reflective of a largely C3 based terrestrial diet (Iacumin et al. 1996; Thompson et al. 2005). As expected this does not appear to have changed significantly from the Badarian Period through to the Christian era, suggesting any dietary shift is likely to be very slight. Although sample numbers are currently very small, there is some indication that slight variations in the source of dietary protein may be distinguishable. The $\delta^{13}C$ values obtained by Iacumin et al (1996) and Thompson et al. (2005) show a greater spread of results during the Naqada Period, with the subsequent First Intermediate Period and Late Period results being more tightly grouped. Further analyses will help determine the statistical significance of these patterns, which may in the long-term help identify the development of agriculture and the shift away from a hunter-gatherer society in the country.

Some potential indicators of social and/or regional variations can also be determined, although again as the number of samples is small, further work is needed to clarify the results. Iacumin et al. (1996) analysed the $\delta^{13}C$ values of bone samples from two different towns during the First Intermediate Period – Asyut and Gebelein. The results demonstrate that more dietary variation was experienced at Asyut and the average $\delta^{13}C$ value indicated a slightly higher C3 component to the diet at Asyut (Table 1). Results were also provided for the Naqadan population of Gebelein. These suggest a largely similar diet in Gebelein in the two periods, but with greater variability between individuals in the First Intermediate Period.

Location	Period	$\delta^{13}C$ range	$\delta^{13}C$ average
Gebelein	Naqada	-19.1 to -19.6 ‰	-19.4 ‰
Gebelein	FIP	-18.8 to -19.7 ‰	-19.4 ‰
Asyut	FIP	-19.3 to -20.3 ‰	-19.8‰

Table 1: $\delta^{13}C$ values from Asyut and Gebelein (taken from Iacumin et al. 1996)

The First Intermediate Period is one characterised by social instability caused by both environmental and political problems in the country. Being able to study the diet of specific regions or towns during this time may provide important information about the availability of food to different areas, which may in turn be linked to factors such as political importance, centres of trade, the productivity of an area etc. Differences between individuals from the same area may provide evidence of social ranking, the movement of individuals and personal choice e.g. food prohibitions. It is possible that greater variation during famine periods may be indicative of the search for any available food source, with individuals consuming food that was outside of their usual dietary range.

Conclusion

It can be concluded that historical and archaeological evidence can provide a good overview of the ancient Egyptian diet, but unfortunately many sources are subject to bias. Research into this area has tended to be fairly general, thus little obvious progress can be seen. Identification of indicators of dietary discrimination over both time and space is possible, making further understanding in this area attainable. Combining more traditional resources with analytical techniques can provide a new and detailed understanding of the ancient Egyptian diet.

References

Bassett, E.J., Keith, M.S., Armelagos, G.J., Martin, D.L. and Villanueva, A.R. (1980) Tetracycline-labelled Human Bone from Ancient Sudanese Nubia (A.D. 350). *Science* 209, pp. 1532-1534.

Bhat, R.V. and Miller, J.D. (1991) Mycotoxins and Food Supply. In *Food, Nutrition and Agriculture. FAO Corporate Document Repository*: http://www.fao.org/docrep/u3550t/u3550t0e.htm [Accessed 19 January 2009]

David, A.R. (1992) Natsef-Amun's Life as a Priest. In David, A.R. and Tapp, E. (eds) *The Mummy's Tale.* Michael O'Mara Books, pp. 65-79.

David, A.R. (1996) *The Pyramid Builders of Ancient Egypt: A Modern Investigation of Pharaoh's Workforce.* Routledge.

Darby, W.J. (1977) *Food: The Gift of Osiris.* Academic Press.

Hassan, F. (2007). Extreme Nile floods and famines in Medieval Egypt (AD 930–1500) and their climatic implications. *Quaternary International* 173–174, pp. 101–112.

Iacumin, P., Bocherens, H., Mariotti, A. and Longinelli, A. (1996). An isotopic palaeoenvironmental study of human skeletal remains from the Nile Valley. *Palaeogeography, Palaeoclimatology, Palaeoecology* 126, pp. 15-30.

Kemp, B. (1987) *Ancient Egypt. Anatomy of a Civilisation.* Routledge.

Larsen, C.S. (2000) Dietary Reconstruction and Nutritional Assessment of Past Peoples. In Kiple, K.F. and Ornelas, K.C. (eds) *The Cambridge World History of Food.* Cambridge University Press, pp. 13-33.

Miller, R.L (1991). Counting Calories in Egyptian Ration Texts. *Journal of the Economic and Social History of the Orient* 34 (4), pp. 257-269.

Nunn, J. (1996) *Ancient Egyptian Medicine.* British Museum Press.

Rutherford, P. (2008) The Use of Immunocytochemistry to Diagnose Disease in Mummies. In David, A.R. *Egyptian Mummies and Modern Science.* Cambridge University Press, pp. 99-115.

Stathakopoulos, D. (2004) *Famine and Pestilence in the Late Roman and Early Byzantine Empire.* Birmingham Byzantine and Ottoman Monographs Vol 9.

Thompson, A., Richards, M.P., Shortland, A. and Zakrzewski, S.R. (2005). Isotopic palaeodiet studies of Ancient Egyptian fauna and humans. *Journal of Archaeological Science* 32, (3), pp. 451-463.

Zakrzewski, S.R. (2003) Variation in Ancient Egyptian Stature and Body Proportions. *American Journal of Physical Anthropology* 121, pp. 219-229.

World Health Organisation (2005). *Report on the Regional consultation towards the development of a strategy for optimizing fetal growth and development.* http://www.who.int/nutrition/publications/FinalRepmjortRegCons.pdf [Accessed 19 January 2009]

SUPPORTING EVIDENCE: THE POTENTIAL ROLE OF STABLE ISOTOPE DATA IN INVESTIGATING THE ANCIENT EGYPTIAN PHARMACEUTICAL TRADITION

J.A. Cockitt

KNH Centre for Biomedical Egyptology, The University of Manchester, UK

Abstract: *This paper seeks to highlight the potential of using scientific methods, in particular stable isotope analysis, to advance our understanding of the ancient Egyptian pharmaceutical tradition. The inextricable links between human diet and localised climate and the development of a pharmaceutical tradition can be exploited to support or enhance what can be learned from the medical papyri. The very nature of studies on ancient Egypt with the associated problems makes alternative sources of information all the more important. Some of the potential applications of this technique are discussed to highlight the growing importance of work in this area, not just for its intended purpose but also more novelly for studying ancient Egyptian pharmacy.*

Key words: Stable isotopes, diet, resource availability, medical papyri.

Introduction

There have been numerous investigations into the ancient Egyptian pharmaceutical tradition based mainly on the translation and subsequent interpretation of the remedies preserved in the surviving medical papyri. Although these have gone a considerable way towards identifying which plants were available to and used by the ancient Egyptians, there remain significant problems with the translation of many plant names. Progressing from the current state of knowledge is likely therefore to require the use of other, more novel, sources of information. The "Pharmacy in Ancient Egypt" project at the KNH Centre for Biomedical Egyptology, The University of Manchester is the first of what is likely to be many attempts to further our understanding of the population's pharmaceutical knowledge, using scientific methods such as DNA and Gas Chromatography-Mass Spectrometry (GCMS). This paper seeks to highlight another analytical technique - stable isotope analysis - that has the potential to support studies in this area.

Stable isotope analysis is a growing field in archaeological science, being used to reconstruct the diets of past human populations and provide indicators of ancient environments, supporting climatological and migration and population studies (Schoeninger and Moore 1992; Van Strydonck et al. 2005). Data from research into both of these areas can potentially help support and progress ancient Egyptian pharmaceutical studies – food and medicine are inextricably linked. Being able to understand what resources were available to the population and what governed their selection of food stuffs and in turn medicinal products could help scholars to understand further the ethos of the pharmaceutical tradition.

There are several advantages to the application of this particular technique to ancient Egyptian pharmaceutical studies: firstly, it has already been applied to human remains from Egypt and Nubia, providing not only proof that reliable results can be obtained but also some preliminary data for study; secondly, the technique is minimally destructive which makes the availability of suitable sample material much higher; and finally, the relatively low cost of analysis makes this type of study much more affordable.

Food for the Pharmacy

One glance at the medical papyri will establish that a significant proportion of the remedies contained the staples of the ancient Egyptian diet: bread and beer or their constituents, wheat and barley. For example, the Ebers papyrus contains over 100 remedies which include beer (Ghalioungui 1987). The dependence of this society upon grain is well-established and has been documented many times (e.g. Brewer et al. 1994 and references therein). All available evidence to date suggests that the ancient Egyptians consumed only C3 type cereals like wheat and barley.

The stable isotope analysis conducted to date on human bone supports this view with $\delta^{13}C$ values being in the range of -18.0 to -20.0 ‰ (Iacumin et al. 1996; Thompson et al. 2001). It appears that, although C4 cereals such as millet and sorghum would grow naturally in the region, they were not favoured by the Egyptians who preferred to raise the more resource intensive wheat and barley. This is also reflected in their use of cereals or cereal-based products; there is only one translation in the Ebers papyrus (*mjmj, mm*) that has been translated as a C4 cereal. Lefebvre in 1956 translated this as sorghum; however, as Ghalioungui (1987, 270) points out this is more consistently translated by other scholars as emmer, casting doubt on the earlier translation. Although some of the remedies do incorporate some unusual ingredients that would be unlikely to form a serious component of the diet, e.g. urine, it seems that there is no deviation as regards cereal. Without tangible evidence it is impossible to determine the reasoning behind this, although it is possible that this was due to the religious link between wheat and Osiris. The sacred nature of this grain would ensure its preferred use in remedies.

Studies conducted by Thompson et al. (2005) to determine the $\delta^{13}C$ and $\delta^{15}N$ of animal bone from various periods of Egyptian history has identified that the consumption of meat was largely restricted to small cattle, such as sheep and goats, and pigs. Based on the comparison of rations between humans and animals, it appears unlikely that any social group or period saw the consumption of significant quantities of beef. This is in accord with the views of Egyptologists, who attest that beef was likely to have been restricted only to consumption by priests following the offering of the meat to the gods. Despite this, a large number of the pharmaceutical remedies preserved involve the use of cattle parts – meat, blood, fat, spleen, bile and milk. It seems likely that this would have made the remedies containing cattle products very expensive. It is known that doctors, and therefore presumably those producing remedies, received remuneration for their services. It is not known however if treatment was in anyway stratified according to social status. Given the ancient Egyptian's notion of the sacred role of cattle, it is sensible to assume that these remedies were considered to be extremely powerful, evoking the power of the bull. Although efficacy from many remedies has been suggested (e.g. Campbell and David 2010), it must not be forgotten that magic and religion played a very important role in the understanding of the causes of disease and its cure.

The small amount of data available for pig bone has proved extremely interesting and warrants further work. The isotope ratios for pigs are consistent with their inclusion in the ancient Egyptian diet. This supports the archaeological evidence for pig consumption found at Amarna. However, there has been considerable discussion about whether the Egyptians ate pigs or whether they were considered taboo. Darby (1977) discussed the available historical evidence and concluded that pigs were taboo for two periods – the Early Dynastic period during the Unification and Dynasties 21-27 – and then this applied mostly to priests. Pig products are found in eight of the remedies in Ebers, although in none of these are they actually consumed. A similar pattern is also noted with fish. The taboos regarding both of these animals are thought to be related to the Osiris myth – the pig is associated with Seth, whilst certain fish species were thought to have consumed the phallus of Osiris. Both of these taboos have positive and negative connotations, for example supporters of Osiris may believe the pig to be a symbol of Seth and therefore dangerous, whilst supporters of Seth may believe it a sin to consume the flesh of Seth himself. In either case, it may have been considered beneficial to use the products in topical applications, but too dangerous to consume them.

It can be determined from this that there were very carefully thought out rules regarding the use of food stuffs in medical remedies. Many of the ingredients included had powerful magic associations that would help the patient to a full recovery. Restrictions on the consumption of some foods for religion reasons may have led to their inclusion in remedies in the first place as the power of a god was invoked. In contrast, food that was not usually eaten or associated with certain taboos was also not usually consumed via the ingestion of a remedy.

It is difficult to understand the ethos behind the development of the pharmaceutical tradition, but by comparing the ancient Egypt diet with the medical remedies, a small degree of comprehension can be achieved. Further dietary work in this area may add more detail; information about the consumption versus the medical use of fish may be obtained, for example.

Environmental Change and Resource Availability

Globally, the late Holocene period is identified as a period of considerable climatic variability (Mayewski et al. 2004). In North Africa, the climatic optimum established in the early Holocene gave way to rising temperatures and declining precipitation. The effects of this environmental change were progressive, being felt earlier in the north of the continent, with evidence of regional ecological variation appearing (Kuper and Kröpelin 2006). There is considerable discussion between scholars as to precisely when the effects of this shift would have been felt in Egypt; suffice to say, it appears to have begun c. 5300 – 5000 BC, with the current climate being largely established by c. 2000 BC.

This will, naturally, have had an effect upon the plants that were available to the ancient Egyptians. It is difficult to ascertain when the pharmaceutical tradition began to develop in ancient Egypt; the oldest extant medical papyrus dates to the Middle Kingdom (the Kahun papyrus from year 29 in the reign of Amenemhat III). However, as Nunn (1996, 11) highlights, numerous scholars believe that many of the medical papyri had their origins in the Old Kingdom. Assuming this supposition to be correct, or at least accepting that the pharmaceutical tradition was developing during this time, then it appears likely that the ancient pharmacists saw the plants available to them beginning to change in response to the environmental shift.

It is particularly difficult to identify trends in the appearance of plant species in ancient Egypt using actual botanical remains. There is a lack of secure contexts in the archaeological remains in many parts of Egypt. Many sites were occupied over long periods or reoccupied at later dates. As structures often remained usable for considerable lengths of time due to the climate of Egypt, new occupation layers were not always formed, so the material remains from different periods are mixed. Problems are also caused by the disturbance of sites by a variety of people including grave robbers, tourists and the local populations, and poor excavation techniques until the late 18th and early 19th centuries. As a result, caution must be advised when identifying the appearance of plant species in this manner. Likewise, the absence of plant remains from the archaeological record cannot be considered definitive proof of that plant's absence from a given site or era. It would however aid the study of ancient Egyptian pharmacy to be able not only to identify if the prevailing climate of the time would support the growth of specific plant species, but also if localised microclimates could be identified from where particular plant species, inhabiting an ecological niche, may have been collected. Attempts to do this would certainly benefit from stable isotope studies, especially oxygen isotope analysis ($\delta^{18}O$) that may allow insight into climatic conditions.

Oxygen isotope analysis has been employed successfully to study the precipitation levels of ancient populations. The oxygen component of an individual's tissues comes almost entirely from the water consumed; this can provide information regarding the water source and the temperature levels in a given area. There is a distinct advantage in applying these types of studies to human, and in a smaller number of instances animal, gastropod and plant, remains; many can be accurately dated to a specific dynasty or even the reign of an individual pharaoh. This would make it possible to refine the current understanding of environmental change in the area, providing a historical rather than a geological timeline. If sufficient sample sets could be identified from a region, then this analysis could also be used to examine the local environment. The only published $\delta^{18}O$ data for ancient Egypt – obtained from human remains from the Dakhleh Oasis during the Roman period – suggests that this type of localised study is feasible (Dupras and Schwarcz 2001). Very specific information regarding temperature and water levels in an area can then be related back to the available botanical information for Egyptian plant species.

The work of the Medicinal Plant Project, Sinai (Batanouny 2005; 2006) and that of scholars such as Boulos (1983) have gone a long way towards identifying the species that are prevalent in North Africa and the conditions they require or can adapt to. Isotope data has the potential to help refine these patterns, and allow further insight into the plant species that could have been grown or deliberately cultivated in the right conditions during the pharaonic period. This in turn may provide information about the availability of plants to the ancient pharmacists and indicate where plants may have needed to have been traded or cultivated, either throughout the pharaonic period or during specific times when environmental conditions may not have supported their growth.

Conclusion

This paper represents an overview of some, but probably not all, of the benefits of stable isotope research to the study of ancient Egyptian pharmacy. Although both areas have been the subject of some work, neither has by any means reached its peak. The evolution of the Egyptian pharmaceutical tradition is as inextricably linked to the diet of the population and the environment of the country as it is to the development of a complex medical system and the belief system of the country. As such, much of the work being undertaken in these areas can potentially benefit those studying the medical papyri. Although the application of some scientific techniques to this area may at times seem slightly abstract, they can provide a great deal of supporting evidence unavailable from other sources.

References

Batanouny, K.H. (2005) *Encyclopedia of Wild Medicinal Plants in Egypt Vol 1.* Project of Conservation and Sustainable Use of Medicinal Plants in Arid and Semi-arid Ecosystems in Egypt.

Batanouny, K.H. (2006) *Encyclopedia of Wild Medicinal Plants in Egypt Vol 2.* Project of Conservation and Sustainable Use of Medicinal Plants in Arid and Semi-arid Ecosystems in Egypt.

Boulos, L. (1983) *Medicinal Plants of North Africa.* Reference Publications.

Brewer, D., Redford, D.B and Redford, S. (1994) *Domestic Plants and Animals. The Egyptian Origins.* Aris and Phillips.

Campbell, J.M. and David, A.R. (2010) The Application of Archaeobotany, Phytogeography and Pharmacognosy to Confirm the Pharmacopoeia of Ancient Egypt, 1850-1200 BC, in Cockitt, J. and David, A.R. (eds.) *Proceedings of the 'Pharmacy and Medicine in Ancient Egypt' Conferences, Cairo (2007) and Manchester (2008).* BAR Publishing, pp. 20-29.

Darby, W.J. (1977) *Food: The Gift of Osiris.* Academic Press.

Dupras, T.L. and Schwarcz, H.P., 2001. Strangers in a Strange Land: Stable Isotope Evidence for Human Migration in the Dakhleh Oasis, Egypt. *Journal of Archaeological Science* 28, pp. 1199-1208.

Ghalioungui, P. (1987). *The Ebers Papyrus.* Academy of Scientific Research and Technology.

Iacumin, P., Bocherens, H., Mariotti, A. and Longinelli, A. (1996). An isotopic palaeoenvironmental study of human skeletal remains from the Nile Valley. *Palaeogeography, Palaeoclimatology, Palaeoecology* 126, pp. 15-30.

Kuper, R. and Kröpelin, S. (2006) Climate-Controlled Holocene Occupation in the Sahara: Motor of Africa's Evolution, *Science* 11 (313), pp. 803-807.

Mayewskia, P.A., Rohling, E.E., Stager, J.C., Karlén, W., Maasch, K.A., Meeker, L.D., Meyerson, E.A., Gasse, F., van Kreveld, S., Holmgren, K., Lee-Thorp, J., Rosqvist, G., Rack, F., Staubwasser, M., Schneider, R.R. and Steig, E.J. (2004). Holocene Climate Variability. *Quaternary Research* 62 (3), pp. 243-55.

Nunn, J. (1996) *Ancient Egyptian Medicine.* British Museum Press.

Thompson, A., Richards, M.P., Shortland, A. and Zakrzewski, S.R. (2005). Isotopic palaeodiet studies of Ancient Egyptian fauna and humans. *Journal of Archaeological Science* 32 (3), pp. 451-463.

Van Strydonck M., Boudin M. and Ervynck A. (2005). Possibilities and Limitations of the Use of Stable Isotopes (δ13C and δ15N) from Human Bone Collagen and Carbonate as an Aid in Migration Studies. In Marian Scott, E., Alekseev, A.Y. and Zaitseva, G. (eds) *Impact of the Environment on Human Migration in Eurasia.* Nato Science Series.

THE X-RAY PLATES OF TUTANKHAMEN: A REASSESSMENT OF THEIR MEANING AND SIGNIFICANCE

R.C. Connolly

Department of Human Anatomy and Cell Biology, University of Liverpool, UK

Abstract: *Of the 100 or so X-ray plates of the 18th Dynasty mummies taken by the late Professor R.G. Harrison during the 1960s and 1970s, very few have been published. This study considers some of the cranial and post-cranial X-ray images of Tutankhamen, with special reference to the very extensive damage or injury to the body and some aspects of mummification. No evidence is presented for a cause of death, but some suggestions are proposed with regard to the possible condition of the body when embalming started and the probable haste with which the process was enacted.*

Key words: Tutankhamen, X-ray plates, Skeleton, Soft Tissue, Embalming.

Introduction

Attempts to determine the cause of death of the young pharaoh started on 11th November 1925 when Professor Douglas Derry performed his famous 'Autopsy of Tutankhamen'. The disappointing condition of the unwrapped mummy, charred almost to destruction in some places, probably caused by an exothermic reaction resulting from over-zealous application of resins by the embalmers, rendered detailed analysis at the time impossible. Fortunately, the restricted oxygen supply in the sarcophagus probably prevented the whole tomb and contents going up in smoke! Although the thermal destruction is very extensive, much of the skeleton and soft tissue, albeit badly damaged, is still intact.

It was not until 4th December 1968 that a group similar to that which attended Prof. Derry's autopsy re-examined the mummy. This group consisted of, amongst others, Professor R.G. Harrison and his radiographer /photographer Mr L. Reeve from the Department of Anatomy at the University of Liverpool, UK, Dr Z. Iskander, Mr A. Taher and Mr S. Osman from the Department of Antiquities in Cairo. The main reason for Professor Harrison's examination of Tutankhamen on this occasion was not to determine a cause of death, but it was an anthropological investigation attempting to establish Tutankhamen's possible family relationship with Smenkhare. Having considered that the remains in Tomb 55 were not those of Akhenaten, but were of Smenkhare (Harrison 1966) he wished to establish a physical comparison between the two individuals. Cause of death was a secondary consideration. So now, over forty years later, in Manchester, we are reviewing the mummy of Tutankhamen.

Materials and Methods

Five X-ray plates are under consideration: lateral, frontal and basal images of the head and neck – plates 1, 2 and 3, and images of the thorax and abdominal pelvis – plates 5 and 6.

Despite the extremely cramped and very difficult circumstances in the tomb under which the radiographs were taken, using a ca. 1930 portable Siemens-Reiniger-Veifa X-ray unit and developed in a bathroom in the Winter Palace Hotel in Luxor, some excellent results were obtained by Mr Reeve. One lateral image has been widely published (Harrison and Abdalla 1972, 8-14; Reeves 1990, 118; Boyer et al. 2003, 1142-7) amongst others, but the one now under consideration is a digitally enhanced image of one of the many originals showing much more detail.

X-ray images of the whole body were obtained, but unfortunately the plates of the feet have all 'temporarily gone missing'.

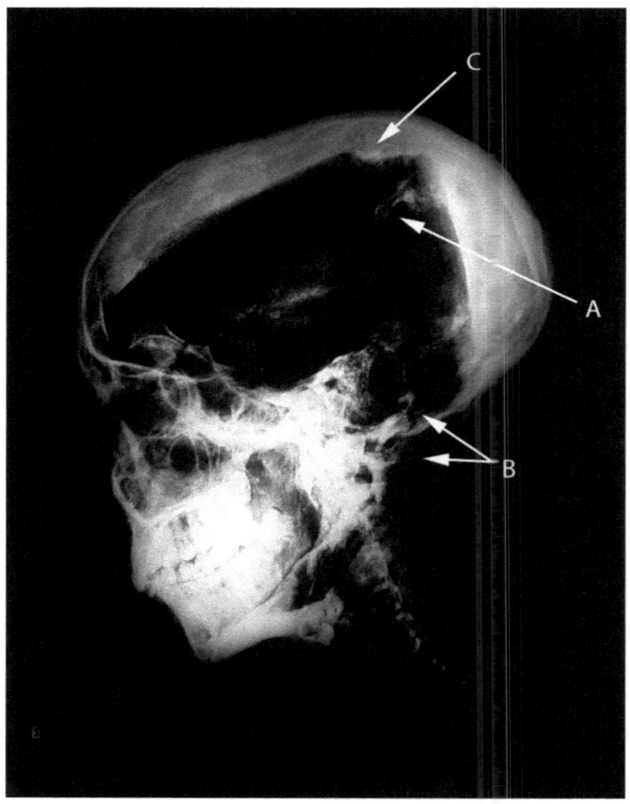

Plate 1: Lateral view of skull. A – Bone fragment. B – Occipital double image. C – Implement.

Results – The Head and Neck

Plate 1 is the digitally enhanced image of the lateral aspect of the skull and cervical spine, the original being the only widely published X-ray plate of Tutankhamen. The most obvious feature of this image is the two levels of X-ray opaque material in the cranial cavity. One occupying the superior cranial fossa which, as molten resin, must have been introduced with the head spinally extended over the end of the embalming table and the other filling the occipital region, presumably with the body lying flat, ventral surface uppermost. Residual layers of resin in the cranial cavity of mummies is not common, but does occur, for instance the mummy of Amenophis III (Amunhotep III) shows a very large occipital pool although no pool in the upper cranial vault.

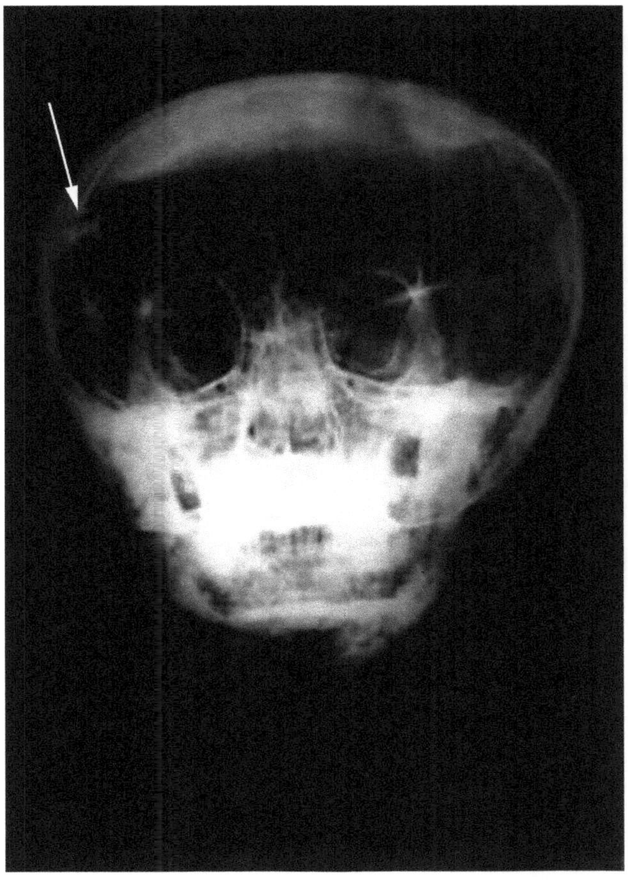

Plate 2: Frontal view of skull. Arrow – Large bone fragment. Shows intact nasal region and nasal packing.

The second feature is the two bone fragments, one large in the upper cranial quadrant – Plate 1A and Plate 3A – and one very small one in the lower quadrant – Plate 3B. These have been widely interpreted as fragments of the ethmoid bone destroyed by the embalmers removing the brain through the nose (Harrison and Abdalla 1972). In that publication, Harrison says 'On closer analysis, however, after further X-rays were developed and became available for study, several main objections to this theory were apparent and an alternative explanation suggests itself. This additional analysis will be discussed in future publication' Sadly he did not live to produce that publication. The enhanced images show quite clearly that the two fragments are the left lateral process of the first (atlas) cervical vertebra. The large fragment is the distal arm of the process, and in plate 3B, the small fragment is identifiable as the proximal portion of this process. They are both loose in the cranial cavity appearing in different places and in different orientations in different X-ray plates. They are not embedded in the resin as they would have been if introduced during the embalming process.

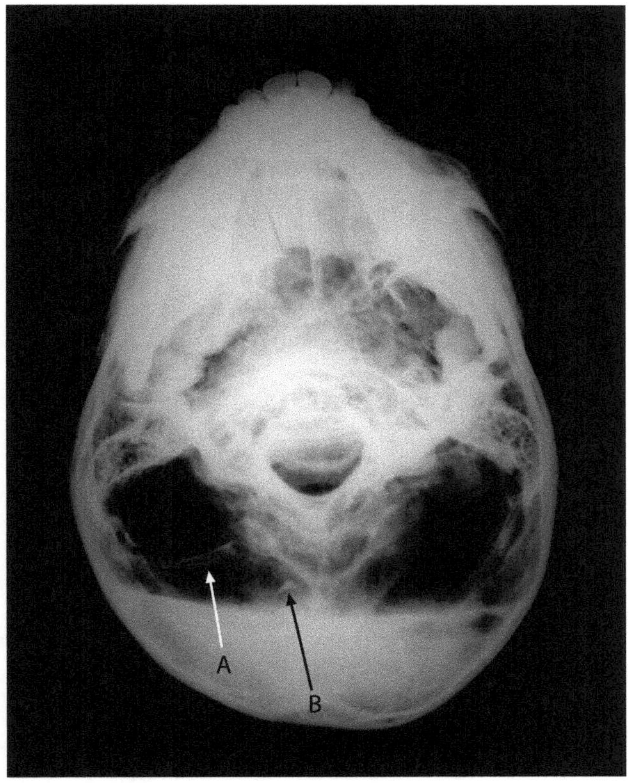

Plate 3: Basal, sub-mental view. Arrows – A: large and B: small bone fragments.

The third significant observation relates to the occipital bones themselves. They are of normal appearance with no pathological thinning or thickening, and what has been grossly misinterpreted as calcified tissue (Brier 1998) is nothing more than both the left and the right occipitals being projected simultaneously on the plate. This is the result of the desperately cramped conditions under which the X-ray pictures were taken with this final image being slightly oblique (Plate 1B).

Interestingly, the posterior corner of the superior resin layer shows an intensely X-ray opaque object embedded in the resin, closely resembling an embalming instrument which was in use at this period of Egyptian history (Janot 2000). This was first noticed in one of the digitally enhanced X-ray plates by Mr Drew Norris working with the author in 2003. Being embedded in the resin indicates that it was lost during embalming and not subsequently.

How did the cervical spine become damaged releasing bone fragments into the cranial cavity? This could not have occurred during mummification, nor from any injury preceding death; otherwise they would have been embedded in the resin, not as has been noted previously, loose in the cranial cavity. As is clear from Plate 2, the bones of the nasal region including the cribriform plate of the ethmoid bone are completely intact around the linen packing inserted by the embalmers, so the usual method of removing the brain through the nose was not employed in this case. The overall general hurry associated with Tutankhamen's mummification and burial has suggested that he had already been dead for some considerable time before embalming started. If this was the case then the brain would have liquefied and could easily have been drained out through the foramen magnum in the base of the skull by separation of the cervical spine from its articulation with the base of the skull. This could have been followed by some minor scraping of the inside of the skull (hence the residual implement) and introduction through the foramen magnum of the hot, liquid resin. An altogether malodorous procedure!

Did Howard Carter or Douglas Derry find that the skull was loose on the cervical spine and ease them apart to inspect the contents of the skull? This could easily have resulted in the – by then – fragile lateral process of the atlas vertebra being broken off and left in the cranial vault. In addition to the embalmers' resin on the cervical spine, Harrison (unpublished) thought there was glue present which Carter or Derry may have applied in addition to wax and apparently newly applied resin (Harrison and Abdalla 1972).

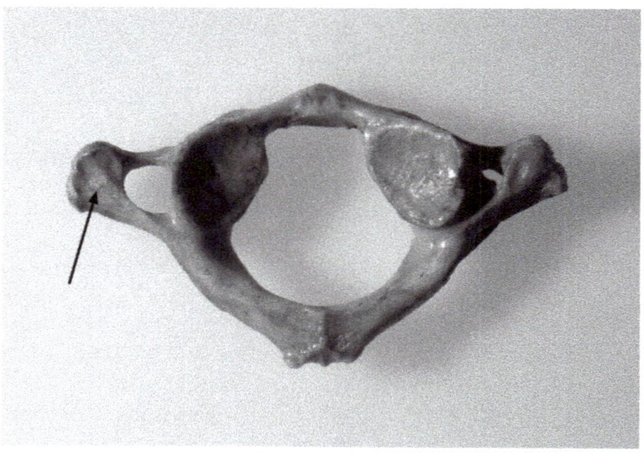

Plate 4: First cervical vertebra (Atlas) lateral process marked with arrow.

The Post Cranial Skeleton

Plate 5 is the thorax and upper abdomen. Much of the unguent-soaked packing is still present as are several small circular faience beads – presumably from a necklace worn before embalming. Similar beads are apparent on the X-ray plates of the upper arms. Notably the sternum is absent as are many of the ribs. Some ribs have been broken off, whereas others have been cut. Such extensive damage was an unheard-of practice for the Royal Embalmers, so who did it? If, as has been widely suggested, Tutankhamen had been dead for some considerable time before embalming was started, it is reasonable to assume that the embalmers would have adopted the easiest and quickest procedure to remove the decomposing viscera and preserve the all-important heart (the whereabouts of which is not now known). Simply removing the entire anterior thoracic wall and some of the anterior abdominal wall would have been the obvious solution. But why are some of the ribs broken and some cut? It would have been much easier simply to cut away the thoracic wall rather than breaking some of the ribs – which is much more difficult than cutting. So, was Tutankhamen seriously injured prior to death, with several broken ribs and possibly an injured sternum? Perhaps a fall from a moving chariot or a hunting accident? Possibilities. But why did the embalmers – if indeed they removed it – not replace at least the sternum? Alternatively, did Howard Carter or Douglas Derry open the thoracic cavity, for scientific enquiry or perhaps hoping to find gold? If so, why did they not replace the thoracic wall, and where is it?

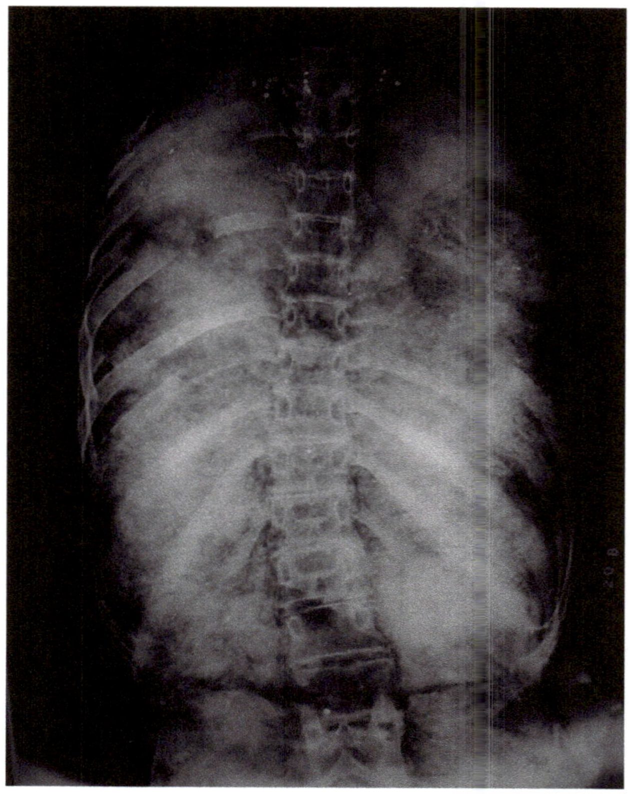

Plate 5: The thorax.

Plate 6 shows the lower thorax and the abdominal and pelvic regions. The two most striking features of which are the complete transection of the body at the level of, and right through, the third lumbar vertebra, and the intense packing of the entire pelvic cavity. It was Howard Carter who cut the body in half ostensibly to remove it from the base-plate to which it was securely attached with a solid resinous substance. At the same time, separating the limbs and head and neck from the torso (conservation procedures have fortunately changed since 1922!). Everything is normal except for very extensive destruction of the pelvis – presumably, but not certainly post-mortem damage. The pubic bones are missing and much of the ilium and adjoining parts of the left side are also destroyed. The greater sciatic notch on the right side is clearly visible, with as Harrison noted a 'very small angle of about 50°' (Harrison and Abdalla 1972). Most of the pelvic girdle appears to have been broken rather than cut. This damage does correspond with the unusual position of the embalming wound as described by Reeves (1990, 117), but it is in no way a normal pattern followed by Royal Embalmers. Was this then the result of a rushed and very hasty embalming or part of the same possible trauma suggested in the analysis of the thorax?

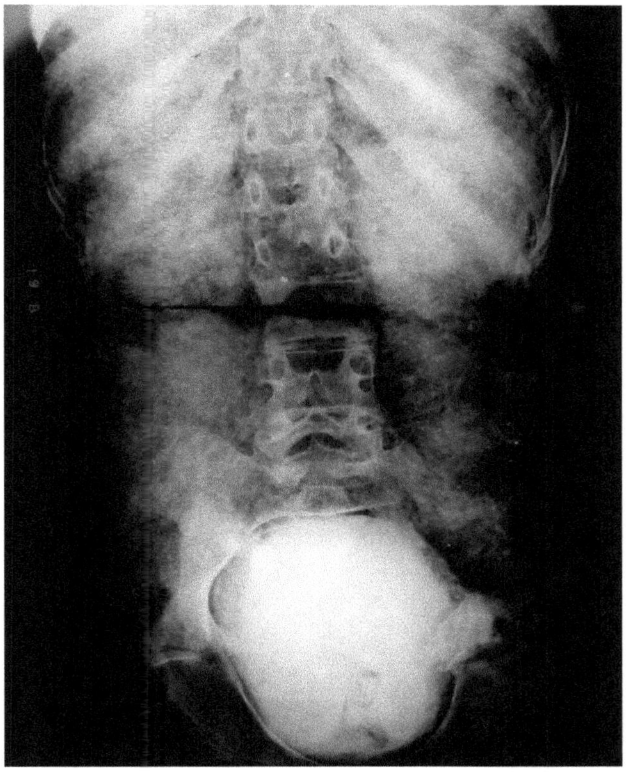

Plate 6: Lower thorax, abdomen and pelvic regions.

Discussion

Nothing on these X-ray plates points to a definitive cause of the death of Tutankhamen, but only a very, very small proportion of the fatal circumstances will leave indicators on an X-ray plate – particularly perhaps 3293 years after death. Several proposals have been made mainly in the popular media for the cause of death of Tutankhamen. Professor Harrison at the conclusion of the BBC TV documentary made in 1969 declared 'there is some thinning of the occipital bone which could have been caused by a blow to the back of the head'. He was pressurised into making a definitive statement for the film and I believe, regretted it to his dying day. I am sure he never really seriously considered the 'blow to the back of the head' as a likely situation; he was far too good an anatomist. This and the 'calcified membrane' previously noted as decidedly absent and the possibility of a sub-dural haemorrhage are not upheld by the evidence. Similarly the thorax shows no bone-related evidence for tuberculosis, although this does not confirm that he did not suffer from this disease. The slight curvature of the vertebral column, designated by some as scoliosis, is due simply to the alignment of the body at laying-out during embalming. There is no evidence of 'wedging' of any of the perfectly normal vertebrae to suggest he had scoliosis. Suggestions of Klippel-Feil Syndrome - fusion of the cervical vertebrae - is simply again, poor analysis of the X-ray plate. The apparent fusion is due to the fact that the vertebrae are stuck together with resin or glue and wax (Harrison and Abdalla 1972). The X-rays of the feet are not currently available for publication but they show no abnormalities and certainly no evidence for club-foot, as has been proposed to explain the collection of walking sticks in Tutankhamen's tomb. The demonstration (Hawass 2005) of a femoral fracture which could have caused a fatal septicaemia is still an open question. Certainly a fracture is visible on Harrison's flat plate X-rays as well as apparently on the CT scans taken by Hawass et al., but this requires much further consideration.

Summary

The partial destruction of the body by the heat presumably generated by the winding of the bandages too soon after the over-liberal application of the hot resin, combined with Howard Carter heating the base-plate on a row of paraffin stoves is a disaster for future study. Some blood-group substances, which fortunately are known to be highly resistant to thermal degradation are still present and undegraded (Connolly 1969, 325; Harrison et al. 1969, 325-6). It is however extremely unlikely that intact DNA will ever be isolated. DNA is very heat-labile and no really deep tissue is available which is not contaminated with the DNA of countless modern investigations. Similarly the prospect of light or electron microscopy of tissues or identification of parasites or pathogenic microbial antigens or toxins is most unlikely to be convincingly achieved.

The age at death determined by Derry is still considered to be accurate. However we are all using the same modern dental criteria. We do not know whether dental eruption or for that matter appearance of ossification centres or fusion of epiphyses occurred at the same developmental age in antiquity as it does now. It may have been earlier, it may have been later. It may have even fluctuated over time. Also whether these bone-changes occurred in the same anatomical sequence in antiquity as they do now is not known. We really need X-rays of several pre-adult mummies of both sexes whose age at death is known with certainty from contemporary textual evidence. This is important and urgent!

There is then no clear evidence of cause of death from radiological studies of Tutankhamen but there is evidence of considerable haste in executing the embalming process. I do consider that a fatal accident involving the chest and possibly pelvic-region, perhaps inflicted some distance away from his home and therefore several days journey before embalming commenced, remains a possibility.

Only new textual evidence will definitively support or disprove this theory.

Acknowledgments

Acknowledgments are due to Dr Philip Cox and Mr Bob Read, University of Liverpool for image-management and production, but especially to Dr Jenefer Cockitt, University of Manchester for her care in the final production of this manuscript and her long tolerance of my entropic hysteresis.

References

Boyer, R.S., Rodin, E.A., Grey, T.C. and Connolly, R.C. (2003). The Skull and Cervical Spine Radiographs of Tutankhamun: A Critical Appraisal. *American Journal of Neuroradiology* 24, pp. 1142-1147.

Brier, B. (1998). *The Murder of Tutankhamun: A True Story*. Putnam.

Connolly, R.C. (1969). Microdetermination of Blood Group Substances in Ancient Human Material. *Nature* 224, pp. 325.

Harrison, R.G. (1966). An Anatomical Examination of the Pharaonic Remains Purported to be Akhenaten. *Journal of Egyptian Archaeology* 52, pp. 95-119.

Harrison, R.G., Connolly, R.C. and Abdalla, A. (1969) Kinship of Smenkhare and Tutankhamun Affirmed by Serological Micromethod. *Nature* 224, pp. 325-326.

Harrison, R.G. and Abdalla, A.B. (1972). The Remains of Tutankhamun. *Antiquity* XLVI, pp. 8-14.

Janot, F. (2000) *Les instruments d'embaumement de l'Egypte ancienne*. Bibliothèque d'étude; t. 125. Institut Français d'archéologie orientale.

Reeves, N. (1990). *The Complete Tutankhamun*. Thames and Hudson.

BLUE LOTUS: ANCIENT EGYPTIAN NARCOTIC AND APHRODISIAC?

D.J. Counsell

Consultant Anaesthetist, Maelor Hospital, Wrexham, North Wales.
Research Associate, KNH Centre for Biomedical Egyptology, The University of Manchester.

Abstract: *The importance of the Blue Lotus Flower (Nymphea caerulea) in the religious iconography of ancient Egypt is well described. Suggestions that the plant was used in a secular context as a narcotic or aphrodisiac remain unproven, but warrant further investigation.*

Narcotic Potential: It is suggested that alkaloids in the flower of N. caerulea were extracted in wine to produce a narcotic beverage. Review of the evidence for alkaloids demonstrates considerable confusion between Nymphea and Nelumbo plant species and provides no proof of alkaloids being present in the plant or the flower. Analysis of modern N. caerulea failed to demonstrate the presence of alkaloids. The fragrance contains benzyl alcohol which may produce narcosis when inhaled in sufficient concentration. The possibility that inhalation of the fragrance led to intoxication has yet to be examined scientifically.

Aphrodisiac Potential: The flower of N. caerulea contains high levels of bioflavonoids which increase peripheral blood flow. Limited evidence suggests Ginkgo biloba has a benefit in male impotence though this may be due to the unique ginkgolides rather than the bioflavonoids. Nelumbo nucifera (Persian or Pink Lotus), known to the Egyptians, contains apomorphine which is now used therapeutically to enhance sexual arousal.

Key words: Egypt, narcotics, blue lotus, Nymphea caerulea, aphrodisiac.

Introduction

It is reported that Nymphaea spp. water lilies were used as sexual stimulants and narcotic intoxicants in sacred rituals by the ancient Maya and ancient Egyptians (Bertol et al. 2004; Dobkin de Rios 1974; Emboden 1978; 1979a; 1979b; 1981; 1989; Emboden and Dobkin de Rios 1981). It is also claimed that the ancient Egyptians used N. caerulea water lilies as an intoxicant in secular celebrations (Harer 1985), the presence of several alkaloids in the Nympheae spp. being key to these effects. The alkaloids in question are apomorphine (Bertol et al. 2004), nymphaeine, nuciferine, nupharidine and alpha (or deoxy) nupharidine (Harer 1985). Harer (1985) suggests that these alkaloids can be extracted from the plant by immersion of the flower in wine, citing as evidence the widespread depiction of N. caerulea in New Kingdom banqueting scenes and the common use of the flower as decoration on drinking bowls and goblets. He also suggests that filtered drinking straws, a lead example of which is in the British Museum (BM 55149), were used to consume the wine. The possibility that N. caerulea, known to Egyptologists as the Blue Lotus, is narcotic was explored in two television documentaries. The first, 'Sacred Weeds' (Channel 4, UK, 1998) used a scientific approach feeding lotus enhanced wine to volunteers who then underwent psychometric testing. The second documentary, 'Private Lives of the Pharaohs' (TV6 for Channel 4, UK, 2000) followed our work on N. caerulea in Manchester but reinterpreted our findings making the first suggestion that N. caerulea was used as an aphrodisiac by the ancient Egyptians, citing the Turin 'Erotic' Papyrus (Turin 55001) as supporting archaeological evidence (Tyldesley 2000, 171). Other archaeologists have since supported this theory (Manniche 2002; Schumann, Antelme and Rossini 2001, 119). This paper re-explores the archaeological and scientific evidence for the use of water lilies, and in particular, Nympheae caerulea as a narcotic and aphrodisiac in ancient Egypt.

Water Lily and Lotus Terminology

Nymphaeales, the water lily order of flowering plants, contains eight genera and over 70 species in five families of which two are of interest: Nymphaeaceae comprising over 50 species and Nelumbonaeaceae with two species. Family Nymphaeaceae contains five genera including Nymphaea and Nuphar spp. The two species of Nelumbonaeaceae are the Asian Nelumbo nucifera (Persian or Sacred Lotus) and Nelumbo lutea or Nelumbo pentapetala (American Lotus) from eastern USA and Central America. Correctly the word 'lotus' applies only to these two species of water lily but the situation is confused by use of the word in other botanical contexts and in particular in Egyptology by naming the Nymphaea water lilies Nymphaea caerulea and Nymphaea lotus as blue and white 'lotus' respectively.

Water Lilies in Ancient Egypt

Three types of water lily were known to the ancient Egyptians (Harer 1985). Nympheae caerulea (blue) and Nympheae lotus (white), being native to Egypt, were known from the earliest periods of Egyptian history. The third species Nelumbo nucifera (pink), the aforementioned 'Persian Lotus' was introduced during the 1st Persian Period of the 27th Dynasty (525-404 BCE) (Harer 1985).

There is little doubt regarding the importance of these water lilies and of N. caerulea in particular to the ancient Egyptians. As the plant emblem of Upper Egypt, N. caerulea is often found entwined with the Papyrus plant, the symbol of Lower Egypt, in symbolism expressing the unity of the 'Two Lands'. The Blue Lotus was also associated with creation myths, rebirth and solar imagery and as the emblem of the god Nefertum; indeed these four aspects are inextricably linked. According to creation myths, the sun was born 'in the beginning' above the primeval waters of chaos (known as Nun) from a water lily, red in colour according to Lurker (1974, 77), blue according to Emboden (1981; 1989). The Egyptians observed that their native blue water lily raised its flowers above the water and faced the sun at dawn and came to associate this natural behaviour with the daily re-emergence or re-birth of the sun; thus solar deities are often shown appearing on a lotus flower from the primeval waters. Nefertum, originally the god of fragrance, is described in the Pyramid Texts (No 266) as 'the lotus-bloom which is at the nose of Re' (Lurker, 1974, 85); later he became recognised as a solar deity in his own right, as one who 'dwelled each day with Re'. A famous depiction of Tutankhamen shows the king as the god Nefertum, his head emerging from a blue lotus flower. Similar vignettes are common in copies of the Book of the Dead; for example, the Papyrus of Ani accompanying Spell (or Chapter) 81, the 'Spell for being transformed into a Lotus' (Faulkner 1972, 79).

Water Lily Analysis

Key to the arguments regarding narcotic and aphrodisiac effects is the presence or otherwise of alkaloids in these plants and in N. caerulea in particular. Three blooms of N. caerulea were obtained due to the kindness of Stapeley Water Gardens in Staffordshire, UK. A further bloom, reputed to be N. caerulea was obtained from the Cairo Botanical Gardens. Upon its delivery it was immediately apparent that this was not N. caerulea but a Nelumbo spp., most probably N. nucifera. The blooms were individually subjected to different extraction techniques. Bloom 1 Stapeley was used for head space analysis of the fragrance, sampled using a solid phase micro extraction (SPME) needle. Bloom 2 Stapely was extracted using a supercritical extraction technique with Freon gas, the resulting extract being re-suspended in 1ml of dichloromethane (DCM). Bloom 3 Stapeley and the Cairo Nelumbo were extracted using a 50:50 methanol:DCM mixture with the resulting extracts dried under nitrogen and re-suspended in 1ml of DCM. The extracts were then analysed using 2 systems of Gas Chromatography-Mass Spectrometry (GCMS) and additional Liquid Chromatography-Mass Spectrometry (LCMS). All systems were controlled by and the results analysed, using MassLynx software (Waters, Micromass, Wythenshaw, Manchester).

GCMS system A was a basic Fisons GC8000 gas chromatograph linked to a Fisons MD800 quadrupole mass spectrometer using Electron Ionisation (EI) and an electron multiplier detection system. GCMS system B was a highly sensitive Hewlett Packard 5890 Series II gas chromatograph linked to a Micromass Autospec tri-sector mass spectrometer using EI and a cone detection system. The LCMS system was a Micromass LCT, a combined liquid chromatography and 'time of flight' (TOF) mass spectrometer with Z-spray ionisation interface and electron multiplier detection system.

The results were analysed using selective ion chromatograms for specific target compounds including *m/z* 138 as a general screen for quinolizidine alkaloids and specific ions for apomorphine (*m/z* 266), deoxynupharidine (*m/z* 98, 233), nymphaeine (*m/z* 237) and nuciferine (*m/z* 295). No alkaloids were detected in either N. caerulea extract using GCMS. LCMS demonstrated the presence of several flavonoids confirmed by comparison with kaempferol and quercitin. This confirms the identification of flavonoids in N. caerulea by Fossen et al. (1999) who interestingly also make no mention of the presence of any alkaloids in the flower (Fossen and Anderson 1999; Fossen et al. 1999). GCMS analysis of the Nelumbo bloom demonstrated the presence of several alkaloids including the dimethyl derivative of apomorphine (CAS# 38291-33-7) and n-nornuciferine (CAS# 4846-19-9) (Counsell 2006, 254). Head space analysis also revealed that benzyl alcohol and cinnamyl alcohol were the principle components of the fragrance (Counsell 2006, 250).

The lack of alkaloids in the flower of N. caerulea does not exclude the presence of alkaloids elsewhere in the plant or in other Nympheae spp. but suggests that a full review of the evidence for alkaloids in these plants is warranted.

Nymphaeaceae and Nelumbonaceae Alkaloids

The nuphar alkaloids are quinolizidine alkaloids with 15-carbon atoms derived initially from Nuphar spp (Wróbel 1977; Hesse 1981). Raffauf (1970) lists 16 nuphar alkaloids including naturally occurring C_{30} thio (sulphur containing) variants. In his review on the nuphar alkaloids, Wróbel (1977) lists 33 including nupharidine, and alpha-nupharidine from Nuphar spp. and nympheine from the rhizome of Nymphea alba. The discovery of nuphacristine by Cybulski et al. (1988) adds to this total. Southon and Buckingham (1989) in fact report 37 alkaloids. According to Hesse (1981), deoxynupharidine is the fundamental type for the class. Nupharidine (MW 249) is the oxidised derivative of deoxynupharidine (MW 233) and is one of the four alkaloids reported to be in N. caerulea (Harer 1985). It was originally isolated from the rhizome of Nuphar luteum in 1910 (Merck Index 1969). Another alkaloid reported by Harer (1985) to be in N. caerulea is alpha-nupharidine (MW 233), which despite having the same molecular weight and base formula ($C_{15}H_{23}ON$) as deoxynupharidine, has different physical characteristics, such as a higher boiling point (Southon and Buckingham 1989). Nympheine is a third alkaloid reported by Harer (1985) to be in N. caerulea, it being a C_{14} alkaloid with a molecular weight of 237 and a base formula of $C_{14}H_{23}O_2N$ (Southon and Buckingham, 1989). Dr Duke's Phytochemical and Ethnobotanical database reports the presence of nuciferine, nornuciferine and N-nornuciferine in leaves of Nelumbo nucifera; this has been verified using LCMS by Xubiao et al. (2005).

Nuciferine was first isolated from Nelumbo lutea but is also found in a number of other species; it is also known as 1,2,-Dimethoxy-aporphine (Southon and Buckingham 1989), and is the fourth alkaloid reported by Harer (1985) in N. caerulea. It is a C_{19} structure with a molecular weight of 295 and a basic structure of $C_{19}H_{21}NO_2$ and unlike the other alkaloids its structure is known (Southon and Buckingham 1989). Overall, of the alkaloids reported to be from N. caerulea, only three clearly belong to plants from the Nymphaea family and only one has been conclusively demonstrated in a close relative of N. caerulea, that being nympheine from the rhizome of N. alba which is the only alkaloid reported to be found in the genus Nymphaea (Southon and Buckingham 1989). In short, there is no scientific evidence for the presence of any alkaloids in any part of N. caerulea or N. lotus to support their use as narcotics or aphrodisiacs.

Emboden (1978; 1979a; 1979b; 1981; 1989), an ethnopharmacologist of some standing, is clearly convinced of the narcotic properties of the Nymphea spp. and of N. caerulea and N. ampla in particular, yet despite writing subsequent to the publication of much of the sources cited above, he relies in his work on much earlier studies. Grunning (1883) is credited with the discovery of 'nupharine' from Nymphaea alba rhizomes, which was demonstrated by Delphaut and Balansard (1943) to have anticonvulsant activity and to be sedating. In 1941 Nupharine was found to compose of nelombine, nupharidine, nymphaeine and α-nupharidine (Raymond-Hamet 1941). Emboden admits that 'most (of these early chemists) did not know the source of their material and were unsure of genera and species', often working from 'anonymous dried fragments of rhizomes' but insists that the discovery of the nupharine mixture in all parts of Nymphea alba, except the seeds, by Pizzetti (1908) is reliable. Emboden cites some more recent work, particularly that by Diaz (1975) who reported the identification of aporphine in the bulbs and roots of N. ampla, which he suggests to be pschodysleptic, because of its chemical similarity to apomorphine. Nowhere does Emboden justify his conclusions regarding the alkaloid content of N. caerulea; in essence he infers their presence in N. caerulea from results in related species, particularly Nuphar spp. This we know to be a hazardous conclusion given that not all members of a plant family necessarily contain the same alkaloids, the Papaver spp. being a good example. Nothing in Emboden's work prompts a change to the original conclusion, supported by Southon and Buckingham (1989), that the only alkaloid proven to come from a Nymphea spp. is nymphaeine and even that not from N. caerulea.

Pharmacology of the Nuphar Alkaloids and Apomorphine

The pharmacological effects of the Nuphar alkaloids, if any, are largely unknown, though Dr Duke reports that nuciferine has antispasmodic activity. Confusingly, Chiej (1984) claims the presence of nympheine and nymphaline in both the rhizome and flower of Nymphaea alba. He gives no references and no other published evidence of the existence of nymphaline has been found to date. He further claims, surprisingly, given the theories under consideration, that these alkaloids have anaphrodisiac properties and are tranquilizing due to their effects upon the parasympathetic nervous system.

The scientific investigation included in the TV documentary 'Sacred Weeds' claims to demonstrate psychometric changes, over and above that produced by the alcohol alone, if N. caerulea is soaked in the wine. This study bears little critical analysis, using only four subjects with no blinding of either subjects or observers to exclude bias.

The appearance of the blue water lily in the Turin Erotic Papyrus, and the suggestions regarding its use as an aphrodisiac, warrant further consideration. Two clear mechanisms exist where drugs can be used to enhance sexual performance. Best known is the mechanism of sildenafil (Viagra) and similar drugs, which produce a specific vasodilator effect to help produce and sustain the male erection. Research has suggested a benefit from the use of Ginkgo biloba in male impotence (Sikora 1989) though this research is limited and whether the effect is due to the bioflavonoid or ginkgolide content is unclear. Certainly, bioflavonoids produce vasodilatation but this non-specific effect is not proven to effect the male erection specifically; therefore no aphrodisiac properties can be ascribed to plants that contain them. Though it is tempting to interpret the appearance of the blue lotus as an aphrodisiac in conjunction with the erotic scenes of the Turin Erotic Papyrus, this association cannot be supported by any scientific evidence of alkaloids in the flower. That said, many substances still used in modern times, and believed to be aphrodisiacs, similarly contain no active ingredients, yet their use continues. Perhaps the same pertains to the blue water lily in ancient Egypt.

More interesting is the Persian Lotus, N. nucifera. Dr Duke reports the presence of apomorphine derivatives in N. nucifera and we have demonstrated the presence of two apomorphine derivatives in its flower. Differing from Viagra in action, small doses of apomorphine are known to act centrally to increase libido, that is the desire for sex, rather than enhancing the ability to perform (Dula et al. 2001; Montorsi et al. 2003). This raises the possibility that Nelumbo spp. might act in this way though there is no archaeological evidence in Egypt to support their use as aphrodisiacs.

Intoxication by Inhalation?

Inhalation of volatile substances can lead to intoxication and, if potent enough, to anaesthesia. The phenomenon is employed by 'solvent abusers' to cause intoxication or inebriation. The potential of a volatile chemical to cause central nervous system effects is due in part to physical characteristics such as lipid solubility. The toxicity of an inhaled substance is determined by its potential to cause adverse effects when inhaled such as heart irregularities. Toxicity data for benzyl alcohol reports that the vapour can be narcotic in high concentration though whether it is possible to achieve that concentration from sniffing blue lotus is untested. With this in mind, further discussion of Harer's 'drinking straw' is warranted. It can be seen from the illustration (Figure 1) that the filter device is of significant diameter and that if attached to a hollow tube of similar girth would make a very inefficient device of high volume that would be difficult to drink through. Alternatively, the pipe would make a very efficient system for inhaling from an enclosed vessel where the vapours of a flower such as N. caerulea had been allowed to accumulate.

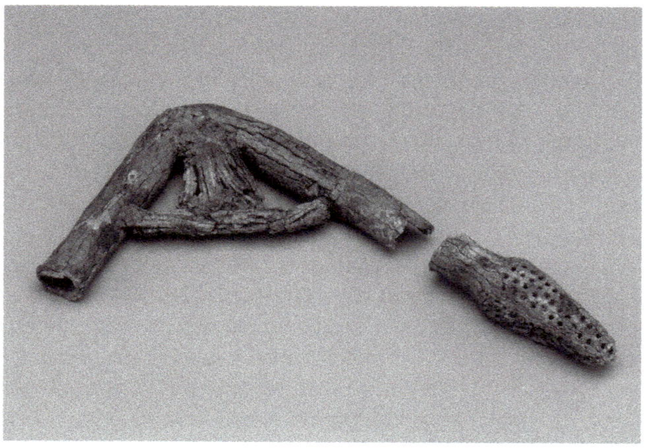

Figure 1: Lead drinking or inhalation straw with filter, BM55149. © Trustees of the British Museum

Conclusions

Despite the extensive literature claiming a narcotic role for Nymphaea water lilies in Egypt, there is no scientific evidence to support this. N. caerulea had a significant role in the religious life of the Egyptians but not as a shamanistic intoxicant as has been suggested. Similarly there is no evidence for aphrodisiac properties in Nymphaea lilies, though Nelumbo spp. might be effective in increasing sexual libido. The possibility that intoxication may be achieved by the inhalation of blue lotus fragrance warrants further investigation.

References

Bertol, E., Fineschi, V., Karch, S.B., Mari, F. and Riezzi, I. (2004). Nympheae cults in ancient Egypt and the New World: a lesson in empirical pharmacology. *Journal of the Royal Society of Medicine* 97, pp. 84-85.

Chiej, R. (1984). *The MacDonald Encyclopaedia of Medicinal Plants.* MacDonald and Co.

Counsell, D.J. (2006). *Intoxicants in Ancient Egypt: The Application of Modern Forensic Analytical Techniques to Ancient Artefacts and Mummified Remains in the Evaluation of Drug Use by an Ancient Society; a Historical and Scientific Investigation.* PhD Thesis, University of Manchester Faculty of Life Sciences.

Cybulski, J., Bąbel, K., Wojtasiewicz, K., Wróbel, J.T. and MacLean, D.B. (1988) Nuphacristine – An Alkaloid from Nuphar luteum. *Phytochemistry* 27, pp. 3339-3341.

Delphaut, J. and Balansard, J. (1943) Recherches pharmacologiques sur le Nénuphar blanc (*Nymphaea alba L). Revue de Phytotherapie* 7, pp. 83-85.

Diaz, J.L. (1975) Ninfaceas: Una lilia acuatica alucinogena entre los Mayas? In Diaz, J.L. (ed) *Ethnofarmacologia de Plantas Alucinogenas Latinoamericanas.* Estud Farmacodependencia.

Dobkin de Rios, M. (1974) The influence of psychotropic flora and fauna on Maya religion. *Current Anthropology* 15, pp. 147-164.

Dr Duke's Phytochemical and Ethnobotanical Databases. http://www.ars-grin.gov/cgi-bin/duke/farmacy2.pl. [accessed Oct 2009]

Dula, E., Bukofzer, S., Perdok, R. and George, M. (2001). Double-blind, crossover comparison of 3mg apomorphine SL with placebo and with 4 mg apomorphine SL in male erectile dysfunction. *Eur Urol* 39, pp. 558-564.

Emboden, W. (1978). The sacred narcotic lily of the Nile: Nymphea caerulea. *Economic Botany* 32, pp. 395-407.

Emboden, W. (1979a). *Narcotic Plants: Hallucinogens, Stimulants, Inebriants and Hypnotics, their Origins and Uses.* Studio Vista.

Emboden, W. (1979b). *Nymphea ampla* and other narcotics in Maya drug ritual and religion. *Mexicon* 1, pp. 50-52.

Emboden, W. (1981). Transcultural Use of Narcotic Water Lillies in Ancient Egyptian and Maya Drug Ritual. *Journal of Ethnopharmacology* 3, pp. 39-83.

Emboden, W. (1989). The sacred journey in dynastic Egypt: shamanistic trance in the context of the narcotic water lily and the mandrake. *Journal of Psychoactive Drugs* 21, pp. 61-75.

Emboden, W. and Dobkin de Rios, M. (1981). Narcotic ritual use of water lilies among ancient Egypt and the Maya. In Meyer, G.G., Blum, K. and Cull, J.G. (eds) *Folk Healing and Herbal Medicine.* Charles C. Thomas.

Faulkner, R.O. (1972). *The Ancient Egyptian Book of the Dead.* The Limited Editions Club.

Fossen, T. and Andersen O.M. (1999) Delphinidin 3'-galloylgalactosides from the blue flowers of Nymphea caerulea. *Phytochemistry* 50, pp. 1185-1188.

Fossen, T., Larsen, A., Kiremirec, B.T. and Andersen, O.M. (1999). Flavenoids from blue flowers of Nymphea caerulea. *Phytochemistry* 51, pp. 1113-1137.

Gruning, W. (1883). Sur la nupharine (Nymphaceae). *Pharmaceutische Zeitschrift feur Russland* 23, pp. 115-120.

Harer, W.B. (1985). Pharmacological and Biological Properties of the Egyptian Lotus. *Journal of the American Research Centre in Egypt* 22, pp. 49-54.

Hesse, M. (1981). *Alkaloid Chemistry.* John Wiley and Sons.

Lurker, M. (1974). *The Gods and Symbols of Ancient Egypt.* Thames and Hudson.

Manniche, L. (2002). *Sexual Life in Ancient Egypt.* Kegan Paul.

Merck Index, The. (1969). *An Encyclopedia of Chemicals, Drugs and Biologicals: 12th Edn.* Budavari, S. (Ed.) Merck and Co

Montorsi, F., Perani, D. and Anchesi, D. (2003). Apomorphine–induced brain modulation during sexual stimulation: a new look at central phenomena related to erectile dysfunction. *International Journal of Impotence Research* 15, pp. 203-209.

Pizzetti, M. (1908). The distribution of alkaloids in Nymphea alba. *Malpighia* 8, pp. 108.

Raffauf, R.F. (1970). *A Handbook of Alkaloids and Alkaloid-Containing Plants.* Wiley Interscience.

Raymond-Hamet, M. (1941) Sur un alcaloide à action excito respiratoire. *Competes Rendus Hebdomadaires des Séances de l'Académie des Sciences* 213, pp. 386-388.

Schumann Antelme, R. and Rossini, S. (2001) *Sacred Sexuality in Ancient Egypt: The Erotic Secrets of the Forbidden Papyrus.* Inner Traditions International.

Sikora, R. (1989) Ginkgo Biloba Extract in the Treatment of Erectile Dysfunction. *Journal of Urology* 141, pp. 188A.

Southon, I.W. and Buckingham, J. (1989). *Dictionary of Alkaloids.* Chapman and Hall Ltd.

Tyldesley, J. (2000) *The Private Lives of the Pharaohs.* Channel 4 Books, Macmillan Publishers Ltd.

Wróbel, J.T. (1977). Nuphar Alkaloids. In Manske, R.H.F. (ed). *The Alkaloids.* vol XVI. Academic Press, pp. 181-214.

Xubiao, L., Bo, C., Jingjing, L. and Shouzhou, Y. (2005). Simultaneous analysis of *N*-nornuciferine, *α*-nornuciferine, nuciferine and roemerine in leaves of Nelumbo nucifera by high-performance liquid chromatography-photodiode array detection-electrospray mass spectrometry. *Analytica Chimica Acta* 538, pp. 129-133.

COCAINE AND NICOTINE IN ANCIENT EGYPT?

D.J. Counsell

Consultant Anaesthetist, Maelor Hospital, Wrexham, North Wales.
Research Associate, KNH Centre for Biomedical Egyptology, The University of Manchester, UK

Abstract: *The widely reported discovery of cocaine and nicotine in Egyptian mummies caused considerable controversy during the mid 1990s and has yet to be adequately explained. Reviewing this discovery in the light of new evidence from our own work and that of others allows conclusions to be drawn that cast doubt on the findings of these researchers and the subsequent theories regarding a transatlantic drug trade in the 2nd millennium BC.*

Nicotine: Review of the nicotine levels reported in the original studies show comparability with those found in later studies and are consistent with nicotine consumed in the diet from plants known to the ancient Egyptians, for example, celery.

Cocaine: Although found in almost all samples in the original studies, more recent studies, including our own work on samples from 12 mummies, from a variety of sources, has failed to demonstrate cocaine. The levels originally reported were at the limit for reliable detection applying analytical standards for the time and are at levels considered inconclusive by other laboratories. The trace levels reported are most likely due to contamination either of the mummies themselves or from the laboratory.

Key words: narcotic, cocaine, nicotine, mummies, Egypt, Peru.

Introduction

The reported discovery of Cocaine and Nicotine in Egyptian mummies from the collection of the Munich Museum (Balabanova et al. 1992; Parsche et al. 1993) raised the possibility of transatlantic trade in the second millennium B.C. Although nicotine is not exclusive to the tobacco plant, being found in a number of plants from the eastern Atlantic land mass, the levels discovered were considered by Balabanova to be too high to have been derived from a dietary source, implying by default the chewing or smoking of tobacco. Cocaine on the other hand is not found elsewhere and could only be obtained from the South American Coca plant (Erythroxylum coca). Certainly, there is no clear evidence in the Egyptian archaeological record of regular transatlantic trade at this time, though critics might claim that is because no one has looked properly. If trade did exist, it would certainly seem strange that it be limited to just two plants given the potential opportunities that such a trade route would produce. One would expect therefore other evidence of cultural exchange between the two areas in terms of artifacts and even written records on both sides of the Atlantic that clearly do not exist. If it is assumed from this basic analysis that Dr Balabanova's results are incorrect, then an explanation is required as to how these results came about.

Hair Analysis for Cocaine and Nicotine: Problems and Pitfalls

Standard techniques for drug analysis use hair samples of about 100 milligrams that are first washed in methanol to remove surface materials such as cosmetics and oils. Extraction is by acid or alkali digestion or using organic solvents, followed by analysis using Radioimmunoassay (RIA) or Gas Chromatography-Mass Spectrometry (GCMS) with quantification against known concentrations. Alkali digestion is the most efficient method but cannot be used for cocaine as it completely degrades the drug. Methanol is the preferred solvent for cocaine extraction. RIA is popular for screening due to the high sensitivity of commercial kits working in nano or picogramme per milligram concentrations. GCMS is then used for confirmation and quantification (Henderson et al. 1995). Given the potential for contamination in archaeological samples, one must question if the rigour of standard techniques is adequate in the more complex situation seen in Egyptian mummies.

Mummified material from complete mummies to various body parts resides in museum collections around the world. Much of this material is unprovenanced, having found its way from Egypt via many circuitous routes over recent centuries, often through early tourists and private collectors. It is quite possible that some of this material is not genuinely ancient beyond a few decades there having been a thriving trade in fake mummies during the 19th century, when real mummies were becoming scarce. It is quite likely therefore, that positive results for cocaine and nicotine would be obtained from these post-Columbian individuals.

Contamination of samples can occur from many sources (Cartmel and Weems 2001). Mummification involved the application, both internally and externally, of plant material as packing and the use of gums and resins. The hair of Egyptian mummies is often densely matted by these ancient unguents. Further contamination of the mummy could occur from spillage or leaching of other grave goods during burial or during the subsequent millennia of interment when vermin, insects bacteria and moulds were free to take up residence on the body or in the wrappings. After excavation, exposure to environmental factors or poor storage could lead to further contamination. It is, for example, a relatively recent innovation to stop people smoking in our museums and it is likely that many of our esteemed archaeologists of the past and present used tobacco; for example, David and Archbold (2000, 90) show two illustrations of Aidan Cockburn, 'his ever present cigar in hand', standing over the mummy of PUM-II, during the autopsy of said mummy in Detroit in the early 1970s. This mechanism may also explain the report of tobacco fibres being found on the mummy of Ramesses II which have not been radiocarbon dated (Bucaille 1990).

The wealth of available organic compounds from the mummy itself and from the mummification and other contaminating processes will, with time, undergo a process known as diagenesis. Degradation of the compounds present by oxidation, fermentation and other processes, including cross reactivity between compounds, takes place, producing new materials and compounds not necessarily present on the mummy to begin with, making interpretation fraught with difficulty and increasing the chances of a false positive result with RIA and High Performance Liquid Chromatography (HPLC).

In addition to these problems, contamination of samples in the laboratory cannot be excluded; for example, hair samples are described as being pulverized but no detail was given as to how this was done or how the equipment was cleaned. Assuming they used a pestle and mortar or similar, one wonders how many other hair samples had been crushed in it, prior to the archaeological samples, and how thoroughly it was cleaned between times.

Cocaine and Nicotine in Ancient Populations

Not surprisingly, cocaine has been detected in Peruvian mummies (Cartmell et al. 1991; Balabanova et al. 1992). In 1992 Balabanova's team published their first identification of drugs in Egyptian mummies. This was followed in 1993 by a further paper (Parsche et al. 1993) reporting the detection of nicotine, cocaine and hashish in a variety of tissues from ancient populations from Peru and Egypt, with nicotine, but not cocaine or hashish, detected in bone from ancient Sudan and members of the ancient 'Bell' culture from Germany. More recently, Cartmell and Weems (2001) have reported the detection of nicotine, but not cocaine, in Egyptian mummies from the Dakhleh Oasis. The reported levels for hair samples in the Parsche and Cartmell papers adjusted to micrograms per milligram of material are summarised in Table 1.

Cartmell and Weems (2001) suggest a cut off point of 2 ng/mg to distinguish between regular tobacco smokers and those exposed passively to smoke or ingesting nicotine in the diet, with levels greater than 20 ng/mg, being reported in previous studies on South American mummies. This is consistent with the range reported by Parsche et al. (1993) in modern addicts. It seems clear therefore that the nicotine found in Egyptian mummies is from a dietary source, the original confusion regarding high levels being due to the unusual units of nanogrammes per gram quoted in the German studies which falsely inflates the results. The ubiquitous presence of nicotine in all the populations tested, all at dietary levels, supports the validity of these results. Dr. Duke's Phytochemical and Ethnobotanical Database lists 23 nicotine containing plants in addition to tobacco (Nicotiana tabacum). Of these, two, Withania somnifera (Ashwaganda or Winter Cherry) and Apium graveolans (Celery) were known to the Egyptians (Manniche 1993), the latter, celery, being the most likely to be used as a food. It is certainly popular in modern-day Egypt.

	Parsche (1993)	Cartmell (1991 and 2001)
Cocaine in Hair Egypt	0.024 – 0.2 ng/mg	nil
Cocaine in Hair Peru	0.22 – 13.9 ng/mg	0.02 – 15.8 ng/mg
Nicotine in Hair Egypt	0.14 – 0.9 ng/mg	0.7 – 2.2 ng/mg
Nicotine in Hair Peru	0.028 – 1.4 ng/mg	Not measured.

Table 1 Comparison of Hair Analysis for Cocaine and Nicotine in Egypt and South America. Data given in papers corrected to ng/mg.

In 1994, as a result of the 'Cocaine Mummies' television documentary (Schaffer Library of Drug Policy 2005), seven samples (6 tissue and 1 hair) from mummies in the Manchester Museum collection were sent for analysis at the Medical Toxicology Laboratory at Guy's and St Thomas' Hospital in London, UK, where they were tested for cocaine and nicotine. Of these, three samples tested positive for nicotine and none for cocaine. Concentration levels were not reported. Of the nicotine positive samples, all were taken from disarticulated heads of unknown provenance. Further investigation and closer inspection demonstrated that two, 7700/ES8(10p) and 7700/ES6(4p), were originally from the collection of Sir Grafton Elliot Smith, former Professor of Anatomy in both Cairo and Manchester. Neither of these show any evidence of embalming; environmental contamination could be a factor in these results. The third, 7700/1981.575(3p), is clearly ancient, being attributed to the Ptolemaic period and shows signs of resin use on the hair and residual traces of gilding on the face consistent with mummies from that period. Without a level for the reported nicotine, it is impossible to say for sure but one would speculate that these too were at a level consistent with diet. Re-testing, albeit of small samples, has failed to confirm the presence of nicotine in these samples. This is further support for the levels present being low as otherwise we would have been more likely to find it even with small samples. There is no record of the size of the samples sent to Guy's Hospital.

The level of cocaine found in Peruvian hair is reassuringly consistent in the two studies (See Table 1), with significantly lower levels detected in the Egyptians. Assuming that the identification of cocaine is correct, this difference might be explained either by a lower level of exposure during life, or greater deterioration of the cocaine present in the hair in the Egyptian sample, over the additional centuries since death. In addition to the seven earlier samples tested at Guy's Hospital, we have tested a variety of hair, bone and tissue samples from another five mummies in the Manchester and Leicester collections, none of which have tested positive for cocaine. If the theory of transatlantic trade were correct, and given the almost 100% positive test rate in Egyptians in the controversial studies, one might expect some of these subjects or those in Cartmell's work to have corroborated the discovery of cocaine in at least one of the Egyptian mummies tested so far. This suggests that either Dr Balabanova and her associates are misinterpreting their results, or that the sample of mummies tested by them has been mysteriously exposed to cocaine from an unknown source.

The cocaine levels recorded for South American mummies in these studies compares favourably with levels in modern coca chewers, in the range of 1.0-28.9 ng/mg (Henderson et al. 1992) and 1.4 and 50.6 ng/mg (Möller et al. 1992). By comparison, the levels in the Egyptian mummies are very low and close to the 0.1 ng/mg limit of detection reported by many investigators at the time of the study (Henderson et al. 1992; 1995). Cartmell et al. (1993) suggest a 3 ng/mg cut off point 'to differentiate a 'negative' and a 'positive' result consistent with previous hair studies'. It appears that they have made a decimal point error as this figure is inconsistent with their results, a figure of 0.3 ng/mg being more sensible. By this interpretation, all the results for cocaine reported by Parsche and Balabanova are negative.

Critique of Dr Balabanova's Work on Drug Analysis in Mummies

It is clear from the general literature on hair analysis for drugs that Dr Balabanova was one of the pioneers of hair analysis. She was the first to report the determination of cocaine in human hair using GCMS and in so doing demonstrated that the primary analyte in hair is cocaine itself, rather than the metabolite benzoylecgonine (BZE) as previously thought (Henderson et al. 1995; Balabanova and Homoki 1987). Clearly, she has some expertise in this area in the context of modern forensic analysis. Reading Dr Balabanova's papers reporting the discovery of cocaine in hair from Egyptian mummies, one is left with a sense of disquiet by the lack of detail, contained therein, concerning the methodology used. One speculates that the method used is similar to that reported in her original work but overall the reports exhibit a deficit in important detail, particularly relating to the GCMS analysis, in terms of retention times in the chromatography phase, use of control samples and whether identification was based on detection of a molecular ion or the full mass-spectrometric profile. Parsche reports using samples weighing 1 gram which is fine for tissue samples but amounts to a significant amount of hair (the norm being 100 mg) to remove from a mummy. Without proven experimental rigour, it is difficult to accept Balabanova's findings, particularly as the concentrations are so low in the presence of heavy contamination when such small quantities of a drug can be difficult to detect against the background contamination even when using modern computer programmes to facilitate interpretation. Analytical methods that have proven accurate and reliable in modern uncontaminated samples must be applied and interpreted with caution when applied to ancient samples, particularly mummified samples, which frequently contain vast quantities of unknown materials. Even hair from a typical Egyptian mummy is heavily coated in, and often glued to, the skull by gums and resins. Compounds from the decaying embalming materials inevitably penetrate the hair shaft as they do the rest of the body.

Cocaine: An Alternative Explanation

If Balabanova's results are indeed correct, and without re-evaluation of her extracts or re-testing of the original mummies she worked on this is difficult to accept, one must consider other possible explanations. The evidence for transatlantic trade, as presented by the Cocaine Mummies documentary, is at best poor. Even the demonstrated possibility of ancient transatlantic travel, such as the voyages of Thor Heyerdahl (1971), is not proof of the reality of such travel. Is there therefore a much simpler explanation; could the Munich mummies have been inadvertently contaminated either in the lab or at some earlier point in their history?

Historically the coca leaf has been a gift of nature, fuelling the extraordinary high altitude achievements of the Inca Empire. It is only as a result of its identification and extraction into the pure form by Gaedcke (1855) and later Niemann (1860), who improved on the earlier technique, that cocaine in its powdered and highly concentrated form became available. In the late 19th and early 20th centuries cocaine, devoid of its modern social stigma, was widely used by members of the upper social classes across Europe and America, eventually finding its way into popular 'pick me up' products such as 'Coca Cola' and 'Forced March' (reputedly used by Ernest Shackleton during his famous polar expedition). Other famous users are said to include Sarah Bernhard and Sigmund Freud. Sherlock Holmes' description of the mind clearing effects of cocaine suggests a familiarity with its effects by the author Sir Arthur Conan Doyle. Along with opium and its refined alkaloids, cocaine can be seen as a stimulant to the success of many of our literary, musical and artistic heroes from Coleridge to Hendrix. It is not implausible that the mummies were contaminated with cocaine at some time in their more recent history

References

Balabanova, S. and Homoki, J. (1987). Determination of cocaine in human hair by gas chromatography/mass spectrometry. *Z. Rechtsmed.* 98, pp. 235-240.

Balabanova, S. Parsche, F. and Pirsig, W. (1992). First identification of drugs in Egyptian mummies. *Naturwissenschaften* 79, pp. 358.

Bjorn, L.O. (1993). First Identification of drugs in Egyptian mummies (Letter). *Naturwissenschaften* 80, pp. 244.

Brothwell, D. and Spigelman M. (1993). Drugs in ancient populations (letter). *The Lancet* 341, pp. 1157.

Bucaille, M. (1990). *Mummies of the Pharaohs: Modern Medical Investigations*. St. Martin's Press.

Cartmell, L.W., Aufderhide, A.C. Springfield, A., Weems, C. and Arriza, B. (1991). The Frequency and Antiquity of Prehistoric Coca Leaf Chewing Practices in Northern Chile: Radioimmunoassay of a Cocaine Metabolite in Human Mummy Hair. *Latin American Antiquity* 2, pp. 260-268.

Cartmell, L.W. and Weems, C. (2001). Overview of Hair Analysis: A report of Hair Analysis From Dakhleh Oasis, Egypt. *Cungarc, Revista de Antropologia Chilena* 33, pp. 289-292.

Cartmell, L.W., Aufderhide, A.C., Witmers, E. and Weems, C. (2003). The Predictive Value of Cocaine Hair/Visceral Ratios in Andean Mummies – A Pilot Study. In Mummies in the New Millenium, *Proceedings of the 4th World Congress on Mummy Studies. Greenland National Museum and Archives and Danish Polar Centre*, pp. 79-81.

David, R. and Archbold, R. (2000). *Conversations with Mummies.* Harper Collins.

Dr Duke's Phytochemical and Ethnobotanical Databases. http://www.ars-grin.gov/cgi-bin/duke/farmacy2.pl [accessed Oct 2009]

Gaedcke, F. (1855). Ueber das Erythroxylin, dargestellt aus den Blättern des in Südamerika cultivirten Strauches Erythroxylon Coca. *Archiv der Pharmazie* 132 (2), pp. 141–150.

Harkey, M.R. Henderson, G.L. and Zhou, C. (1991). Simultaneous quantitation of cocaine and its major metabolites in human hair by gas chromatography/ chemical ionisation mass spectrometry. *Journal of the Annals of Toxicology* 15, pp. 260-265.

Henderson, G.L., Harkey, M.R., Zhou, C. and Jones, R.T. (1992). Cocaine and metabolite concentrations in the hair of South American coca chewers. *Journal of the Annals of Toxicology* 16, pp. 199-201.

Henderson, G.L., Harkey, M.R. and Jones, R.T. (1995). Analysis of hair for Cocaine. In Cone, E.J., Welch, M.J. and Grigson, M.B. (eds) *Hair Testing for Drugs of Abuse: International Research on Standards and Technology.* NIH Publication No 95-3727, pp. 91-120.

Heyerdahl, T. (1971) *The Ra Expeditions.* George Allen and Unwin.

Niemann, A. (1860). Ueber eine neue organische Base in den Cocablättern. *Archiv der Pharmazie* 153 (2), pp. 129–256.

Parsche, F., Balabanova, S. and Pirsig, W. (1993). Drugs in ancient populations. *The Lancet* 341, pp. 503.

Schaffer Library of Drug Policy (2005) Transcript of the video: Mystery of the Cocaine Mummies. http://www.druglibrary.org/schaffer/Misc/mummies.htm [accessed Oct 2009]

DEAD MEN TELL TALES: WHAT WE CAN LEARN FROM THE COURTIER SKELETON. A MULTI-DISCIPLINARY STUDY

B.L. Dement

KNH Centre for Biomedical Egyptology, University of Manchester, UK

Abstract: *There is a wealth of information that can be garnered from human skeletal remains. This investigation examines many aspects of a courtier skeleton, discovered by Flinders Petrie in one of the Tombs of the Courtiers. This multi-disciplinary study starts with a look into the past, which reveals the site from which the skeleton was found and the role he might have played in the royal court. Following that, there is a full osteological report that reveals his ancestral affinity, sex, age, and stature. A bone sample was taken from the distal end of the left femur and histological analysis was performed. Finally, there is a statistical study using discriminant function analysis to examine ancestral affinity by comparing cranial measurements from the courtier to those from various ethnic groups. Through these tests, the story of the courtier emerges and highlights the value of scientific techniques on archaeological specimens.*

Key words: Osteology, Egyptology, Histology, Abydos

History

The courtier skeleton, now housed at the Manchester Museum, was found at Abydos by Flinders Petrie at the site known as the Tombs of the Courtiers, which dates to the First Dynasty. The skeleton is almost complete and devoid of any remaining soft tissue. Based on the location of this site, in relation to the Royal Tombs found nearby, Petrie believed that individuals found in the Tombs of the Courtiers were court officials (Petrie 1925, 1-3), while later archaeologists have suggested they may have been artisans or funerary priests who were sacrificed so that they may serve King Djer in the afterlife. The latter suggestion is supported by the position of the bodies within the tombs (Kemp 1966).

Osteology

A full osteological investigation was carried out to the standards of modern forensic analysis (Stewart 1979; Buikstra and Ubelaker 1994). Both visual and metric techniques employed on the skull and pelvis revealed the courtier to be a male between 15-25 years of age. The courtier stood approximately 167.5 to 174.1 cm tall during life, which would make him slightly taller than average based on a study which found the ancient Egyptian male to be between approximately 152.9 and 166.1 cm tall (Zakrzewski 2003).

Cranial metric and cranial morphological analysis revealed characteristics present in the Courtier's skull that shared certain affinities with Caucasoid, Negroid, and Mongoloid ancestries. This suite of traits is not unexpected due to the high amount of variation present in Egyptian crania (Wilkinson 2004).

Originally, the taller than average stature combined with the comparatively small circumference of the femoral head caused the author to suspect some sort of hormonal abnormality, such as that experienced by a eunuch. Literary evidence for the presence of eunuchs in Egypt can be found in the Joseph narrative in Genesis chapters 37-48 (Tougher 2002). However, due to a lack of analytical data the suspicion cannot be confirmed.

Histology

One interesting feature that stands out on this skeleton is the twisted and cracked femora. A number of ailments, including nutritional deficiencies and taphonomic influences may be responsible for this. A histological study was conducted to try and shed light on the cause of this condition. A core sample was taken from the distal end of the left femur. It was not decalcified due to the fragile nature of the sample. The sample was embedded in resin, sectioned, and stained using 0.005% Toluidine Blue to highlight the cellular structure (An and Martin, 2003, 205; Bancroft and Stevens 1982, 385). Unfortunately, there were not enough histological features remaining to support any kind of diagnoses or conclusions about the condition of the femur. Both fungi and bacteria were identified visually in the bone section, although resources did not allow for any further stains to be carried out.

Cranial Comparisons

A statistical study was performed using cranial measurements from the courtier skeleton, the Duckworth collection of skulls from the Tombs of the Courtiers, and other measurements of skulls taken from literature. Measurements taken from the literature included groups from The Royal Tombs of Abydos, Nepal, Tibet, Sakkara, Anglo Saxons, Thebes, Kerma, and Naqada (Collett 1933; Morant 1924; 1925; 1926; Batrawi and Morant 1947; and Fawcett 1902). The aim of the study was to assess the geographical affinity of the Courtier skull using discriminant function analysis. An analysis was run using all groups discussed above, leaving the courtier skull ungrouped. The courtier skull was classified with the Anglo Saxons, not with other individuals recovered from the Tombs of the Courtiers as expected. This analysis was substantiated by a significant Wilks Lambda value.

Conclusion

The results obtained from this study have come together to tell the story of the Courtier Skeleton. Osteological profiling revealed the age, sex, ancestral affinity and stature, while histological tests attempted to reveal nutritional and taphonomic abnormalities, and statistical analysis related the courtier to other groups from around the world.

As to whether or not the Courtier was a eunuch, further tests could be carried out to look for hyperossification of the bones, which would indicate increased levels of estrogen, and thus lend support to this theory (Gardner and Pfeiffer 1943).

The twisted and cracked femurs were one of the most intriguing aspects of the Courtier Skeleton. Further osteological and histological study could provide a definitive explanation for this condition, whether caused by pathological or taphonomic factors. One possible approach would be the use of gram positive and gram negative stains which could help characterize the microbes found.

Many previous studies conducted on Egyptian crania have demonstrated a suite of cranial characteristics associated with various racial groups. The Courtier skull's statistical affinity to an Anglo Saxon population can be seen as an example of such diversity and does not necessarily disprove its relationship to other members of the Tombs of the Courtiers. An in-depth statistical study of individual crania from the Tombs of the Courtiers could provide a more appropriate comparison.

The application of modern forensic techniques to archaeological specimens has allowed researchers to develop a more complete reconstruction of past individuals and cultures. The information obtained during this study of the Courtier Skeleton could not have been accomplished through historical research alone.

References

An, Y.H. and Martin, K.L. (Eds). (2003). *Handbook of Histology Methods for Bone and Cartilage*. Humana Press.

Bancroft, J.D. and Stevens, A. (1982). *Theory and Practice of Histological Techniques.* Churchill Livingston.

Batrawi, A. and Morant, G.M. (1947). A Study of a First Dynasty Series of Egyptian Skulls from Sakkara and of an Eleventh Dynasty Series from Thebes. *Biometrika* 34 (1/2), pp. 18-27.

Buikstra, J.E. and Ubelaker, D.H. (1994). *Standards for Data Collection from Human Skeletal Remains.* Arkansas Archeological Survey Research Series 44.

Collett, M. (1933). A Study of Twelfth and Thirteenth Dynasty Skulls from Kerma (Nubia). *Biometrika* 25 (3/4), pp. 254-284.

Fawcett, C. D. and A. Lee (1902). A Second Study of the Variation and Correlation of the Human Skull, With Special Reference to the Naqada Crania. *Biometrika* 1 (4), pp. 408-467.

Gardner, W.U. and Pfeiffer, C.A. (1943). Influence of Estrogens and Androgens on the Skeletal System. *Physiological Reviews* 23, pp. 139-165.

Kemp, B.J. (1966). Abydos and the Royal Tombs of the First Dynasty. *Journal of Egyptian Archaeology* 52, pp. 13-22.

Morant, G.M. (1924). A Study of Certain Oriental Series of Crania Including the Nepalese and Tibetan Series in the British Museum (Natural History). *Biometrika* 16 (1/2), pp. 1-105.

Morant, G.M. (1925). A Study of Egyptian Craniology from Prehistoric to Roman Times. *Biometrika* 17 (1/2), pp. 1-52.

Morant, G.M. (1926). A First Study of the Craniology of England and Scotland from Neolithic to Early Historic Times, with Special Reference to the Anglo-Saxon Skulls in London Museums. *Biometrika* 18 (1/2), pp. 56-98.

Petrie, F. (1925). *Tombs of the Courtiers and Oxyrhynkhos.* British School of Archaeology in Egypt 37.

Stewart, T.D. (1979). *Essentials of Forensic Anthropology.* Charles C. Thomas.

Tougher, S. (2002). *Eunuchs in Antiquity and Beyond.* Gerald Duckworth and Co. Ltd.

Wilkinson, C. (2004). *Forensic Facial Reconstruction.* Cambridge University Press.

Zakrzewski, S.R (2003). Variation in Ancient Egyptian Stature Proportions. *American Journal of Physical Anthropology* 121, pp. 219-229.

HISTOLOGICAL EXAMINATION OF ANCIENT POMEGRANATE AND WHEAT

J. Denton and S. Wassef

KNH Centre for Biomedical Egyptology, The University of Manchester, UK

Abstract: *Samples of modern and ancient wheat and pomegranate have been examined histologically. Tissues were processed to paraffin wax and sectioned in the newly formed Ancient Tissue Histology Laboratory (ATHL) within the KNH Centre, University of Manchester. The histological analysis showed a remarkable preservation of external and internal microscopic structure of the ancient tissues when compared with contemporary seeds. The investigation reinforces the multi-disciplinary approach to the investigation of ancient tissues.*

Introduction

Histology is one of the oldest techniques used in the examination of ancient tissues and is the foundation of modern pathology. It can be used for both plant and animal tissues. Plants have been used as pharmaceuticals since man developed the awareness that they helped alleviate disease symptoms and in some cases, cured disease. Wheat and pomegranate are amongst many plants that are described as being used as pharmaceutical agents in the ancient Egyptian hieroglyphs and papyri, particularly in the Ebers papyrus. Histological examination of samples of ancient wheat and pomegranate has demonstrated that the preservation of the seeds is broadly comparable to that of modern samples despite the age of the specimens.

Materials and Methods

Single seeds of ancient Emmer wheat and pomegranate found as burial offerings in ancient Egyptian tombs were compared to modern sourced samples. One of the problems associated with the histological examination of ancient plant tissues is that they are desiccated and using standard processing schedules they would be difficult, if not impossible, to section at the required 5 micron thickness. In order to allow sectioning, the tissues must be rehydrated in an attempt to regain the normal architecture of the tissues. Various methods for rehydration have been devised but following the unpublished method of K. Currie - a solution of a 0.1% solution of sodium laureth sulphate in neutral buffered formalin at pH 7.2 - has been determined as the optimum for the rehydration of human tissues. The method was used without adaptation for the plant seeds other than extending the time to 5 days to allow penetration of the rehydrating solutions through the relatively impermeable outer cellulose seed coat. The modern seeds were not rehydrated but fixed in neutral buffered formalin at pH 7.2. One problem that was encountered was that the pomegranate seed was surrounded by a sugary capsule which inhibited conventional processing. The sugary component had to be washed out by a 7 day immersion in neutral buffered formalin. Both sets of seeds were processed by dehydration in ethanol followed by the removal of the ethanol by xylene and infiltration by paraffin wax. Sections were cut at 5 micron and mounted onto glass microscope slides. The wax was removed by immersion in xylene which was then removed by immersion in ethanol prior to hydration in water.

Staining is a necessary part of the technique of histology as the tissue has no inherent colour or contrast. Stains are used to specifically colour individual tissue types or macromolecules. In this investigation a 0.005 % aqueous solution of toluidine blue at pH 4.0 (Johansen 1940) was used as a stain for general cellular and matrix architecture, Safranine and alcian blue (SAB) (Berlyn 1976) was used for the demonstration of cellular components, a 'one step MSB' stain as a multicolour visualisation of the individual tissue components, Lugols iodine (Berlyn 1976) for the presence of starch and calcafluor optical brightener (Hageage 1984) for the specific demonstration of cellulose.

Following staining, the sections other than the Lugols iodine stained section were dehydrated in ethanol and then immersed in xylene after which they were encapsulated with a coverslip using permount as the adhesive. The Lugols iodine stained section was mounted with glycerine based mounting media as the iodine starch complex was hydrocarbon soluble.

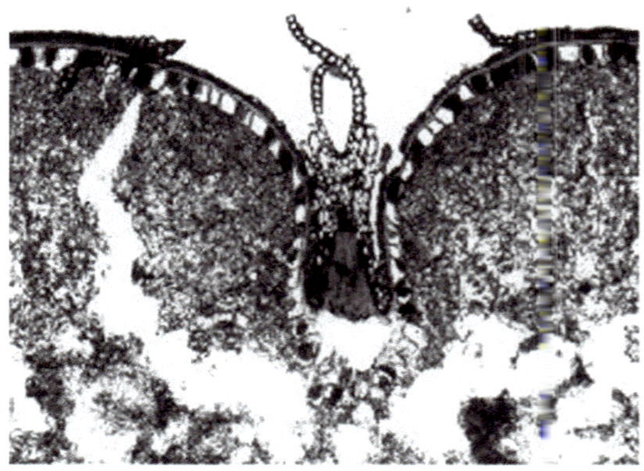

Figure 1.

Simple microscopic examination of the stained sections showed that preservation of the ancient seeds was remarkable, as there was very little difference in the architecture between ancient and the modern equivalent in both the wheat and pomegranate. Iodine staining demonstrated starch grains as dark blue grains in both ancient and modern wheat. This was confirmed by examination of unstained sections by polarising microscopy, where the classical 'Maltese cross' pattern of four bright quadrants interspersed by four dark quadrants was evident. The Safranine and alcian blue stain technique clearly segregated tissue types particularly where the outer pericarp, the spermoderma and the aleuron layer were present in the wheat.

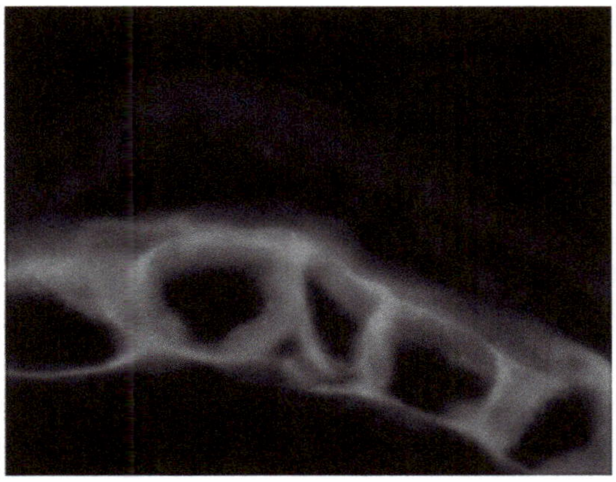

Figure 2.

Of the techniques used, the trichrome stain proved to be the most useful for the examination of both modern and ancient plant tissues demonstrating the different tissues and tissue components in individual colours (Figure 1). However, iodine staining was the most specific for the identification of starch in the wheat seed where the iodine reacted with the starch producing a deep blue staining pattern. Excellent demonstration of the cellulose walls of the seeds was demonstrated by the calcafluor optical brightener technique when examined by fluorescence microscopy (Figure 2).

Conclusion

In conclusion, histological examination of ancient plant seeds demonstrates excellent preservation of the remains when compared to the modern equivalent which allows an insight into ancient Egyptian funerary rites.

References

Berlyn, G.P. and Miksche, J.P. (1976) *Botanical Microtechnique and Cytochemistry*. Iowa State University Press.

Hageage, G.J. and Harrington, B.J. (1984) The Use of Calcofluor White in Clinical Mycology. *Laboratory Medicine* 15, pp. 109-112

Johansen, D.A. (1940). *Plant Microtechnique.* McGraw Hill.

POROTIC HYPEROSTOSIS IN ANCIENT EGYPTIANS FROM THE BAHRIYAH OASIS, GRAECO-ROMAN PERIOD

M. Erfan Zaki, A. El-Sawaf, M. Al-Tohamy Soliman and A. Azab

Biological Anthropology Department, Medical Research Division, National Research Centre, Egypt

Abstract: *Porotic hyperostosis is a palaeopathological condition which is characterised by small and localised perforations on the surface of cranial bones. Cribra orbitalia and cribra cranii are considered good indicators of the health and nutritional status of ancient populations. The main goal of the present study is to identify cribra orbitalia/cribra cranii in order to assess the health status of ancient Egyptians living around the Bahriyah Oasis during the Roman rule. The study also attempts to analyse environmental living conditions and detect the possible etiological factors that might play a significant role in the development of porotic hyperostosis.*

The sample consisted of 171 skulls (95 males, 59 females and 17 sub-adults). They were recovered from Bahriyah Oasis, belonging to the Graeco-Roman period (332 BC - 395 AD). Cribra orbitalia and cribra cranii are quite frequent in this sample, being present in 46.8% and in 54.4% of all subjects. Our results showed that cribra orbitalia and cribra cranii are often associated with each other. Males and females were equally affected. Comparative data with other Egyptian populations showed similar patterns; however, they displayed a lower prevalence than the data from Bahriyah. The differential analysis suggests that the porotic hyperostosis lesions are due to chronic acquired anemia, probably caused by various environmental stressors.

Key words: porotic hyperostosis; health status; ancient Egyptians; Bahriyah Oasis

Introduction

Cranial porotic hyperostosis has been of interest to researchers since the mid-19th century (Stuart-Macadam, 1987). The term 'porotic hyperostosis', coined by Angel (1966), refers to a condition characterised by lesions found on the parietal and occipital bones, and on the superior orbital plates; the latter condition is referred to as cribra orbitalia. The lesions appear as areas of porous and thickened bone, thinning of the outer cortical bone, and exposure of the inner trabecular bone. Such bony modifications initially appear in the orbital cavity and then spread to the other areas of the skull. Cribra orbitalia represents an osseous evidence of marrow hyperplasia (Ortner et al. 1999; 2001; Schultz 2001). Porotic lesions of the cranial vault, also known as cribra cranii, are attributed to an increase in the cranial diploe at the expense of the outer table resulting in a thinning and porosity of the cortex (Ortner and Putschar 1985; Stuart-Macadam 1985; Hershkovitz et al. 1997). The etiological association of these two bone pathologies has been confirmed in many studies (Stuart-Macadam 1989; Facchini et al. 2004). Such lesions appear on radiographs, as a 'hair-on-end' pattern of trabeculation (Lallo et al. 1977; Stuart-Macadam 1985; 1989). The thickening of the flat bones of the skull and the roof of the orbits may be due to several etiological factors such as hypoxia, acquired or genetic anemia (Steinbock 1978; Stuart-Macadam 1989; Hill and Armelagos 1990). The body responds to decreased oxygen levels by increasing its production of red blood cells and large immature cell precursors. Thus, a marked increase in the production of these cells results in the expansion of the marrow cavity to accommodate diploe proliferation. Skeletal and radiographic data indicated that porotic hyperostosis in adults is always in a healed state and studies suggested that porotic hyperostosis in adults reflect a childhood episode of anemia (Ortner et al. 2001; Schultz 2001).

Porotic hyperostosis of acquired origin has a multifactorial etiology (e.g., dietary stress, growth-related stress or health condition). Hence, several factors were suggested as causes for porotic hyperostosis such as anemia, syphilis, rickets, scurvy, and pressure exerted on the cranium due to carrying heavy loads (El-Najjar 1976; Hill and Armelagos 1990; Hill 2001). Moreover, many authors have attributed porotic hyperostosis to iron-deficiency anemia, nutritional deficiencies (e.g. folic acid, vitamin C), and parasitic infection (El-Najjar et al. 1976; Steinbock 1976; Ortner and Putschar 1985; Walker 1986; Stuart-Macadam 1992; Grauer 1993; Ortner et al. 1999; Wapler et al. 2004; Deborah et al. 2005). In the Mediterranean region (e.g., Cyprus and Greece), cribra orbitalia and porotic hyperostosis were attributed to a genetic anemia, thalassemia (Angel 1971; Hershkovitz et al 1991; Keenleyside and Panayotova 2006). Yet, this can not explain their high prevalence in past populations that lived in places where there has been no malaria (Facchini, et al. 2004).

The etiology of porotic hyperostosis, in ancient skeletal materials for various populations, can be clearly understood when related to several stressors. Thus information about living conditions and life-styles will be very useful for interpretation (Benfer 1990; Larsen 2002).

The Bahriyah Oasis is located in the Libyan Desert, 180 km west from the Nile Valley, 350 km southwest of Cairo. Archaeological literature indicated that ancient Egyptians living in Bahriyah Oasis in the Graeco-Roman period were engaged in many activities, such as agriculture, wine and textile production (Fakhry 1999). Pharaonic Egypt was also famous throughout the ancient world for the production of linen which was well known during Roman times (Redford 2001). The Roman period was characterised by political instability, socioeconomic and cultural transformations with a climate of tension. The human skeletal remains from Bahriyah Oasis, Egypt, are a unique sample set due to the geographical position of this region. The main goal of the present study is to account for cribra orbitalia/cribra cranii in order to assess the health status of the ancient Egyptians who lived in the Bahriyah Oasis during Roman rule. Also, the study attempts to analyse environmental living conditions and detect the possible etiological factors that might play a significant role in the development of porotic hyperostosis.

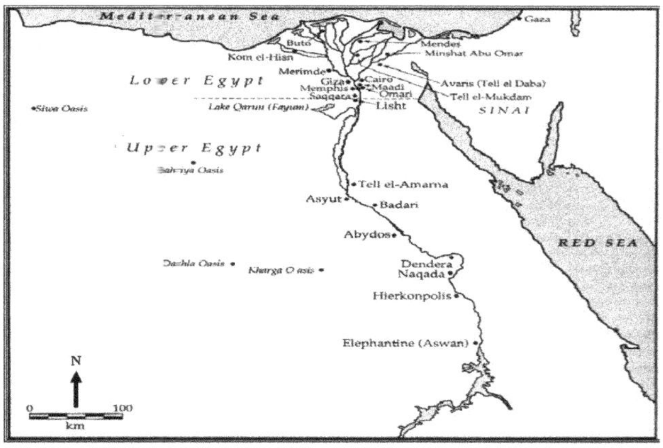

Figure 1: A map of Egypt showing the Nile Delta and Oases. Modified after Fakhry (1974, 23).

Material and Methods

The material of the present study consisted of 171 skulls (95 males, 59 females and 17 sub-adults) that were well-preserved. These skulls were collected from the Bahriyah oasis from two sites, Al-Hayz and Al-Bawiti (Figure 1). They belong to the Graeco-Roman period, dating back to 332 BC - 395 AD. They were recovered during the excavation seasons between 1991 and 1994 by the Supreme Council of Antiquities (SCA). The following studies were performed on the collection:

1- Sex determination of the adult skeletons was done using standard morphological criteria of the crania (Bass, 1987; Ubelaker, 1989).

2- Sub-adult's age at death was estimated using dental formation (Moorrees et al. 1963a; b) and dental eruption. Adult age estimation was based on ectocranial suture closure (Meindl and Lovejoy 1985). The total sample was classified into five age groups: (10-19 y), (20-29 y), (30-39 y), (40-49 y) and (50-60 y).

3- The samples were examined macroscopically for cribra orbitalia and porotic hyperostosis. The presence/absence and severity of cribra orbitalia were assessed in all individuals with at least one orbital roof preserved and cribra cranii were recorded using the scale of Stuart-Macadam (1982; 1991). In this scale, the severity of porotic lesions is quantified as:

Degree 1: presence of small, scattered holes.
Degree 2: presence of small and large scattered holes.
Degree 3: presence of holes that join within the trabecular structure.
Degree 4: marked development of the trabecular part of the bone surface, which protrudes toward the outside.

4- Statistical analyses were conducted (to interpret the epidemiological profile of both cribra orbitalia and cribra cranii) on the basis of sex, age, the severity of lesions and the combined presence of the two conditions. The differences in the prevalence of lesions between the five age groups as well as between males and females were tested. The correlation between cribra orbitalia, cribra cranii was also carried out.

Results

Table 1 shows the prevalence of cribra orbitalia and cribra cranii by sex. Our results revealed that cribra orbitalia and cribra cranii are quite frequent in this sample, being present in 46.8% and in 54.4% of all subjects, respectively. There are no significant sex differences in the frequencies of either cribra orbitalia or cribra cranii. Subadults present slightly higher frequency of cribra orbitalia than males and females, but the differences are not significant. Similarly, females show slightly higher frequency of cribra orbitalia than males. Males show a slightly higher frequency of cribra cranii than subadults and females.

Sex	No. observed	Cribra orbitalia No. affected / %		Cribra cranii No. affected / %	
Females	59	31	52.5	26	44.1
Males	95	39	41.1	57	60.0
Sub-adults	17	10	58.8	10	58.8
Total	171	80	46.8	93	54.4

Table 1: Prevalence of cribra orbitalia and cribra cranii by sex.

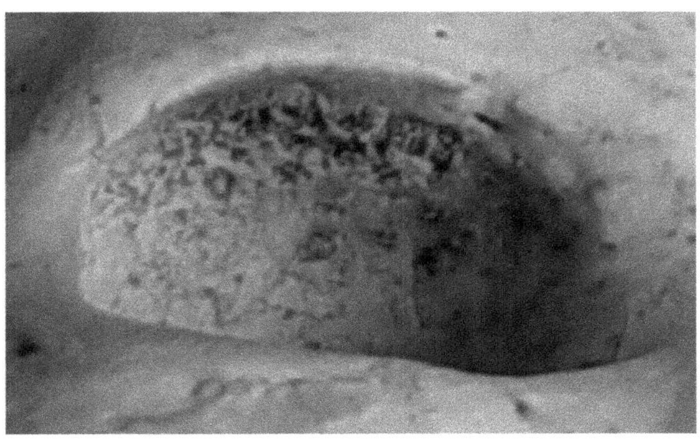

Figure 2: Cribra orbitalia (degree 3) in an adult female, 30-35 years old

With regard to severity of the pathology, Tables 2 and 3 show the degrees of severity of cribra orbitalia and cribra cranii according to sex. Cribra cranii is presented by mild lesions (degree 1 and 2), while cribra orbitalia is presented from degree 1 to degree 4. There is a significant difference ($p < 0.002$) in the severity degrees of cribra orbitalia between the examined groups, females, males and subadults (Table 2). The highest degree of severity (degree 4) of cribra orbitalia occurred in the subadults (35.3%). Degree 4 of cribra orbitalia is significantly more prevalent in subadults than males. Also, females show slightly higher frequency of cribra orbitalia with degrees 3 and 4 than males, but the differences are not significant. With regard to severity of cribra cranii (Table 3), degree 1 is more prevalent in subadults than both males and females, but the differences are not significant.

Sex	Degree			No.
	2	3	4	
	No. affected / %	No. affected / %	No. affected / %	
Female	0 0	21 35.6	10 16.9	59
Male	2 2.1	28 29.5	9 9.5	95
Sub-adult	1 5.8	3 17.6	6 35.3	17
Total	3 1.7	52 30.4	25 14.6	171

P< 0.00

Table 2: Severity of cribra orbitalia by sex.

Sex	Degree		No. observed
	1	2	
	No. observed / %	No. affected / %	
Female	19 32.2	7 11.9	59
Male	54 56.8	3 3.2	95
Sub-adult	10 58.8	0 0	17
Total	83 48.5	10 5.8	171

Table 3: Severity of cribra cranii by sex

Tables 4 and 5 present the prevalence of cribra orbitalia and cribra cranii according to age. Generally, we observed a decreasing trend of both cribra orbitalia and cribra cranii with age. Significant differences were found between the different age groups ($p < .002$). The first and the second age groups (20-29 years) had significant higher frequencies of cribra orbitalia than the fifth age adults (50-60 years).

Age group (years)	Cribra orbitalia		%
	No. observed	No. affected	
10-19	17	10	58.8
20-29	60	38	63.3
30-39	41	12	29.3
40-49	38	17	44.7
50-60	15	3	20

P< 0.002

Table 4: Prevalence of cribra orbitalia by age groups.

Age group (years)	Cribra cranii		%
	No. observed	No. affected	
10-19	17	10	58.8
20-29	60	37	61.6
30-39	41	21	51.2
40-49	38	19	50
50-60	15	6	40

Table 5: Prevalence of cribra cranii by age groups

Tables 6 and 7 show the distribution of the combined presence of cribra orbitalia and cribra cranii according to sex and age, respectively. With regard to sex both lesions occur together in 27 of the 95 males (28.4%), in 18 of the 59 females (30.5%) and in 5 of the 17 subadults (29.2%), but the differences are not significant. The highest prevalence of both lesions has been observed (Table 7) in the first and the second age groups, with statistical significant differences as compared to other age groups ($p < .05$).

Sex	Cribra orbitalia and cribra cranii		No. observed
	No. affected	/ %	
Females	18	30.5	59
Males	27	28.4	95
Sub-adults	5	29.4	17
Total	50	29.2	171

Table 6: Distribution of combined cribra orbitalia and cribra cranii according to sex.

Age group (years)	Cribra orbitalia and cribra cranii		%
	No. observed	No. affected	
10-19	17	5	29.4
20-29	60	26	43.3
30-39	41	8	19.5
40-49	38	8	21.1
50-60	15	3	20

P< 0.05

Table 7: Distribution of combined presence of cribra orbitalia and cribra cranii according to age groups.

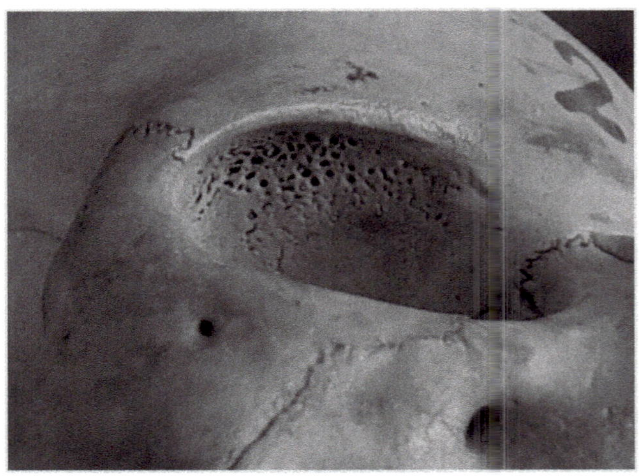

Figure 3: Cribra orbitalia (degree 2) in a subadult

There is significant positive correlation between cribra orbitalia and cribra cranii in the present sample ($p < .01$) Figures 2 and 3 show cribra orbitalia lesions found in an adult female and a sub-adult from the Bahriyah Oasis, respectively. Figures 4 and 5 show lesions of cranial bones (parietals and occipital) found in an adult male. Figures 6 to 7 are skull radiographs (lateral and anterior-posterior views respectively) of adult female with cribra orbitalia. Figure 6 (lateral view) shows orbital roof thickening, and Figure 7 (anterior-posterior view) shows orbital rim changes including thinning, flattening and obscuring of the normal rim outline. Figure 8 is a lateral radiograph of a male with porotic hyperostosis, showing diploic thickening of the parietal bone.

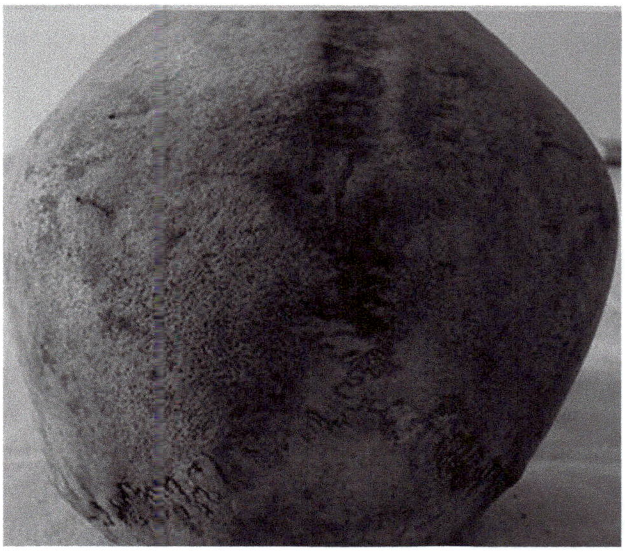

Figure 4: Porotic hyperostosis in the parietal and occipital bones (degree 2) in an adult male 30-35 years old.

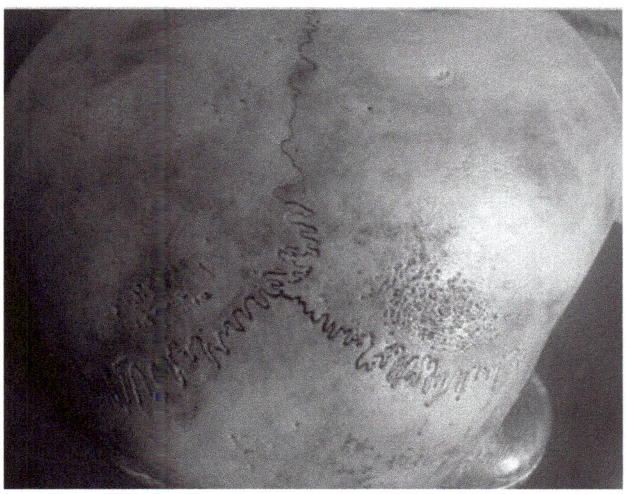

Figure 5: Porotic hyperostosis in the parietal bones (degree 2) in an adult male 30-35 years old.

Discussion

The osteological material of the present study dates to a particularly important and interesting historical period - the Graeco-Roman period. Therefore, the cultural context of this sample must be taken into consideration. In this study, cribra orbitalia and cribra cranii were used to evaluate the health status of this population as their presence are considered as good indicators of the health and nutritional status of past populations.

The development of some sort of anemia in this skeletal sample could be suggested because of the geographic position of the Oasis, i.e., the individuals were potentially susceptible to various environmental stressors that could favor the development of some sort of anemia. The possible factors include parasitic infestations, infectious diseases and potentially low bioavailability of iron in the diet. Although evidence of indigenous parasites was not found, this alone does not negate the possibility. Nonetheless, the possibility exists that the isolation of the Bahriyah oasis from the Nile Valley represents a filter which reduced many parasitic infections. Other possible factors of chronic acquired anemia could include the weaning diet which might be rich in carbohydrates with only low levels of iron, but also contains phosphorus and phytates which inhibit its intestinal absorption. Cribra orbitalia can also be attributed to folic acid deficiency; that results in megaloblastic anemia, due to weaning of infants on goat's milk which was a known practice in ancient Egypt (Scott and Molto 2000). Gastrointestinal infections, causing gastrointestinal bleeding could also be suggested. Hence, nutritional deficiencies and exposure to infectious diseases probably played an equally, if not more, important role in the development of these lesions (Keenleyside and Panayotova 2006). In addition, skeletal evidence of genetic anemia is absent in this region although it was reported on the Dakhleh skeletons (Ortner and Putschar, 1985; Hershkovitz et al. 1997; Aufderheide and Rodriguez-Martin, 1998). Also, malaria has been considered a real factor in this region as it was documented in the Kharga Oasis; however, Hrdlicka (1912) noted that 'malaria is not very frequent'. On the other hand, other studies reported that these lesions may also be indicative of other metabolic disorders such as scurvy and rickets (Ortner and Ericksen 1997; Ortner and Mays, 1998; Ortner et al. 1999, 2001; Ortner, 2003).

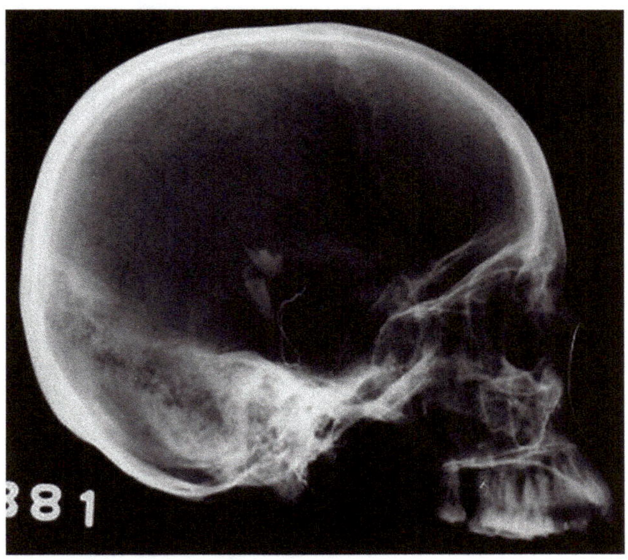

Figure 6: A lateral cephalogram for an adult female with cribra orbitalia

Our results showed slightly higher frequency of cribra orbitalia in female than males, but the differences are not significant. Generally we observed a decreasing trend of cribra orbitalia with age. Growing children need diets rich in iron (Dallman 1986; Ryan 1997); hence, a diet lacking a sufficient amount of bioavailable iron, after initial iron stores are depleted, is regarded as a common cause of iron-deficiency anemia (Mitchem 1998; Ortner et al. 2001). Moreover, iron-deficiency anemia may result due to prolonged breast-feeding or weaning using iron-poor diets such as maize, wheat and lupins (El-Najjar et al. 1976; and Mensforth et al. 1978). Ancient Egyptians in this region favoured maternal breast feeding and weaning on crumbled bread, honey and goat's milk. It was concluded that porotic hyperostosis is much more frequent and severe in populations that depend on maize agriculture (Mensforth et al. 1978; Cohen and Armelagos 1984; Holland and O 'Brien 1997). Also, populations depending on both marine and agricultural resources may also have a greater prevalence of iron-related anemia, since the high content phosphorus in marine foods reduces iron absorption (Lallo et al. 1977; Walker 1986). The current population of the Oasis is agriculturally based, growing vegetables, fruits (dates, apricots, oranges, and olives) and cereals (rice, sorghum, and wheat). The vegetables are grown for local consumption and are supplemented from the Nile Valley in the hot weather (Mills, 1979).

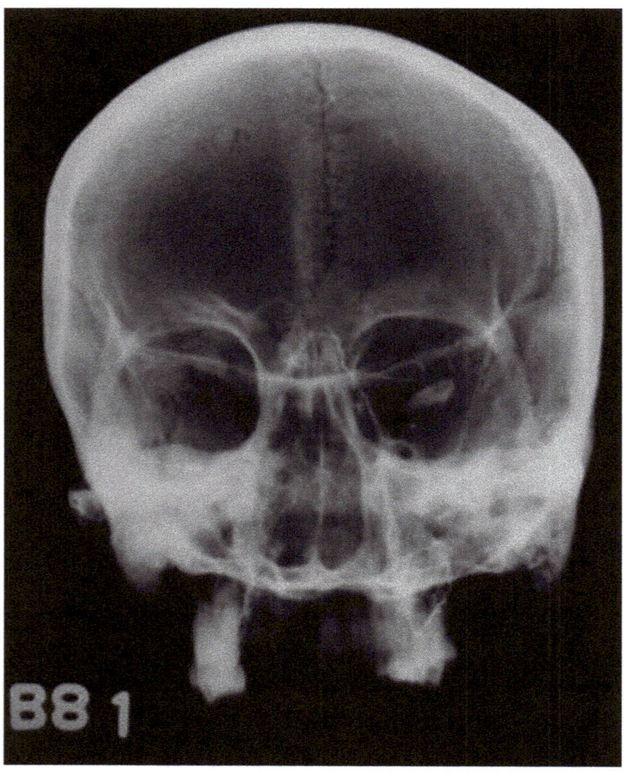

Figure7: A postero-anterior cephalogram for an adult female with cribra orbitalia

The significantly higher frequency of degree of severity of cribra orbitalia in sub-adults in the Bahriyah Oasis compared to adults is in agreement with results reported by Aufderheide and Rodriguez (1998) and Keenleyside and Panayotova (2006). Scott and Molto (2000) have demonstrated significant relationships between the prevalence and degree of severity of cribra orbitalia and age of the individual. On the contrary, no significant relationships were found between the prevalence and degree of severity of cribra orbitalia and the sex of the individual. However, in adults, the severity of both cribra orbitalia and cribra cranii were less because once the anemia and its causes disappear the lesions are repaired, except in cases of genetic anemia, associated with high levels of medullary hypertrophy throughout life, or when living conditions favouring anemia persist.

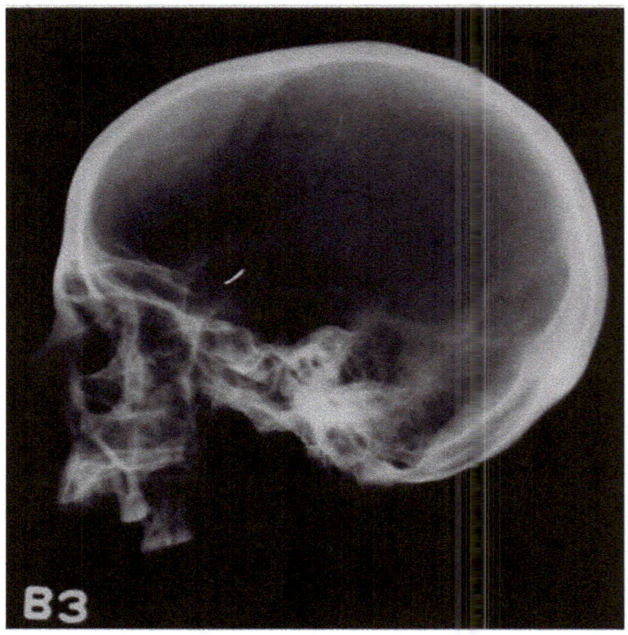

Figure 8: A lateral cephalogram for an adult male with porotic hyperostosis in the parietal bones

Various studies reported the combined presence of the two conditions, cribra orbitalia and cribra cranii (Stuart-Macadam 1989; Facchini et al. 2004). Our results revealed that cribra orbitalia and cribra cranii are often associated with each other, in agreement with the results of other studies (Hrdlicka 1914; El-Najjar et al. 1976; Stuart-Macadam 1989).

It is well known that the prevalence of cribra orbitalia and cribra cranii vary among different populations. Scott and Molto (2000) reported that cribra orbitalia occurs in 67% of the crania (N = 296; 'pre-Roman' n = 153 and 'Roman period' n = 143) from the Dakhleh Oasis which is adjacent to the Bahriyah Oasis, Egypt. Other areas of Egypt and Sudan have yielded studies of skeletal remains with variable rates of porotic hyperostosis (Strouhal and Jungwirth 1980; Mittler and Van Gerven 1994). Rose (2006) reported that cribra orbitalia was seen in 23% of cases living in the capital city, Tell Amarna, which is located between the previous capitals of Memphis (near Cairo) in the north and Thebes (modern Luxor) in the south. Zink et al. (2000) reported that the rate of cribra orbitalia was 29.2% in New Kingdom to Late Period Nobles from Thebes. Rates from early and late Christian cemeteries at Kulubnarti, Nubia, ranged between 18 and 50% (Van Gerven et al. 1995) and Late Period and Early Christian adults from Dakhleh Oasis, Egypt, vary between 39 and 84% (Scott and Molto 2000). Buzon (2006) reported that the rate of cribra orbitalia was 11% in Tombos, a cemetery in Upper Nubia. None of these reports would serve as an appropriate comparison due to the geographic context as well as the cultural structure of the Oasis.

In comparison with other European populations, most studies display lower rates than the Egyptian population; in a Greek colonial population (5th to 3rd Centuries BC) the rate of cribra orbitalia was 28% (Keenleyside and Panayotova, 2006) and in central Italy it was 19.4% (Salvadeli et al. 2001). If some of the cases of cribra orbitalia in these samples do, in fact, represent iron deficiency anaemia or other metabolic diseases rather than thalassemia, the variability in the prevalence of these lesions may reflect varying environmental conditions, dietary differences, and differential exposure to infectious disease.

Conclusions

It is very probable that the observed lesions in our skeletal sample were caused by acquired chronic anemia, since in this type the most affected areas are the parietal bones and the orbital roofs with no involvement of other facial bones In addition, the higher frequency of the cribrotic lesions in sub-adults than in adults led us to exclude genetic anemia. The presence of cribrosity of the orbits and cranial bones in both adults and subadults suggest nutritional stresses and parasitic infections during growth. Moreover, as a potential cause of porotic hyperostosis in this sample, it is important to consider not only iron deficiency, but also folic acid and vitamin C deficiencies. The generally poor living conditions can be attributed to the general conditions of the Roman period, i.e. continual wars and political instability which led to collapse of trade and agriculture and causing socioeconomic crisis. Cereals were the basic element of the diet of the poor class, while meat was not a primary food item. Thus, the inhibition of intestinal absorption of iron by phytates could be suggested. Cultural differences in the diet of this population could include different weaning practices and a change of dietary components or proportions of dietary constituents. Thus, porotic hyperostosis should not be seen as a single bit of evidence but should be analysed within the framework of other indicators in the sample.

References

Angel, J.L. (1966) Porotic hyperostosis, anemias, malarias, and marshes in the prehistoric eastern Mediterranean. *Science* 153, pp.760-762.

Angel, J.L. (1971) *The People of Lerna: Analysis of a Prehistoric Aegean Population.* Smithsonian Institution Press.

Aufderheide, A.C. and Rodrıguez-Martın, C. (1998) *The Cambridge Encyclopedia of Human Paleopathology.* Cambridge University Press.

Bass W.M. (1987) *Human Osteology: A Laboratory and Field Manual of the Human Skeleton* (3rd. edn.). Special Publication No. 2. Missouri Archaeological Society.

Benfer, R.A. (1990) The preceramic period site of Paloma, Peru: bioindications of improving adaptation to sedentism. *Latin American Antiquity* 1, pp.284-318.

Bharati, P. and Basu, A. (1990) Fertility, mortality and maternal anaemic status in a village population of West Bengal, India. *Annals of Human Biology* 17, pp.331-335.

Buzon, M.R. (2006) Health of the Non-Elites at Tombos: Nutritional and disease stress in New Kingdom Nubia. *American Journal of Physical Anthropology* 130, pp.26-37.

Cohen, M.N. and Armelagos G.J. (1984) *Paleopathology at the origin of agriculture.* Academic Press.

Dallman, P. (1986) Biochemical basis for the manifestations of iron deficiency. *Annual Review of Nutrition* 6, pp. 13-40.

Blom D.E., Buikstra, J.E., Keng, L., Tomczak, P.D., Shoreman, E. and Stevens-Tuttle, D. (2005) Anemia and Childhood Mortality: Latitudinal Patterning Along the Coast of Pre-Columbian Peru. *American Journal of Physical Anthropology* 127, pp. 152-169.

El-Najjar, M.Y. (1976) Maize, malaria and the anemias in the preColumbian New World. *Yearbook of Physical Anthropology* 20, pp. 329-337.

El-Najjar, M.Y., Ryan, D.J., Turner, C.G. and Lozoff, B. (1976) The Etiology of Porotic Hyperostosis among the Prehistoric and Historic Anasazi Indians of Southwestern United States. *American Journal of Physical Anthropology* 44, pp. 477-488.

Facchini, F., Rastelli, E. and Brasili, P. (2004) Cribra orbitalia and cribra cranii in Roman Skeletal Remains from the Ravenna Area and Rimini (I-IV Century AD). *International Journal of Osteoarchaeology* 14, pp. 126-136.

Fairgrieve, S.I. and Molto, J.E. (2000) Cribra Orbitalia in Two Temporally Disjunct Population Samples From the Dakhleh Oasis, Egypt. *American Journal of Physical Anthropology* 111, pp. 319-331.

Fakhry, A. (1974) *The Oases of Egypt. Bahriyah and Farafra oases.* Vol. II. American University in Cairo.

Fakhry, A. (1999) Egyptian Deserts, Part 2. Bahriyah and Farafra Oasis. In Gaballah, G.A. (ed) *Development of Contemporary Cultural Awareness series of scientific and historical Culture 100 Book Project.* Supreme Council of Antiquities Press.

Grauer, A.L. (1993) Patterns of anemia and infection from medieval York, England. *American Journal of Physical Anthropology* 91 (2), pp. 203-13.

Hershkovitz, I., Ring, B., Speirs, M., Galili, E., Kislev M., Edelson, G. and Hershkovitz, A. (1991) Possible congenital hemolitic anaemia in Prehistoric coastal inhabitants of Israel. *American Journal of Physical Anthropology* 85, pp. 7-13.

Hershkovitz, I., Rothschild, B.M., Latimer, B., Dutour, O., Leonetti, G., Greenwald, C.M., Rothschild, C. and Jellema, L.M. (1997) Recognition of sickle cell anemia in skeletal remains of children. *American Journal of Physical Anthropology* 104, pp. 213-226.

Hill, M.C. (2001) *Porotic hyperostosis as an indicator of anemia: an overview of correlation and cause.* Ph.D. Dissertation, University of Massachusetts, Amherst.

Hill, M.C. and Armelagos, G.J. (1990) Porotic hyperostosis in past and present perspective. In Buikstra, J.E. (ed). *A life in science: papers in honor of J. Lawrence Angel.* Center for American Archeology Anthropological Association, pp. 52-63.

Holland, T.D. and O'Brien, M.J. (1997) Parasites, porotic hyperostosis, and the implications of changing perspectives. *American Antiquity* 62, pp. 183-193.

Hrdlicka, A. (1912). The Natives of Kharga Oasis, Egypt. *Smithsonian Misc Collection* 59, pp. 1-153.

Hrdlicka, A. (1914) Anthropological work in Peru in 1913, with Notes on the Pathology of the Ancient Peruvians. *Smithsonian Miscellaneous Collection* 61.

Keenleyside, A. and Panayotova, K. (2006) Cribra Orbitalia and Porotic Hyperostosis in a Greek Colonial Population (5th to 3rd Centuries BC) from the Black Sea. *International Journal of Osteoarchaeology* 16, pp. 373-384.

Lallo, J.W., Armelagos, G.J. and Mensforth, R.P. (1977) The role of diet, disease, and physiology in the origin of porotic hyperostosis. *Human Biology* 49 (3), pp. 471-483.

Larsen, C.S. (2002) Bioarchaeology: the lives and lifestyles of past people. *Journal of Archaeological Research* 10 (2), pp. 119-166.

Mittler, D.M. and Van Gerven, D.P. (1994) Developmental, diachronic, and demographic analysis of cribra orbitalia in the Medieval Christian population of Kulubnarti. *American Journal of Physical Anthropology* 93, pp. 287–297

Meindl, R.S. and Lovejoy, C.O. (1985) Ectocranial suture closure: a revised method for the determination of skeletal age at death based on the lateral-anterior sutures. *American Journal of Physical Anthropology* 68, pp. 57-66.

Mensforth, R., Lovejoy, C.O., Lallo, J. and Armelagos, G.J. (1978) The role of constitutional factors, diet and infectious disease in the etiology of porotic hyperostosis and periosteal reactions in prehistoric infants and children. *Medical Anthropology* 2, pp. 1-59.

Mills A.J. (1979) Dakhleh Oasis Project: report on the first season of survey, October–December, 1978. *J Soc Stud Egypt Antiq* 9, pp. 163–185.

Mitchem, R. (1998) *Testing the maize theory: a case of the biological factors for porotic hyperostosis.* Masters thesis, University of Cincinnati.

Moorrees, C.F.A., Fanning, E.A. and Hunt, E.E. (1963a) Formation and resorption of three deciduous teeth in children. *American Journal of Physical Anthropology* 21, pp. 205-213.

Moorrees, C.F.A., Fanning, E.A. and Hunt, E.E. (1963b) Age variation of formation stages for ten permanent teeth. *Journal of Dental Research* 42, pp. 1490-1502.

Ortner, D.J. (2003) *Identification of Pathological Conditions in Human Skeletal Remains* (2nd edn). Academic Press.

Ortner, D.J. and Ericksen, M.F. (1997) Bone changes in the human skull probably resulting from scurvy in infancy and childhood. *International Journal of Osteoarchaeology* 7, pp. 212-220.

Ortner, D.J. and Mays, S. (1998) Dry-bone manifestations of rickets in infancy and early childhood. *International Journal of Osteoarchaeology* 8, pp. 45-55.

Ortner, D.J. and Putschar, W.G.H. (1985) *Pathological conditions in human skeletal remains.* Smithsonian Institution Press.

Ortner, D.J., Butler, W., Cafarella, J. and Milligan, L. (2001) Evidence of probable scurvy in subadults from archeological sites in North America. *American Journal of Physical Anthropology* 108, pp. 321-331.

Ortner, D.J., Butler, W., Cafarella, J. and Milligan, L. (2001) Evidence of probable scurvy in subadults from archaeological sites in North America. *American Journal of Physical Anthropology* 114, pp. 343-351.

Ortner, D.J.; Kimmerle, E.; Diez, M. (1999) Probable evidence of scurvy in subadults from archeological sites in Peru. *American Journal of Physical Anthropology* 108, pp. 321-331.

Redford, D.B. (2001) *The Oxford Encyclopedia of Ancient Egypt.* Vol. 2. The American University in Cairo Press.

Rose, J.C. (2006) Paleopathology of the commoners at Tell Amarna, Egypt, Akhenaten's capital city. *Mem Inst Oswaldo Cruz Rio de Janeiro* 101 (Suppl. II), pp. 73-76.

Ryan, A.S. (1997) Iron-deficiency anemia in infant development: implications for growth, cognitive development, resistance to infection, and iron supplementation. *American Journal of Physical Anthropology* 40, pp. 25-62.

Salvadei, L., Ricci, F. and Manzi, G. (2001) Porotic hyperostosis as a marker of health and nutritional conditions during childhood: studies at the transition between Imperial Rome and the Early Middle Ages. *American Journal of Human Biology* 13 (6), pp. 709-17.

Schultz, M., Larsen, C.S. and Kreutz, K. (2001) Disease in Spanish Florida: Microscopy of porotic hyperostosis and inferences about health. In Larsen, C.S. (ed.), *Bioarchaeology of Spanish Florida: The Impact of Colonialism*. University Press of Florida, pp. 207-225.

Steinbock, R.T. (1976) *Paleopathological Diagnosis and Interpretation.* Charles C.Thomas.

Steinbock, R.T. (1978) *Paleopathological diagnosis and interpretation.* Charles C. Thomas.

Strouhal, E. and Jungwirth, J. (1980) Paleopathology of the Late Roman-Early Byzantine cemeteries at Sayala, Egyptian Nubia. *Journal of Human Evolution* 9, pp. 61–70.

Stuart-Macadam, P. (1982) *A Correlative Study of Paleopathology of the Skull.* PhD Thesis, Department of Physical Anthropology, University of Cambridge.

Stuart-Macadam, P.L. (1985) Porotic hyperostosis: representative of a childhood condition. *American Journal of Physical Anthropology* 66, pp. 391-398.

Stuart-Macadam, P.L. (1987) A radiographic study of porotic hyperostosis *American Journal of Physical Anthropology* 74 (4), pp. 511-20.

Stuart-Macadam, P.L. (1989) Porotic hyperostosis: relationship between orbital and vault lesions. *American Journal of Physical Anthropology* 80, pp. 187-193.

Stuart-Macadam, P.L. (1991) Porotic hyperostosis: changing interpretations. In Ortner, D.J. and Aufderheide, A.C. (eds). *Human paleopathology: current syntheses and future options.* Smithsonian Institute Press, pp. 36-39.

Stuart-Macadam, P.L. (1992) Porotic hyperostosis: a new perspective. *American Journal of Physical Anthropology* 87, pp. 39-47.

Tung, T.A. (2003) *The health impact of Wari imperialism: a bioarchaeological assessment of communities in the core and periphery.* PhD Dissertation, University of North Carolina.

Ubelaker, D.H. (1989) *Human Skeletal Remains* (2nd edn). Taraxacum.

Van Gerven, D.P., Sheridan, S.G. and Adams, W.Y. (1995) The health and nutrition of a Medieval Nubian population. *American Anthropologist* 97, pp. 468-480.

Walker, P.L. (1985) Anemia among prehistoric Indians of the American Southwest. In Merbs, C.F. and Miller, R.J. (eds). *Health and disease in the prehistoric Southwest.* Arizona State University, Anthropological Research Papers No.34, pp. 139-164.

Wapler, U., Crubezy, E. and Schultz, M. (2004) Is cribra orbitalia synonymous with anemia? Analysis and interpretation of cranial pathology in Sudan. *American Journal of Physical Anthropology* 123, pp. 333-339.

Williams, S.R. (1990) *The skeletal biology of Estu-quina: a Late Intermediate Period site in southern Peru.* PhD Dissertation, Northwestern University.

Zink, N.A., Hagedorn, H.G., Szeimies, U. and Weyss, C. (2000) Anthropological and palaeopathological analysis of the human remains from three Tombs of the Nobles. of the Necropolis of Thebes-west, Upper Egypt. *Anthropologischer Anzeiger* 58, pp. 321-343.

WERE THE DENTISTS IN ANCIENT EGYPT OPERATIVE DENTAL SURGEONS OR WERE THEY PHARMACISTS?

R.J. Forshaw

KNH Centre for Biomedical Egyptology, The University of Manchester, UK

Abstract: *Was there a dedicated dental profession in ancient Egypt? If there was, what exactly was their role – were they operative dental surgeons as we know them today or did they merely prescribe pharmaceutical remedies? This is a topic that has been debated for nearly a hundred years and even today, due to the paucity of evidence, the literature provides little clear consensus. This paper examines the dental problems facing the ancient Egyptians, and reconsiders the evidence for the existence of a dental profession in ancient Egypt.*

Examination of skeletal and mummified remains has shown that tooth wear was widespread whilst caries was infrequently seen. Abscesses and dental infections, predominantly a result of pulp necrosis caused by the tooth wear, were not uncommon. The incidence of generalised periodontal disease may not have been as frequent as once thought.

The case for surgical treatment of dental abscesses, prosthetic appliances and extractions is considered by examination of the skeletal and mummified remains. Reference to the medical papyri indicates dental remedies, and amongst these are prescriptions which attempt to stabilise periodontally involved teeth and others designed to treat ulcers and abscesses. Hieroglyphic inscriptions from tombs and funerary monuments indicate nine known dentists. Ancient writings from other Near Eastern societies make reference to Egyptian medicine and dentistry.

The indication is that little if any operative dentistry was practised. Most of the dental treatment that appears to have been provided was restricted to pharmaceutical preparations that were either applied to the oral tissues or used as mouthwashes. These remedies would only have provided limited relief as it was the symptoms that were being treated and not the causes of the dental problems.

Key words: Dental health, pharmaceutical remedies, ancient Egypt.

Was there a dedicated dental profession in ancient Egypt, and if there was, were the dentists operative dental surgeons as we know them today, or were they pharmacists? This is a subject which has been debated for nearly a hundred years by both Egyptologists and dentists alike, and even today the literature seems to offer little clear consensus.

Perhaps before this subject is considered in detail it is necessary to briefly review the well-documented dental problems from which the ancient Egyptians suffered. This information, together with the surviving documentary and archaeological evidence, has enabled a detailed picture of their dental health to be established, probably more so than for any other civilisation in antiquity.

The most frequent pathological condition identified was that of excessive tooth wear, a condition so widespread that it is found in most of the surviving Egyptian skulls from the dynastic period (Ruffer 1920, 348; Leek 1967a, 51; Hillson 1979, 156; Harris et al 1998, 50). The teeth were rapidly worn down throughout life due to the presence of inorganic particulate matter in the food, chiefly the bread. These particles were present largely as a result of contamination of the grain by wind-blown sand and also as a result of grinding corn with soft sandstone implements. In time this tooth wear became so extensive that the enamel and dentine layers of the tooth were worn away and the pulp chamber became exposed (Fig. 1). As a consequence necrosis of the living tissue inside the tooth occurred and the root canals, now devoid of pulpal tissue, became a source of chronic infection and abscesses. A number of skulls show multiple abscess formation, indicative of how severe the problem of this tooth wear was.

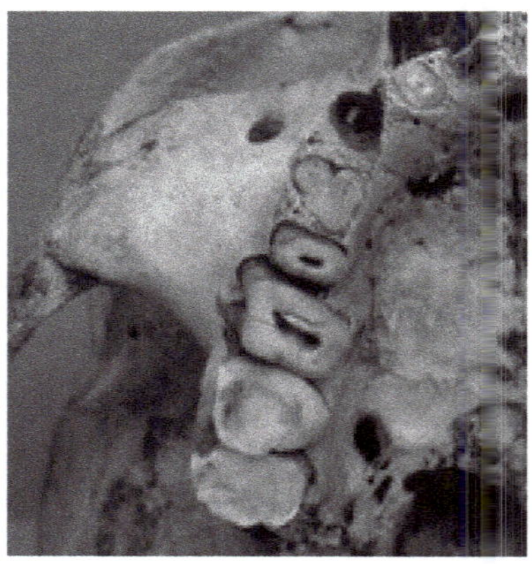

Figure 1: Nubian maxillary teeth (c.2000 BC), showing tooth wear and pulpal exposure

Periodontal disease or gum disease, a disorder frequently found in dentitions today, was also evident in ancient Egypt. The principal cause of periodontal disease is bacterial irritation brought about by deposits of plaque and calculus at the dentogingival junction, which results in inflammation of the gums, tissue destruction and loss of bony support for the teeth. Although generalised bone loss in periodontal disease is often considered to be responsible for the loss of many teeth in antiquity, more recent work questions this assumption. Research by Clarke et al (1986, 175; 1990, 371) concluded that localised vertical bone defects of pulpal aetiology were common and severe, often resulting in infection, abscesses and tooth loss. However, more generalised horizontal bone loss of gingival origin, usually considered to be periodontal disease, was far less frequent and of minor severity.

There is also evidence of caries or tooth decay, a condition caused by bacteria found in plaque breaking down certain fermentable carbohydrates in the diet. This reaction results in acid production which causes tooth destruction and may eventually lead to necrosis of the pulp with subsequent abscess formation. Although prevalent in modern society, caries was infrequently seen in ancient Egypt due to the lack of fermentable carbohydrates in the diet. Another factor was the fibrous abrasive nature of the food, which would tend to inhibit the retention of plaque on the tooth surface (Marion 1996, 15). However, in later periods of ancient Egyptian history caries incidence rose as increasing foreign influence resulted in changes to dietary habits, one of these being an increase in the consumption of fermentable carbohydrates. Interestingly, due to the nature of their diet, caries was more prevalent in the upper echelons of society during most periods of pharaonic history.

These three major dental disorders would have caused considerable pain and discomfort to the populace of ancient Egypt and so the question arises - was there a dedicated dental profession that the population could visit to address these problems? To consider this further, the evidence on the subject from various sources such as human remains, medical papyri, hieroglyphic inscriptions, and ancient writings needs to be examined (Weeks 1980, 100).

Evidence of operative dental surgery in the skeletal and mummified human remains from ancient Egypt is a much debated subject in the medical literature. From the many thousands of remains that have been examined there are only a few cases of possible prosthetic work, some rare instances where a surgical approach for the treatment of dental abscesses is claimed to have been adopted, and some examples where an extraction may have been performed. Much has been made of these cases by some authors (Ghalioungui 1971, 92; Iskander et al. 1979, 112; Blustein et al. 1987, 122; Chohayeb 1991, 69) suggesting that this evidence proves the existence of an operative dental profession, but other researchers (Leek 1967a, 58; Hoffman-Axthelm 1979, 77; Miller 2008, 31; Forshaw 2009, 482) have disagreed with this assumption.

In 1917, Hooton claimed he had found evidence that the ancient Egyptians had treated a dental abscess by surgical means (Hooton 1917, 29). His examination of a Fourth Dynasty mandible revealed two small holes directed towards the root of a worn molar tooth, which had become abscessed following pulpal exposure (Fig. 2). Due to their smooth symmetrical appearance and upward angulation, Hooton claimed that these holes were artificially created, and Breasted later considered that a fire-drill could have been used for such an operation (1930, 9).

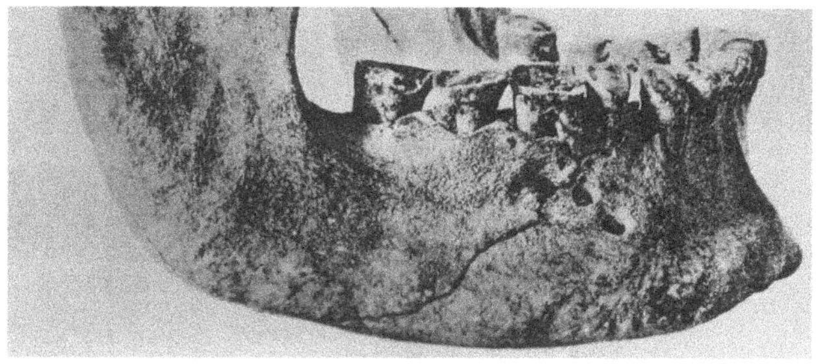

Figure 2: Ancient Egyptian mandible, IVth Dynasty, showing 'borings'

However, the holes are quite possibly the result of a normal pathological process caused by the dissolution of bone by pus from an abscess. Many abscess sinuses, similar in appearance, have often been found in skulls, not only from ancient Egypt but from all civilisations in antiquity. Such sinuses occur frequently, in many different positions and can be associated with any tooth in the dentition. They are often symmetrical, giving the appearance of being artificially created, but are not the result of human intervention

The question of whether dental prosthetic devices were used in ancient Egypt is a difficult subject to address due to the very limited nature of the evidence upon which to base a judgement. The earliest known of only three appliances was found at Giza near Cairo in a burial shaft dating to about 2500 BC. It consists of a fine gold wire connecting a mandibular second molar to a worn third molar, and importantly was not found attached to a skull but unearthed amongst the rubble of the tomb shaft (Fig. 3). The German dental report of 1927 concluded that because the teeth had a similar colour and morphological pattern, they belonged to the same individual (Junker 1929, 256). It has since been asserted in the literature that the original report claimed that the presence of calculus deposited on the teeth and wire indicated that the appliance had been worn during life (Leek 1967a, 55; Weeks 1980, 107).

However, Leek (1967a, 55; 1972, 405) considered that it was impossible to confirm that the teeth belonged to the same individual, as the tooth wear had produced such a considerable change in the tooth form that comparison was impossible. Interestingly, a more recent translation of the original German dental report indicates that calculus was only found on the teeth and not the wire, and so this particular piece of evidence does not provide proof that the appliance was worn during life. This incorrect translation has often been quoted in the literature. Another factor is that the deposits on the teeth might not be calculus but concretions of extraneous/mineral matter formed over a period of 4,500 years. Only a microscopic examination could determine the difference, a procedure that was not carried out at the time and due to subsequent damage to the appliance is now no longer possible.

A more probable explanation is that the device was inserted after death in an attempt to make the body whole for the afterlife, a practice common in ancient Egypt. Alternatively, it is possible that it was worn as an amulet during life.

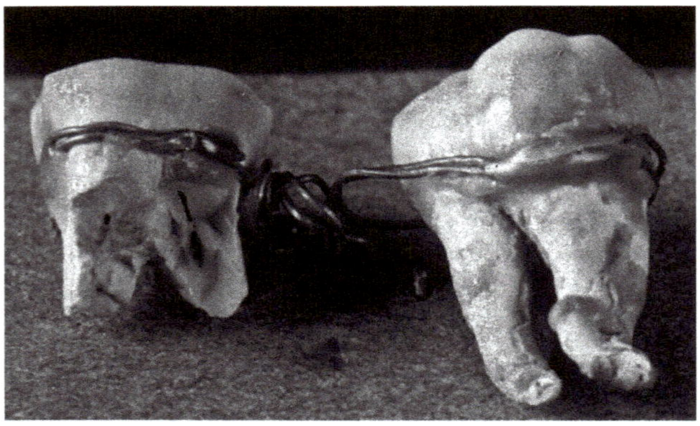

Figure 3: 'Dental appliance/ Teeth connected by wire?' found at Giza (IVth Dynasty)
© Roemer- und Pelizaeus-Museum, Hildesheim

Another appliance, also not found attached to a skull, was unearthed at El-Quatta where three teeth were found linked together by gold wire (Iskander et al. 1979, 108). It was suggested that the device was worn during life because of the artificial modification to the roots of the teeth and again because of the presence of calculus. However, the presence of calculus on the roots of the teeth could indicate periodontal involvement during life, whilst the alteration to the roots was not sufficiently extensive to suggest it being a conventional bridge. Again this device could be a post-mortem attempt at restoring the body in preparation for the afterlife.

It is not certain if extractions were carried out in ancient Egypt, as although this is a relatively simple method of relieving tooth-ache the evidence for this procedure is not unequivocal. The medical papyri are silent on the topic and no ancient Egyptian instrument has ever been identified as being used for the extraction of teeth. However, the appearance and features of the bone in areas where there are missing teeth has suggested to some researchers that extractions did occur (Quenouille 1975, 101; Leek 1986, 37). Nevertheless, there are many examples excavated from Egyptian cemeteries of periodontally involved and carious teeth which have caused extensive tissue destruction, and which could easily have been removed by a simple procedure, but have been left in situ (Ruffer 1921, 314; Miller 2008, 30). This seems rather perplexing when one considers the sophistication of the ancient Egyptian civilisation, their extensive knowledge of medicine, and indeed the painful nature of the condition itself.

Perhaps the most important source of information about dentistry is to be found in the medical papyri - these being the written records that have survived the ravages of time, and been handed down to us from ancient Egypt. Although they are silent on all operative aspects of dental care, four of them include prescriptions for the treatment of dental problems, whilst a fifth papyrus supplies instructions for dealing with fractures and dislocations of the mandible and maxillary regions.

Of the dental prescriptions listed, seven appear to be aimed at avoiding tooth loss by packing various substances in paste form around the teeth and adjacent gums. The theory seems to have been that these would harden and serve as a temporary means of stablising teeth that were mobile due to apical infection or periodontal disease. An example of such a prescription is Papyrus Ebers 739:

> *'Beginning of the remedies to consolidate a tooth; flour of emmer seeds; ochre; honey; made into a mass; and the tooth to be fattened therewith.'*
>
> (Wreszinski 1912, 181).

Emmer wheat used in this prescription is not known to have any pharmacological action, but ochres, which are iron oxides, do have recognised astringent and antiseptic properties. Honey has an antibacterial effect as it kills micro-organisms by drawing water out of them through osmosis (Worth Estes 1993, 69). Such a prescription would therefore have reduced inflammation in the tissues surrounding the teeth, resulting in some pain relief, and helped to splint the mobile teeth. However, it would not have cured the disease process, as for this to happen it would have been necessary firstly to remove the plaque and calculus.

Some translations of Ebers 739 (Ghalioungui 1963, 57; Halioua and Ziskind 2005, 167) suggest that this prescriptive agent was used as a filling material rather than being externally applied to the tooth. For a number of reasons this seems unlikely. Considering the hieroglyphs both in 739 and in similar prescriptions for this type of material, the translations begin by using words such as 'set in place', 'make strong', 'if it wants to fall to the ground' - all these wordings seem to imply a mobile tooth rather than a carious cavity.

At the end of the prescription after the constituents is found: '*... and the tooth to be fattened therewith*'. The ancient Egyptian verb here is *wSA*, with a meaning of fattening or stuffing out, and this would seem to indicate applying the material to the exterior of the tooth. Even if *wSA* is translated as filling, it could perhaps suggest filling a pocket between the tooth and the gum. The existence of such a pocket is not an uncommon result of periodontal disease and one form of treatment, used for this condition today, is the insertion into the pocket of an antimicrobial agent.

Another line of reasoning against this type of compound being used as a filling material is that the placing of it inside a carious tooth is unlikely to provide even a short term solution. Such a substance is quite likely to come adrift with the stresses of mastication and could well dissolve in the oral environment. Additionally, honey is a very cariogenic material and would certainly not be a suitable choice for a filling material.

The second main group of prescriptions appears to be designed to treat various ulcers, abscesses and gum infections. An example of such a remedy, seemingly used as a mouthwash, is Ebers 742:

> *'Another to treat the gums by rinsing of the mouth: bran, sweet beer, Swt DHwti are chewed and spat out'*
>
> (Ebbell 1937, 104)

Some translations of the papyrus suggest that the remedy was used as a masticatory and spat out (Ghalioungui 1987, 190). Among the components is *Swt DHwti,* which is thought to be the herb cinquefoil, and also sweet beer, probably used here as a vehicle for the remedy. Cinquefoil is used by herbalists for alleviating the pain of a toothache; it is used as an herbal gargle for treating oral sores, and has general disinfectant and astringent properties. So as with Ebers 739 there seem to be a rational approach to the problem, with some attempt to provide treatment.

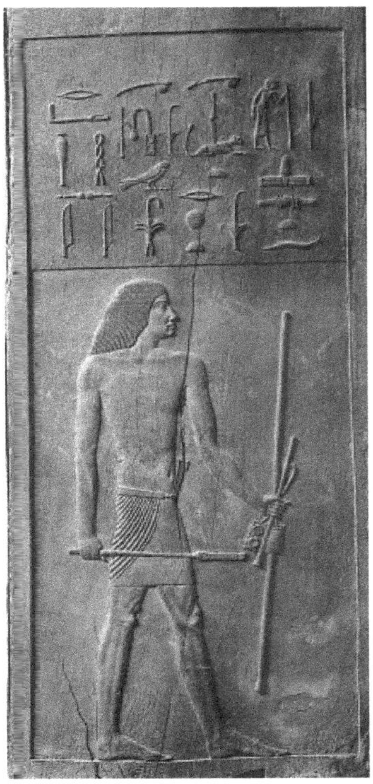

Figure 4: Hesyre - Chief of dentists and physicians. Courtesy of Cairo Museum

Translation of the hieroglyphic inscriptions found in tombs and monuments throughout Egypt has been able to reveal the occupation of the dead person, which in some cases has pointed to a medical or dental title. Of the approximately 150 persons who are recorded as being medical personnel in ancient Egypt, only nine are recognised as dentists. They appear to have been hierarchically ordered with two basic categories 'one who is concerned with teeth', usually regarded as a dentist, and 'one who deals with teeth'. It is not certain how these two titles differ, but possibly they reflect differences in duties and status (Weeks 1980, 114).

The earliest recorded dentist was Hesyre, who is evidenced from six finely carved wooden panels that were found in his tomb at Saqqara, near modern day Cairo (Fig. 4). Hesyre, who lived about 2660 BC, was not only chief of dentists but also chief of physicians, and in addition held a number of other religious and secular titles. Other dentists similarly held multiple titles such as Nyankhsekhmet who again was a chief of physicians. Khuwy was not only a dentist, but elder of the physicians of the palace as well as specialising in gastrointestinal complaints (Jonckheere 1958, 67). Whether these multiple titles indicated that the individual was engaged in several specialities or that the titles were perhaps administrative or ceremonial is unclear, but overall they do indicate an awareness of dental problems.

There are references to ancient Egyptian medicine and dentistry in early texts of other Near Eastern societies. Classical authors such as Homer, Pliny the Elder, and Herodotus describe the celebrated position that Egyptian medicine achieved in the ancient World (Weeks 1980, 99). In particular Herodotus, who was a Greek traveller and historian, visited Egypt in approximately 440 BC, later writing an account of the country and its history. He described how Persian monarchs wished to have Egyptian physicians at their courts, and in an often quoted passage described how the practice of Egyptian medicine was specialised:

> *'The practice of medicine they split into separate parts, each doctor being responsible for the treatment of only one disease. There are, in consequence, innumerable doctors, some specialising in diseases of the eye, others of the head, others of the teeth, others of the stomach, and so on'*
>
> (Herodotus 1972, 114).

Although the above extract mentions specialisation, other translations of the same lines refer to '*undertaking to treat a particular part of the body'* (Weeks 1980, 99), which could imply a division of labour rather than the existence of advanced Egyptian medical knowledge requiring specialised practitioners. However, again there is recognition of some form of dental care.

Perhaps one of the most significant pieces of evidence concerning dentistry in ancient Egypt is provided by an examination of the radiographs of the Royal mummies in Cairo Museum. Several of the pharaohs, particularly some of Egypt's greatest heads of state such as

Amenhotep III and Ramesses II, show severe dental problems involving extensive tooth wear, dental abscesses and advanced periodontal disease (Harris et al. 1980, 329). These conditions must have caused considerable pain, which will undoubtedly have had some bearing on the quality of life of the particular pharaoh, yet nowhere was there evidence of any form of dental treatment. If anyone in Egypt was to receive such treatment surely it would have been these powerful rulers, and this must undoubtedly point to a lack of or at best a very limited knowledge of dentistry.

The evidence would suggest, therefore, that operative dental treatment, if it did exist at all, was very limited, and management of dental conditions seems to have been restricted to the type of pharmaceutical preparation listed in the medical papyri. These remedies were directed towards the symptoms of the problem, rather than the cause, and at best will only have provided some short term relief.

References

Blustein, Y., Stern, N. and Kottek, S.S. (1987). A case of prosthetic dentistry in ancient Egypt. *Bulletin of the History of Dentistry* 35 (2), pp. 120-4.

Breasted, J.H. (1930) *The Edwin Smith surgical papyrus.* Vol 1. Chicago University Press.

Chohayeb, A.A. (1991) The dental heritage of ancient Egypt. *Bulletin of the History of Dentistry* 39 (2), pp. 65-9.

Clarke, N.G., Carey, S.E., Srikandi, W., Hirsh, R.S. and Leppard, P.I. (1986) Periodontal disease in ancient populations. *American Journal of Physical Anthropology* 71, pp. 173-183.

Clarke, N.G. (1990) Periodontal defects of pulpal origin: Evidence in early man. *American Journal of Physical Anthropology* 82, pp. 371-376.

Ebbell, E. (1937) *The Papyrus Ebers.* Levin and Munksgaard, Ejnar Munksgaard.

Forshaw, R.J. (2009) Dental Practice in ancient Egypt. *British Dental Journal* 206 (9), pp. 481-486.

Ghalioungui, P. (1963) *Magic and medical science in ancient Egypt.* Hodder and Stoughton.

Ghalioungui, P. (1971) Did a dental profession exist in ancient Egypt? *Medical History* 15 (1), pp. 92-94.

Halioua, B. and Ziskind, B. (2005) *Medicine in the days of the pharaohs.* Harvard University Press.

Harris, J.E., Ponitz, P.V. and Ingalls, B.K. (1998) Dental health in ancient Egypt. In Cockburn, A., Cockburn, E., Reyman, T.A. (eds.) *Mummies, disease and ancient cultures.* 2nd ed. Cambridge University Press, pp. 59-68.

Harris, J.E., Storey, A.T. and Ponitz, P.V. (1980) Dental disease in the royal mummies. In Harris, J.E., Wente, E. F. (eds.) *An X-Ray atlas of the royal mummies.* University of Chicago Press, pp. 328-345.

Herodotus (1972). *The Histories.* Trans. De Sélincourt A. Revised Ed. Penguin.

Hillson, S. (1979) Diet and dental disease. *World Archaeology* 11, pp. 147-62.

Hoffman-Axthelm, W. (1979) Is the practice of dentistry in ancient Egypt an archaeological fact? *Bulletin of the History of Dentistry* 27 (2), pp. 71-8.

Hooton, E.A. (1917) Oral surgery in Egypt during the Old Empire. *Harvard African Studies* 1, pp. 29-32.

Iskander, Z., Harris, J.E. and Farid, S. (1979) Further evidence of dental prosthesis in ancient Egypt. *Annales du Service des Antiquités de L'Égypte* 63, pp. 93-122.

Jonckheere, F. (1958) *Les médecins de l'Égypte pharaonique.* La Médecine Égyptienne No.3. Fondation Égyptologique Reine Élisabeth.

Junker, H. (1929) *Giza I: Die mastabas der IV Dynastie auf des Alten Reiches.* Holder-Pichler-Tempsky AG.

Leek, F.F. (1967a) The practice of dentistry in Ancient Egypt. *Journal of Egyptian Archaeology* 53, pp. 51-8.

Leek, F.F. (1967b) Reputed early Egyptian dental operation, an appraisal. In Brothwell, D.R. (ed.) *Diseases in antiquity.* Thomas, pp. 702-705.

Leek, F.F. (1972) Did a dental profession exist in ancient Egypt during the 3rd millennium BC? *Medical History* 16 (4), pp. 404-406.

Leek, F.F. (1986) Dental health and disease in ancient Egypt with special reference to the Manchester mummies. In David, A.R. (ed.) *Science in Egyptology.* Manchester University Press, pp. 35-42.

Lipton, J.S. (1982) Oral surgery in ancient Egypt as reflected in the Edwin Smith Papyrus. *Bulletin of the History of Dentistry* 30 (2), pp. 108-114.

Marion, L.R. (1996) Dentistry of ancient Egypt. *Journal of the History of Dentistry* 44, pp. 15-17.

Miller, J. (2008) *An appraisal of the skulls and dentition of ancient Egyptians, highlighting the pathology and speculating on the influence of diet and environment.* BAR Publishing.

Quenouille, J.J. (1975) *La bouche et les dents dans l'antiquité Égyptienne.* Doctorat en chirurgie dentaire thesis, Lyon University.

Ruffer, M.A. (1920) A study of abnormalities and pathology of ancient Egyptian teeth. *American Journal of Physical Anthropology* 3, pp. 335-382.

Ruffer, M.A. (1921) *Studies in the paleopathology of Egypt.* University of Chicago Press.

Weeks, K.R. (1980) Ancient Egyptian dentistry. In Harris, J.E. and Werte, E.F. (eds.) *An X-Ray atlas of the royal mummies.* University of Chicago Press, pp. 99-121.

Worth, W.J. (1993) *The medical skills of ancient Egypt.* Science History Publications.

Wreszinski, W. (1912) *Der papyrus Ebers.* 1 Teil: *Umschrift.* Hinrichs.

SKULL INJURIES DISCOVERED IN THE TOMB OF DJEHUTIMES, THEBES (TT 32)

E. Fóthi and Z. Bernert

Hungarian Natural History Museum, Department of Anthropology, Hungary

Abstract: *Large numbers of skull injuries on individuals emerged during the anthropological examination of Theban Tomb 32, in a typical linear Ramesside tomb including 3 forecourts, cult chapels, a sloping passage and a burial chamber. At the site remains of more than 400 individuals have come to light. In this report two cases of skull injuries are described.*

The neurocranium of a male of mature age from the Ptolemaic age was discovered in Room III. Several injuries can be observed on the skull. Meningitis resulting from a sword-cut of 83 millimetres and otitis media together most probably caused death.

In Tomb B, located in the central court of the Tomb of Djehutimes, a big, thickly bandaged mummy head dated to the Twenty-First Dynasty was discovered. An elliptic clay disk covered the huge injury of 10 centimetres. The young man died most probably of toxaemia caused by his untreated wound.

Key words: Thebes, mummies, skull wounds.

Theban Tomb 32 has been investigated since 1983 by the Hungarian Mission of the Department of Egyptology of Eötvös Loránd University, Budapest. Works were started by László Kákosy. After his death, the project was taken over by Gábor Schreiber. The tomb itself can be found on the western side of the Nile, in the necropolis of ancient Thebes, in the cemetery of nobles, on the Khokha hill (Fig. 1). The monument was constructed for a high-ranking official of Ramesses II, Djehutimes, who bears in his inscriptions a number of titles, e.g., Royal Scribe, Overseer of the Granaries of Amun, Great Steward of Amun, Overseer of the Fields of the Two Lands, Governor of Esna, etc.

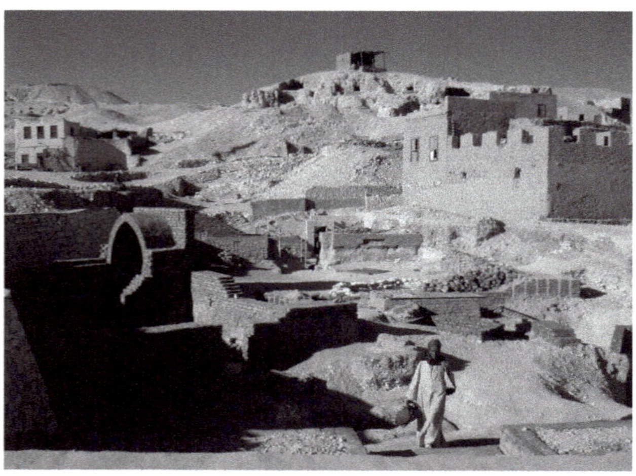

Figure 1: Theban Tomb 32 in Khokha hill.

As far as architecture is concerned, the tomb is a typical linear Ramesside tomb including 3 forecourts, cult chapels, a sloping passage and a burial chamber. The bodies of Djehutimes and his wife (the Songstress of Amun, Iset) were lying in the lowermost chamber of the tomb in their giant sarcophagi made of granite from Aswan. There are several secondary graves both in the internal tomb and the outer courts, especially from the age of the Eighteenth Dynasty (earlier period), the age of later dynasties as well as from the Ptolemaic and Roman periods (Kákosy and Schreiber 2003, 201).

While many anthropologists have seen this tomb, only one study on some anthropological findings of Tomb B has been published (Farkas 1993). Our anthropological study was carried out in 2005-2007 and extended over the entire anthropological material uncovered in TT 32, namely the human remains found in the tomb interior and also the findings of tombs and of trenches excavated in the courtyards.

The preservation of the anthropological material was extremely poor. The tomb was probably plundered during the period until the present, and that resulted in disintegration of the mummies and their parts became redeposited throughout the entire tomb area, and even through the courtyards. All the burials inside the tomb and also in the courtyards were robbed, the remains were scattered and mixed. No findings have been found *in situ*.

The large number of skull injuries found on individuals in this area gives an excellent opportunity to examine the healing practices of the age. We describe two cases:

Case 1: The neurocranium of a male of mature age (50-60 years of age) was discovered in Room III of Djehutimes' Tomb. The lamina cribrosa is intact. The brain has not been removed during the process of mummification as its remains can be seen in the skull. There is no hair on the scalp. A thick layer of bitumen with remnants of coarse-textured fabric covers the nape. The large amount of bitumen is most probably due to the fact that this mummy was made in the Ptolemaic age.

The scalp on the brain-cap is knobbly. Several injuries can be observed on the bone under that. The entire sinciput is bumpy as a result of the injuries, and several cutmarks are observed on the bone below the scalp. On the right side, the traces of a depressed injury can be observed – this injury has healed up. Several healed injuries can be seen on the skull. Most probably, it is because this individual was a soldier.

Another injury can be seen on the right side of the skull, namely on the parietal bone: a long and linear cut of 83 millimetres (Fig. 2). This injury has healed up as the cranial bones joined at several sections whereas gaps remained at others. The external side of the parietal bone is not porotic, there are no signs referring to inflammation. This wound has been carefully treated immediately after the event. However, inflammation resulting from the injury occurred on the internal surface of the skull. Here, a coral like proliferation of the bone can be observed following the line of the cut on the outside.

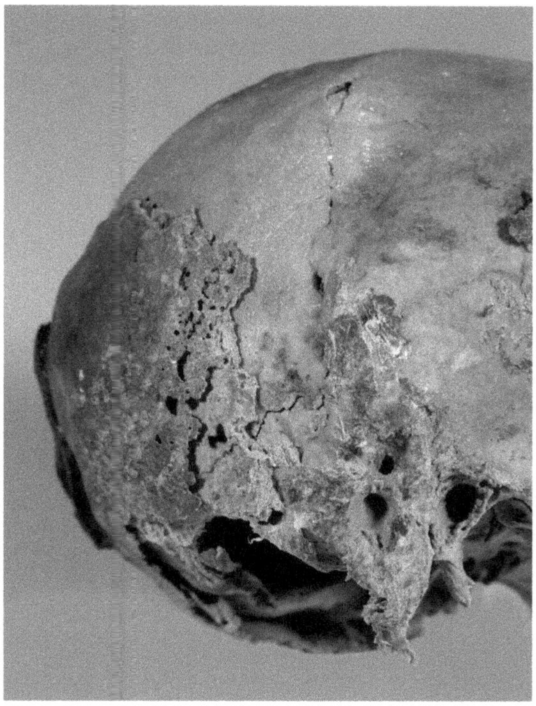

Figure 2: A long sword-cut on the vault and two fissures on the outer surface of the right mastoideum.

In addition to that, two large associated fissures can be seen on the outer surface of the right mastoideum. The fissures are connected to each other. The skin infolds at their openings (Fig. 2). It seems that the pus produced as a result of the otitis was discharged to the outside as the internal surface is intact. Meningitis resulting from the sword-cut and the otitis media together most probably caused death.

Case 2: Tomb B occupies a large area on the southern slope of el-Khokha that partly overlies the first and second forecourts of TT 32. The structure of Tomb B is constituted by two architectural units: the superstructure made entirely of mudbrick, and the underground parts hollowed out from the bedrock (Schreiber and Vasáros 2005, 2, 5). In Tomb B a large, thickly bandaged mummy head was discovered. According to Kákosy (1993, 3), it can be dated to the Twenty-First Dynasty. The bandage is coarse on the outside but it is extremely fine next to the face.

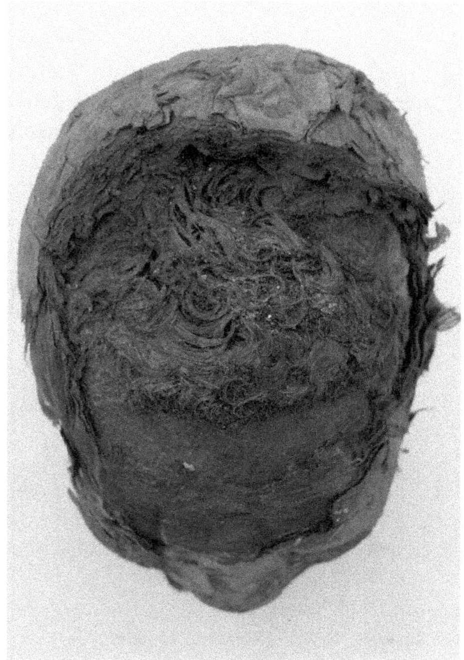

Figure 3: Huge wound of 10 centimetres covered by the mixture of clotted blood and hair, os frontale intact.

The textile layers were gummed with resin. A huge wound of 10 centimetres can be seen on the forehead, covered by the mixture of clotted blood and hair, forming a layer about 10 millimetres thick (Fig. 3). The os frontale was intact. The wound was covered by an elliptic clay disk (thickness: 8 mm, length: 12.5 cm) before the body was embalmed (Fig. 4). The clay was pressed onto the forehead of the man while it was wet. When it dried, it became choppy. Since the injury has not affected the os frontale, this young man died most probably of toxaemia caused by his untreated wound.

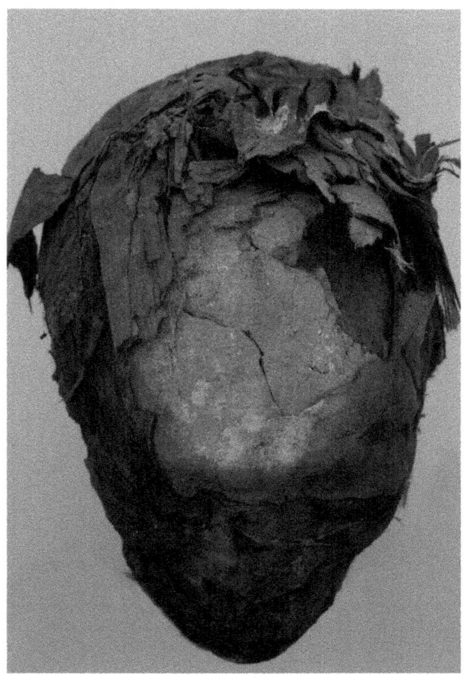

Figure 4: Elliptic clay disk on the forehead.

This inexplicable use of a clay disk is a singular occurrence and as far as we know no similar case is published in the literature. According to Farkas (1993, 24), this orange-coloured 'clay-like' substance has been used to model the frontal area of the head. Assuming the frontal bone is missing due to fatal trauma, the clay disk might have been used as a prosthesis. Since the frontal bone was not broken, this idea has not been substantiated. Most probably this practice was used as cultic custom.

References

Farkas, E. (1993) *Human remains from the Theban Tomb 32.* Acta Archaeologica Academiae Scientiarum Hungaricae.

Kákosy, L. (1993) *Eighth Preliminary Report on the Hungarian Excavation in Theban Tomb 32.* Acta Archaeologica Academiae Scientiarum Hungaricae.

Kákosy, L. and Schreiber, G. (2003) *Use and Re-use. An Overview of the Post-Ramesside Burials in TT 32.* Studien zur Altägyptischen Kultur.

Schreiber, G. and Vasáros, Zs. (2005) *A Theban Tomb of the Late Third Intermediate Period on El-Khokha.* Acta Archaeologica Academiae Scientiarum Hungaricae.

J3dt rnpt OR THE 'PESTILENCE OF THE YEAR'

H. Győry

Museum of Fine Arts, Budapest

Abstract: *The study of the first incantation of the recto of the Smith papyrus is enormously revealing if we are looking for the ancient Egyptian conception of the 'pestilence of the year' in medical terms. First of all, we learn that it can be related at least to three known diseases from those times, namely the ḫ3yt, dnd and dḥrt. Fortunately, we also have their ancient descriptions in the Ebers medical papyrus, used probably at the same time as the Smith papyrus. From here it is clear that they mean different types of well-known endemic febrile illnesses. After comparing the symptoms of the now widespread tropical febrile diseases with the ancient ones, I would like to propose a possible identification for dnd as a collective name for a disease group centred around the mainly food-born typhoid fever and the mosquito induced dengue-like diseases with continuous high temperatures.*

The Beginning of the Year and the Flood

The ancient Egyptian Calender contained 5 epagomenal days, which brought the civil year to 365 days. They considered them remarkably dangerous. They thought that on these days Sekhmet sent her arrows, messengers, errand-boys or knife-carrying demons to fill people with fear and make death dominate at this time of the year. These 'bad and evil things' were called 'the pestilence of the year' (*j3dt rnpt*), feared mostly at the turn of the year. Its general meaning recalls the primeval chaos, the state of the whole disorder, when the evil spirits are free to cause destruction, death and maladies, but in medical-magical texts, as I will show in this paper, it can mean serious, widespread diseases, thus epidemics in a medical sense. The New Year's starting point coincided with the beginning of the innundation. Thus, the not always deadly, but at this time regularly returning severe disease-waves commonly called the 'pestilence of the year' and the innundation seem to be connected. The idea of a connection between plagues and the innundation is not new; Greta Hort (Hoffmeier, 1996, 146-149) thinks that the first 6 out of the 10 plagues of the Bible (Exodus, 4,18 - 5,1. Ps. 78,43-51, Ps. 105) are essentially the results of the flood. The link is also raised by H. Engelmann and J. Hallof (1996, 110-111) in their article on the Sekhmet priests. If so, we have a key to investigate how and why these plagues were established, and their medical identification.

Sekhmet and the Diseases

Whilst the ancient Egyptians fought diseases, they could only perceive diseases that were visible to the naked eye. They could thus only attribute the severe diseases caused by pathogens to supernatural activity. In the case of the epidemics at the end of the year, their sources called this force mostly Sekhmet (or Bastet). They also thought the god who caused evil could fix it in the fastest and safest way, so they hoped to be saved by the same divinity. Therefore, when these diseases appeared en masse, big offerings and various rituals were arranged for her in the whole country. This might also be the reason why more than 300 Sekhmet statues in the Mut precinct in Karnak were erected by Amenhotep III (i.e. they were probably destined to stop a great epidemic). As Legrain noticed, her increased worship is also shown by the strong wear and tear on the legs and left arm of these statues which he attributed to the frequent touch of adherents (Hoenes 1976, 43).

Fatal epidemic diseases (Marr and Malloy 1996, 7-24; Hoyte 1993, 706-708; Miller 1991, 1-24) seem to be handled in some ancient Egyptian sources as one disease-group called *j3dt* /*jdw*. They already had a well-known connection to the goddess Sekhmet in the Middle Kingdom, when the Story of Sinuhe mentioned them as a general explanation:

> '*How will that land be now, without that perfect god (i.e. Amenemhat I) whose fear permeated the lands like Sekhmet's year of pestilence?*'
>
> (pBerlin 3022, 43-45)

Also, the Eloquent Peasant listed a 'mistress of the pestilence' in his 2nd claim during the First Intermediate Period.

Ancient Medical Identification of 'The Pestilence'

The *j3dt*, in earlier texts *jdw*, was used in the common Egyptian language as a general expression, but among medical texts it seems to have a much narrower meaning. The recto of the Smith papyrus contains several utterances against it, which declare that it may bring death (verso, 18,1-11/ end of the 2nd and 7th incantation: *I die not through you! – n mwt.j n.t*), and suggest as a mediator, the *ṯ3w*, translated usually as wind, air or breath. Utterances and amulets were used to fight it. In the 4th incantation the 'flame or heat' / *nsrt* is mentioned as its characteristic feature, while in the 5th incantation the heart, liver, various types of spirits, and the *ḫ3ytjw*-demons are listed. The 6th spell is an incantation for cleansing a fly (*sw*ʿ*b* ʿ*ff*), without its injuring the patient (more exactly his *ḥt*), the 7th is an 'incantation for everything in the pestilence', where the *ḫ3yt* are banished by spells and the *nfrt* and *ḥt-ds* wood was used to help in it, while in the 8th spell the *š3ms* is written as a pestilence repeller plant. The most interesting from this point of view however, is the first utterance, which gives us a hidden medical description of the pestilence:

'Spell for barring the air of the pestilence of the year: Oh, Flame-in-His-face, the foremost of the Akhet! I am speaking to you, to the Foremost of Per-Neith town. Make firm Osiris, the foremost of the land.

Nekhbet, who can lift the land to the sky for her father, come and tie two plumes behind me, that I may live and become sound, for I am that White One.

The first is the elder god in Heliopolis, the second is Isis, the third is Nephthys, and I am after for you (i.e. for Nekhbet?).

Grasper of the Great One (i.e. crown), son of Sekhmet, mighty of the mightiest, son of the god ḫ3yt and god dnd, son of Hathor, lady of the Red Crown, who swells the rivers as you row Nu and sail in the Morning-boat! You have saved me from every dḥrt.

Spell for this year in the breath (nft) of every bad air. Horus, Horus, the son / sound one (w3ḏ) of Sekhmet, be all around my flesh for life!

To be recited over 2 feathers of vulture, put over a man and put as his protection against any place he might walk in.

It is the year's protection; it is a dḥrt repeller in the pestilence of the year.'

(Breasted 1930, 472-476; Allen 2005, 106-107.)

As long as the symptoms of the epidemics are undetermined, we can only speculate. This incantation, however, gives us a clue by denominating three disease-demons who are responsible for bad health, and who are connected to various divinities. It does not say how many disease-demons were feared at that time all together, but possibly the most dangerous are listed: *ḫ3yt*, *dnd* and *dḥrt*. The first two are named as gods. They seem to be connected to Sekhmet and Hathor respectively, but the 3rd one has no divine relationship mentioned, although we learn that the vulture goddess Nekhbet can save the patient from it by the help of her two feathers bound behind the patient. The cry for the help of Horus is again a magical means to survive with one's health intact, and again the choice of the word for his epithet, *w3ḏ*, which can be translated either as the 'son' or the 'sound one', refers also to a common New Year's amulet, the papyrus column. The White Crown was another powerful amulet against the pestilence, as the incantator's wish to live and be sound is justified by his identification with this crown. Thus it helps against all three disease demons, who are, however, mentioned not only in magical texts, but in a medical context, too.

The *ḫ3yt* Disease

The *ḫ3yt* disease is the most common among them; it is mentioned several times, for instance:

In the 'Book of *r3-jb*': Eb 188c, Eb 190a, Eb 190c, Eb 193a, Eb 196, Eb 197a, Eb 203c;

In other paragraphs of the Book of the *ḫt*: Eb 251b = Eb 25;

In the second 'anatomical treatise' in connection with the *mtw*: Eb 854c, Eb 854l, Eb 855q;

Against the *ꜥḫw*: L 24 (8,4-5) where it has the epithet of '*every kind*' (nb);

Or as a *ḫ3yt* demon in other Spells of the Smith papyrus: Sm 18,6 (266/455), 18,12 (266/455), 18,13 (266/455), 19,8 (266/455), 20,7 (266/456), 19,20 (266/456), or of those in the Book of the Dead: ch. 149.

From a medical point of view for instance, in the above prescription of Ebers 188 or Ebers 875l it is used as a summary expression for liver inflammation (Győry 2001, 31), while in prescription Ebers 190 it describes a case where the *ḫ3yt* is felt as a faeces-ball at the ribcage. We can thus conclude that it was a fairly general disease or a dangerous health condition, a sort of disease-group. Its general meaning seems to be supported also by its connection to the notion 'enemy'. The root itself expresses 'torment, suffering', but can be deduced from the verb *ḫ3j* 'to measure' by the passive perfect participle 'what is measured (on somebody)'.

The *dḥrt* Disease

The *dḥrt* 'bitterness' or 'sadness/grief'- disease, which might even be connected to the skin, is described in the 'anatomical treatise' by paragraph Ebers 855k. It says:

'What 'any kind of *dḥrt*-diseases' concerns: it enters through the left eye, and departs through the navel. It is the breath of the activity of the *wꜥb* priest. The *ḥ3tj*-heart gives, that they enter into his *mtw*, and cook in his whole flesh. The *ḥ3tj*-heart is moving down (*nḏḥḏḥ*) because of them, because it comes out cooked. The *mtw* of his *ḥ3tj*-heart are trembling because of [these] things. What their defeat (*d3r*) concerns, it is their covering by the *dḥrt*-diseases. What the lifting of his *dḥrt*-diseases concerns, it is their flooding.'

The symptoms are rather unclear. It is, however, evident that the whole body of the patient trembles sometimes, they experience a very high temperature, but also that in his organs contrary actions are taking place. The first signs appear in the eye, the others are connected to the belly. Again, the heart plays a central role in the Egyptian circulation system, which gives a feeling of pressure all over the body; when the *dḥrt* is apparent the *mtw* are covered, which might mean that they were blocked from outside, as the contrary state is being flooded, thus technically unobstructed or open to the air (as the healthy state of the *mtw*). The origin of these processes was unknown, thus the divine cause is evidenced through the activity of a priest. Another possible interpretation of the role of the *wꜥb*-priest is that he lets the disease depart from the body through his actions (Bardinet, 1996). The *wꜥb* priest might hint at the priests of Sekhmet, who were responsible for the treatment and prevention of epidemics (Engelmann and Hallof 1996, 103-146).

The *dnd* Disease

The *dnd* has a root meaning 'to be angry, furious, raging'. It was already a personified deity by the Old Kingdom, when the Pyramid Texts mention him in the form of *dndn* (Pyr 200d) or *dndnw* (Pyr 1254b). During the New Kingdom, he was represented as a ram-headed god (e.g. Book of the Gates, 12th hour, upper row in tombs of Ramses III, VI, Seti II.). His name might have had also a medical meaning of 'agressive behaviour' or 'fit'. Actually, we also have the ancient Egyptian description of *dnd* as:

'What the 'ball (*swš*) fallen on his *ḥ3tj*-heart' concerns, it means that a ball of the *t3w*-heat has fallen on his *ḥ3tj*-heart, bringing frequent weakness (*3hd*). That means he is faint (*ꜥm-jb.f*) because of the *dnḏ* caused by his *ḥ3tj*-heart being full of blood. This is what makes it happen: The drinking of water causes it, or eating the warm *sbjt* fish causes it to happen.' (Ebers 855v).

Thus, according to this passage, the disease was caused by contaminated food, either water or a special sort of fish as shown by the determinative – both probably increased during the heavy floods, when the staple food was most probably fish.

If nourishment and disease were connected, the cause and effect would have had to be quickly apparent. Otherwise, it would not have been noticed. However, the symptoms seem to be unclear: just a general weak condition, including faintness. The central role of the Egyptian circulation system and the high temperatures are given. In addition, the name probably also describes a typical symptom, the state of mind mentioned above during the disease.

Conclusions

These ancient explanations show that the Pestilence of the Year does not mean one given disease regularly returning and exclusively at the end of the year, or a general term without a direct medical meaning, but it did mean the grouping of several concrete and widespread diseases which were infectious, and thought to be spread by the breath / air, and which could appear scattered at any time of the year. They were feared and severe, but not always fatal, although never to be underestimated. Their most significant common and dangerous conditions were high temperatures and the central role of the heart-system. Although unnamed in ancient Egyptian texts, the presence of these features in pharaonic and even earlier times (and not just as a theorectical case, but we also have proof in ancient Egyptian mummies) led me to wonder if tropical infectious diseases with high temperatures could be the ailments described. As there is not space enough for a detailed discussion of all these ancient diseases, I will now focus on one of them.

Considerations concerning *dnd*

The diseases listed by the World Health Organisation (WHO) for modern Egypt: (http://wwwn.cdc.gov/travel/yellowBookCh3Africa.aspx) have been clinically separated and precisely determined only in terms of modern medicine. Several of them could be considered the same according to pharaonic medicine, while various symptoms of the same disease might be determined as different diseases at that time. Even today, clinical diagnosis is often unreliable concerning febrile diseases, and diagnostic tests might give very different results. In a random inspection of 31 patients with brucellosis identified by diagnostic tests, 26 (87.1%) were treated clinically for typhoid fever, although the former has no rash, but a typically odorous sweating (Crump et al. 2003, 539-544). Both are, however, food-borne, although there are again big differences; for instance, typhoid fever is transmitted by contaminated water and food, while brucellosis is only transmitted through the milk of the infected animals.

If we consider the symptoms of the *dnd*-disease - that is the extreme weariness and great fever which makes the heart and circulation system suffer so much that the patient tends to faint - and do not take into consideration the skin alterations, which might be considered as a separate illness, the given features do not exclude the possibility that this ancient expression comprised the above febrile diseases. It would also explain the 'anger or fury' that the name of the disease meant for the Egyptians, with the help of the typhosus conditions, from where also the communal modern root for the names for typhus and typhoid fever comes. They are now recognised to be two different diseases, but a hundred years ago they were still thought to be two variations of the same one. What speaks against an eventual indentification with a typhoid-like disease-group is the typical diarrhoea and cough in some cases which are missing in the given disease description. As asymptomatic cases however occur fairly often, the ancient Egyptians might not have taken into account these features as obligatory, or could attribute them to one of the several types of the disease.

A similar disease group can again be centered around the dengue fever. Although its antigen is still unidentified in ancient Egyptian mummies, both the virus and the vector are indigenous; thus the disease most probably existed in pharaonic times, but was possibly not separated from other similar febrile diseases. It is still now often misidentified as West Nile or yellow fever in tropical regions if special dengue-testing is not performed. The symptoms share similarities with the typhoid fever/ brucellosis group, and their occurance was increased by high water tables during the floods, when mosquitos were able to reproduce in great numbers. If we take into consideration the fact that typhoid fever and the typhus were for a long time considered to be different variations of the same disease, we cannot exclude the possibility of their ancient forms belonging to the same disease-group.

The common features of the continuous high fever and general weariness in all body parts with a central role of the heart and the frequent occurance at given times may suggest the possibility that all these febrile diseases with a continous high temperature belonged to the same disease group.

References

Allen, J.P. (2005) *The Art of Medicine in Ancient Egypt* (exh. cat.). The Metropolitan Museum of Art.

Bardinet, Th. (1995) *Les Papyrus médicaux de L'Égypte pharaonique*. Penser La Médecine.

Breasted, J.H. (1930) *The Edwin Smith Surgical Papyrus*. University of Chicago Press.

Engelmann, H. and Hallof, J. (1996) Der Sachmetpriester, ein früher Repräsentant der Hygiene und des Seuchenschutzes, *Studien zur Altägyptischen Kultur* 23, pp. 103-146.

Hoenes, S-E. (1976) *Untersuchungen zu Wesen und Kult der Göttin Sachmet*. Bonn.

Hoffmeier, J.K. (1996) *Israel in Egypt. The Evidence for the Authenticity of the Exodus Tradition*. Oxford University Press.

Hoyte, H.M. (1993) The plagues of Egypt: what killed the animals and the firstborn? *Medical Journal of Australia* 158 (10), pp. 285-6.

Győry, H. (2001) 'Négy ere van a májnak' - A májról alkotott anatómiai ismeretek az Ebers papiruszban, *Orvosi Hetilap* 142 (20), pp. 1061-1066.

Crump, J.A., Youssef, F.G., Luby, S. P., Wasfy, M.O., Rangel, J.M., Taalat, M., Oun, S.A. and Mahoney, F. J. (2003) Estimating the Incidence of Typhoid Fever and Other Febrile Illnesses in Developing Countries. *Emerging Infectious Diseases* 9 (5), pp. 536-544.

Marr, J.S. and Malloy, C.D. (1996) *An epidemiologic analysis of the ten plagues of Egypt*. Caduceus 12 (1), pp. 7-24.

Miller, R.L. (1991) Palaeoepidemiology, literacy, and medical tradition among necropolis workmen in New Kingdom Egypt, *Medical History* 35 (1), pp. 1-24.

SIMILARITY OF FRACTURE TREATMENT OF WORKERS AND HIGH OFFICIALS OF THE PYRAMID BUILDERS

F. Hussien, R. El Banna, W. Kandeel and A. Sarry El Din

Department of Biological Anthropology. National Research Centre, Cairo

Abstract: *The present work focuses on the evidence of treatment for fractures and amputation in skeletal remains of the pyramid builders from Old Kingdom Giza. The analysis takes into consideration the social class of individuals to examine whether treatment was available for everybody or to only the élite.*

The material consists of 271 skeletons from workers and high officials Skeletons were examined macroscopically and radiologically for evidence of the treatment of fractures and amputation. The incidence of fractures was 43.75% and 26.41% in male and female workers respectively. It was only 20.73% and 16.66% in male and female high officials respectively. The most affected bone was the right ulna. All healed fractures were realigned and two cases of amputation showed healing. Healed fractures and amputation indicate medical intervention. There was no difference between the lines of treatments in both groups.

Key words: Old Kingdom, pyramid builders, treatment, fracture.

Introduction

Fractures can be defined as the result of any event which leads to a complete or partial discontinuity of bone (Aufderheide and Rodriguez-Martin 1998). Studying these lesions provides important information about an ancient population's practices when dealing with war, interpersonal violence and other aspects of daily life (Ortner and Putscher 1985; Filer 1992). As early as the 17th century BC bone injuries were well described in the Edwin Smith Papyrus (Stiefel et al. 2006). It is useful to look at trauma in the broader context of human behaviour, such as circumstances that produce trauma, the effects on the individuals and populations and medical efforts to heal the results of traumatic stress (Merbs 1989). Of considerable anthropological interest is the evidence provided by massive healed fractures (Aufderheide and Rodriguez -Martin 1998).

Sarry El Din (2003) studied the evidence for healed fractures of the skull and appendicular skeleton in Old Kingdom ancient Egyptians from Giza. The Giza material not only belongs to a very important period, the period of the Pyramid Builders (4th to 6th Dynasty), but also involves two well documented social classes from the same population (the workers and high officials) (Hawass 1996). The incidence of fractures in male workers was highest (43.75%); it was 20.73% in high official males, 26.41% in female workers and 16.66% in female high officials.

The aim of this study is to compare the treatment of fractures in the two social classes from Old Kingdom Giza - the workers and the high officials.

Material and Methods

The material of this study consists of 271 skeletons. It was divided into two main groups: the worker individuals consisting of 117 individuals (64 males and 53 females) which were excavated by the Egyptian Antiquities Organization (E.A.O.) under the direction of Dr Zahi Hawass (1989-1995), from the south east part of Giza plateau, and the high officials (83 males and 72 females) excavated from the western cemetery of the Giza plateau. Parts of this material were excavated by the Hearst Expedition (1941-1945) and the others were excavated by the E.A.O. also directed by Dr. Zahi Hawass (1989-1995). Sexing of the individuals was determined using descriptive measures of the skull and the pelvis (Ubelaker 1978; Stewart 1979). Aging was estimated using macroscopic methods to examine the pubic symphysis and the auricular surface metamorphoses (Miendle et al. 1985; Lovejoy et al. 1985). Macroscopic examinations were conducted to seek evidence of fracture bone injuries. Radiological assessment by antero-posterior and lateral views used Agfa films and Shimadzu Corporation-MD 100P- 11PW X-ray apparatus. The percentage of affected long bones was calculated as the number of affected bones compared to the number of complete bones present.

Results

Table 1 shows the percentage of affected bones for both groups in both sexes. There is a significant difference between the numbers of bones affected in the two male groups, these being higher in the workers. Moreover, a significant difference according to sex can be noticed between workers, while in the high officials there is no significant difference between the two sexes. It can be noticed that among the male workers the most commonly affected area is the ribs, followed by the ulna which is the most commonly affected bone in all groups.

Bone	M.W.	F.W.	M.H.O.	F. H.O.
Skull	6/64(9.37)	3/53(5.66)	2/82(2.43)	0
Clavicle	3/89(3.37)	0	1/125(0.80)	0
Humerus	0	0	0	0
Radius	4/98(4.08)	3/88(3.40)	1/115(0.86)	2/80(2.5)
Ulna	11/96(11.45)	6/83(7.22)	7/122(5.73)	6/88(6.81)
Femur	1/96(1.04)	0	1/124(0.80)	0
Tibia	0	0	0	0
Fibula	3/64(4.68)	1/80(1.25)	1/57(1.75)	0
Ribs	9/61(14.06)	2/53(3.77)	1/82(1.21)	0
Metacarpals	2/64(3.11)	1/53(1.88)	2/82(2.43)	1/72(1.38)
Metatarsal	3/64(4.11)	0	0	0
Phalanges	1/64(1.56)	0	1/82(1.21)	2/72(2.77)

Table 1: Fracture Incidence by Element Bone
M.W.: Male Workers; F.W.: Female Workers; M.H.O.: Male High Official; F. H.O.: Female High Official

Figures 1 and 2 represent the percentage of well-aligned healed fractures which is 90% in workers and 88.7% in high official groups.

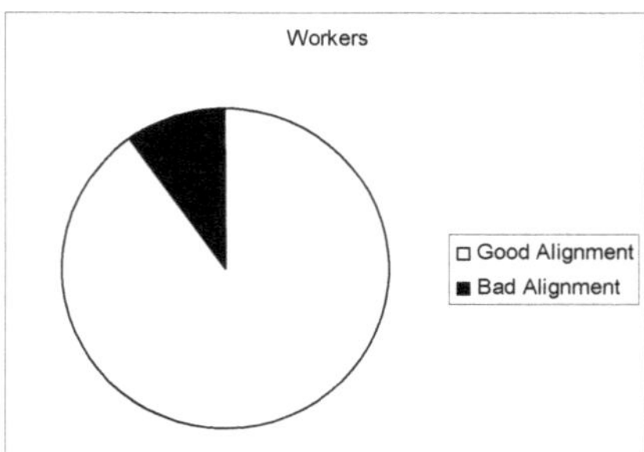

Figure 1: The percentage of good aligned healed fractures in the worker group

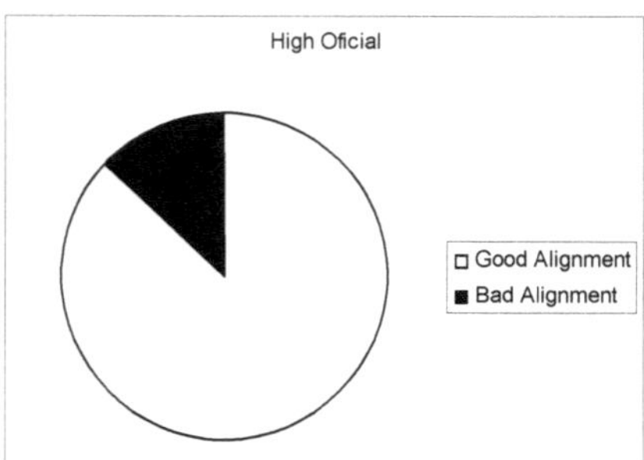

Figure 2: The percentage of good aligned healed fractures in the high officials group

Study of the archaeological data in association with the palaeopathological evidence is essential for understanding the treatment and healing of fractures. A fracture, which is a break in the structure of a bone, can occur in any bone in the skeleton. Environment and hygiene will affect how well and how quickly a fracture heals. The study of trauma and treatment in antiquity has, by necessity, generated many avenues of research to follow. One must consult many sources of evidence to gain an accurate picture of how well cranial and postcranial fractures were treated and how well they healed (Roberts 1991).

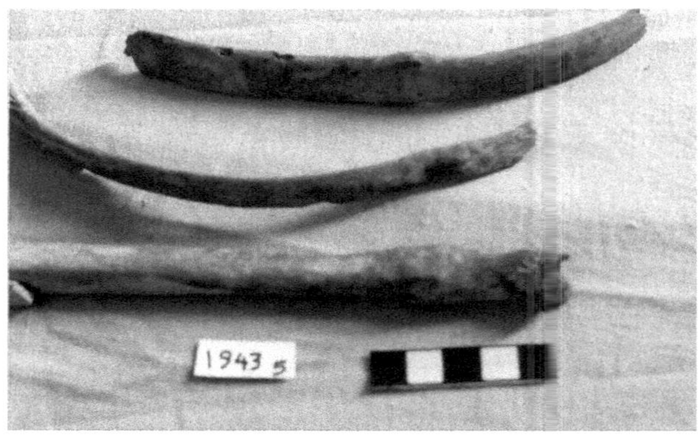

Figure 3: Good aligned healed fractured ulnae from a worker

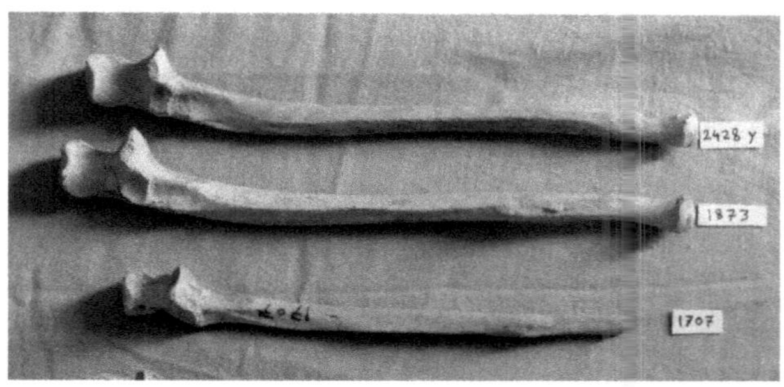

Figure 4: Good aligned healed fractured ulnae from the high officials

Assessment of healing processes enhances our understanding of past ways of life. In conjunction with the gross evaluation, X-rays were used to determine the type and degree of healing and differentiate between well and poorly aligned healed bones (Nystrom et al. 2005).

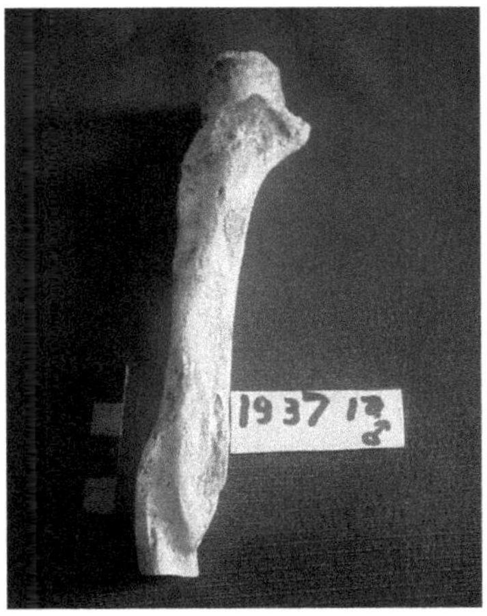

Figure 5: Badly aligned healed fractured ulna from a worker

The sites of fractures evident in the Old Kingdom increase our understanding of ancient ways of life in general and of the nature of social behaviour of the pyramid builders in particular. This research encompasses the skeletal evidence of fractures and splinting, as well as treatment and surgical management. Evidence of healing is the best indicator that a trauma occurred pre-mortem (Aufderheide and Rodriguez-Martin 1998). Similarly, postmortem fractures occurring on dry bone are relatively easy to recognize (Berryman and Haun 1996) because bone needs at least 2 weeks of survival to show signs of healing (Mann and Murphy 1990). Perimortem fractures are very difficult to interpret, but careful excavation and recording of the exact position of every bone fragment can clarify the issue in many cases (Duday 1987; Duday et al. 1990; Roksandic 2002).

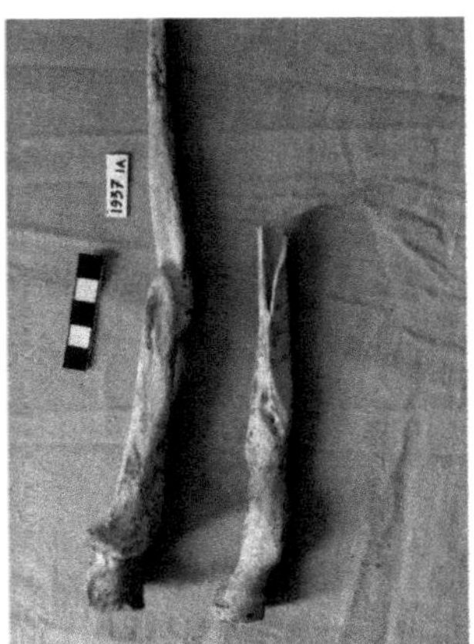

Figure 6: Badly aligned healed fractured ulna from a high official

When a modern fracture has been diagnosed, splinting is the initial treatment for most limb fractures. Padded pieces of plaster or fibre glass are placed over the injured limb and wrapped with gauze and an elastic wrap to immobilize the break. In ancient times strips of wood, padded with linen were used as splints. The bandage is first dipped in powdered beans or honey and resins that stiffen when dry. The joints above and below the injury are immobilized to prevent movement at the fracture site (Stiell et al. 2001).

The ancient Egyptians reduced fractures by manipulation, either unaided or with the help of pads, cushions etc. with great skill. The Egyptians were one of the first civilisations to have practising physicians. Egyptian doctors knew a lot about the human body for their time. They studied the structure of the brain and knew that the pulse was related to the heart. Egyptians were very interested in surgery and rituals to cure their people; most of their cures came from religious beliefs. Egypt had a professional class of doctors as early as the Old Kingdom (Stiefel et al. 2006). Doctors in ancient Egypt usually went through years of hard training at temple schools, usually in the arts of interrogation, inspection and palpation. They could also cure many illness and set broken bones.

Some of the things that doctors used were knives, drills, swords, forceps, or pincers, censers, hokes, bags tied with string, beaked vessels, vases with burning incense and Horus eyes (Redford 2001). A bone setter is a practitioner of joint manipulation who would also reduce joint dislocations and re-set bone fractures. This form of treatment has documented use as far back as Hippocrates, the ancient Egyptians and Asian cultures and was carried out through the ages by families of bone setters. For many years, this type of training was normal practice in these families and communities, being passed on from generation to generation (Aries et al. 2007). Mummified bodies, wall paintings and papyri have shown some of the orthopaedic practices of that time (Redford 2001).

In this study, the skeletons show simple and multiple fractures, mostly at the ulna and radius (forearm bones) and of the fibula (leg). Most of those fractures show signs of complete healing with good alignment, indicating that they had been set correctly with a splint. Although Aufderheide and Rodriguez-Martin (1998) stated that well-aligned long bone healed fractures in ancient humans are not common, the percentage of well-aligned fractures is higher than those poorly aligned in workers and high officials. In this material no differences between sexes were observed in the management of fractures. Moreover, the percentage of well aligned fractures was 90% in workers and 88.7% in high officials; this indicates a similarity of fracture management in both groups.

The most informative medical text from ancient Egypt is that called the Edwin Smith Surgical Papyrus, named after its modern owner. The document describes 48 cases of injury to the face, head, neck and upper spine, all of which were free from any magic or necromancy. In each case, a prognosis is given and if this is favourable, suitable treatment is recommended (Stiefel et al. 2006).

The site of the fracture may provide a clue as to how the injury was caused (Roberts 1991). Injuries to the head are particularly interesting as, whilst they may be accidentally caused, they are often the result of intentional violence. Head injuries in the present study tended to be sustained more in men than in women, as men were engaged in the manual work and military action that could lead to such injuries.

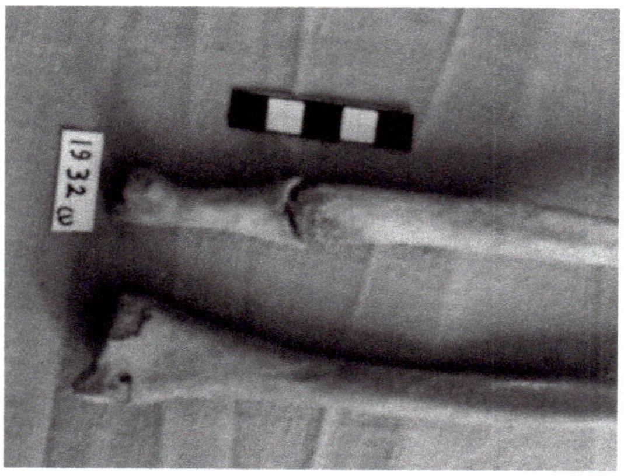

Figure 7: A case of non union in the distal third of the shaft of the ulna in a female worker

Long bone injuries are frequently seen in ancient Egyptian bodies and are more likely to be the result of an accident. Injuries to the femur occurred quite commonly, whilst there is no evidence of tibia fractures which are considered to be caused by going barefoot, especially among agricultural workers (Filer 2002). Fractures of the arms are interesting, as they may be the result of an accidental fall or, as has been suggested for some Nubian injuries, may be the result of using the arms defensively to ward off violent blows to the head. Here the episodes of violent interactions were few and without evidence of a specific temporal pattern. They probably represent sporadic episodes of interpersonal conflict that do not support the notion of endemic warfare (Roksandic et al. 2006).

In contrast, Rose (2006) attributed fractures of the elbow region to accidents. The factors that produce non-union remain somewhat obscure. Repeated disruption of callus results in increased hyline cartilage formation instead of mineralizable osteoid normally expected in callus. This may be a response to reduced blood supply caused by breakage of the developing vessels during movement of the broken ends (El Din 2003). A case of non-union in the distal third of the shaft of the ulna in a female worker aged 30-40 years old was observed. The radius was intact; this makes us think that there was no disruption of the function in the arm. Clinical data suggests that fractures of the radius and ulna are extremely common in modern human populations. Accurate reduction of these fractures is functionally vital; even slight displacement during healing may disturb the relationship between radius and ulna and impair rotation of the forearm. Delayed or non-union of these long bones is also common, especially at the junction of the mid and distal thirds of the ulna shaft. (Grauer and Roberts 1996; Jurmain 1991). In this study, poorly aligned ulnae are 90% (4/5) of all poorly aligned bones.

Another example of similar treatment applied to both social classes is amputation. Two cases of amputation were observed: one of the left leg of a male high official aged (60+years old) and the second of the right arm of a male worker aged (45-50 years old). The sites show successful healing indicating appropriate and similar management in the two classes. Reliefs in the private tombs of the reigns of Khufu and Menkaure show that the builders of their pyramids named themselves the friends of the pharaoh (Hawass 2006).

Conclusion

Similarity of injury management is shown in both high officials and workers which indicates that good medical care was introduced equally to different social classes with no difference between sexes.

References

Aries, M.J., Joosten, H., Wegdam, H.H. and Van der Geet, S. (2007) Fracture treatment by bonesetters in Central Ghana: Patients explain their choices and experiences. *Top Med Int health* 12 (4), pp. 564-74

Aufderheide, A. C. and Rodriguez-Martin, C. (1998) *The Cambridge Encyclopedia of Human Paleopathology.* Cambridge University Press.

Berryman, H. and Haun, S. (1996) Applying forensic technique to interpret cranial fracture patterns in an archaeological specimen. *International Journal of Osteoarchaeology* 6, pp. 2-9.

Duday, H. (1987) Contribution des observations ostéologiques à la chronologie interne des sepultures collectives. In Duday, H. and Masset, C. (eds) *Anthropologie physique et archéologie.* C.N.R.S., pp. 51-61.

Duday, H., Courtaud, P., Crubezy, E., Sellier, P. and Tillier, A-M. (1990) L'anthropologie de 'terrain': reconnaissance et intérpretation des gestes funeraires. *Bull Soc Anthropol* 2, pp. 26-49.

Filer, J.M. (1992) Head injuries in Egypt and Nubia: a comparison of skulls from Giza and Kerma. *Journal of Egyptian Archaeology* 78, pp. 281-5.

Filer, J.M. (2002) *Health hazards and cures in Ancient Egypt.* (Online). Available at: http://www.bbc.co.uk/history/egyptians/health_04.shtml [Accessed 25 November 2008].

Grauer, A.L. and Robert, C.A. (1996) Paleoepidemiology, healing and possible treatment of trauma in the Medieval Cemetery population of St.Helen-on- the-Walls, York, England. *American Journal of Physical Anthropology* 100, pp. 531-44.

Hawass, Z. (1996) The workmen's community at Giza. In *Haus Und Plast in Alten Ägypten.* Wien, pp. 53-67.

Hawass, Z. (2006) *Mountain of the Pharaohs: the Untold story of the pyramid builders.* The American University Press in Cairo.

Jurmain, R.D. (1991) Paleoepidemiology of trauma in a prehistoric central California population. In Ortner D.J. and Aufderheide A.C. (eds) *Human Paleopathology: Current Syntheses and Future Options*, pp. 241-24.

Lovejoy, C.O., Meindle, R.S., Pryzbeck, T.R. and Mensforth, R.P. (1985) Chronological metamorphosis of the auricular surface of the ilium: A new method for the determination of adult skeletal age at death. *American Journal of Physical Anthropology* 79, pp. 117-120.

Mann, R. and Murphy, S.P. (1990) *Regional atlas of bone disease.* C.C.Thomas.

Merbs, C.F. (1989) Trauma. In Iscan, M.Y. and Kennedy, K.A.R. (eds) *Reconstruction of Life from the Skeleton.* A.R. Liss, pp. 161-89.

Miendl, R.S., Lovejoy, C.O., Mensforth, R.P. and Walker, R.A. (1985) A revised method of age determination using the os pubis with a review and tests of accuracy of other current methods of pubic symphyseal aging. *American Journal of Physical Annthropology* 68, pp. 29-45.

Nystrom, K.C., Buikstra, J.E. and Braunstein, E.M. (2005) Radiographic evaluation of two early classic élites from Copan, Honduras. *International Journal of Osteoarchaeology* 15, pp. 196-207.

Ortner, D.J. and Putscher, W., 1985 *Identification of Paleopathological Conditions in Human Skeletal Remains.* Smithsonian Institution Press.

Redford, D.B. (2001) *The Oxford Encyclopedia of Ancient Egypt.* The American University Press in Cairo.

Roberts, C. (1991) Trauma and treatment in the British Isles in the historic period: A Design for multidisciplinary research. In Ortner D.J. and Aufderheide A.C. (eds) *Human Paleopathology: Current Syntheses and Future Options*, pp. 241-24.

Roksandic, M. and Arbeev, K. (2002) *Organic method dealing with really poor preservation.* Paper presented at the second workshop in paleodemography, June 5-8 2002. Max Plank Institute for Demographic Research, Rostock, Germany.

Roksandic, M., Marija D., Zoran, R.C. and Kimberly, S. (2006) Interpersonal Violence at Lepenski Vir Mesolithic /Neolithic complex of the iron gates gorge (Serbia-Romania). *American Journal of Physical Anthropology* 129, pp. 339-348.

Rose, C.J. (2006) *Paleopathology of the commoners at Tell Amarna, Egypt, Akhenaton's capital city.* Mem inst Oswaldo Cruz, Rio de Janeiro, 101 (Suppl.II), pp. 73-6.

Sarry El Din, A.M. (2003) Bone Fractures in ancient Egyptians from Giza Old Kingdom, Egypt. *Med. J. NRC* 2 (2), pp. 1-13

Stewart T.D. (1979) *Essentials of Forensic Anthropology.* Charles C. Thomas.

Stiefel, M., Shaner, A. and Schaefer, S. (2006) The Edwin Smith papyrus. The birth of analytical thinking in medicine and otolaryngology. *Larynoscope* 116 (2), pp. 182-188.

Stiell, I. G. et al. (2001) The Canadian CT head rule for patients with minor head injury. *The Lancet* 5 (I) 357, pp. 1391-6.

Ubelaker, D.H. (1978) *Human Skeletal Remains.* Aldine Publishing Company.

A STUDY OF *PUNICA GRANATUM* L. (POMEGRANATES)

S.W.Y. Lee

KNH Centre for Biomedical Egyptology, The University of Manchester, UK

Abstract: *Punica granatum L. (Pomegranate) is a fruit that has been well-known for millennia and has been used in ancient remedies. It belongs in the Lythraceae family and is a shrub that originated from the Middle East. Many different religions feature pomegranates, including Judaism, Zoroastrianism, Hinduism, Buddhism, Christianity and Islam. It is also used in different coats of arms and is mentioned in important literature. Pomegranate is part of remedies in the medical papyri of ancient Egypt and can be seen on walls of temples and tombs. Modern scientific analyses have uncovered many medicinal properties of different parts of pomegranate, as well as its side effects and interaction with other medication. Pomegranate is also used in beauty products. Phylogenetic study shows that the rbcL region of the gene of the fruit from different countries is the same.*

Key words: Punica granatum, pomegranate, antioxidant, pelletierine, rbcL, phylogeny

Introduction

Pomegranate is a fruit that originated from the Middle East and the Mediterranean (Bajaj 1991, 44) and has been used in remedies to cure illnesses for thousands of years (Pliny The Elder 1991, 237). It is for this reason that it has been regarded as a 'super-fruit'. Recent studies into pomegranate have shown that it has many medicinal properties (Kim et al. 2002, 204; Seeram et al. 2006).

History and Origin

Natural resources have been used for medical purposes since prehistoric times (Anesini and Perez 1993, 119). Ancient Egyptian medical papyri show how different resources were used to treat illness. Organic materials were buried with the dead to prepare them for the journey to the after-life. There are references to the use of pomegranates as an ingredient in medical papyri and in tombs; in some cases the fruit itself was buried with the deceased. Images of pomegranates have also been found on walls of temples (Krymow 2002, 128).

Pomegranates have been found together with medicinal herbs in the ancient sacred animal necropolis at Saqqara (Manniche 1989, 20). This strongly suggests that it was used as a medicinal plant.

Punica is the genus dedicated to pomegranates. It has two species: *Punica granatum* and *Punica protopunica*. The former has an uncertain native origin; the latter is endemic to the island of Socotra.

There are many claims regarding the origin of the *granatum* species. During ancient times, the boundaries of countries were ambiguous. Whilst many nationalities may claim that pomegranates came from their country, they might all be referring to the same region. It must have been an area with a hot, dry and sunny climate, most suitable for the cultivation of pomegranates. Pomegranate has always been an important part of the Middle Eastern diet, and the Middle East is also the geographical origin of three major religions: Christianity, Judaism and Islam, all of which refer to this fruit, strengthening the belief that the pomegranate did originate from this area.

Symbolism

The pomegranate is considered a sacred symbol in many of the world's major religions. It is frequently associated with maidens and maiden goddesses (Agha-Jaffar 2002, 48), because the fruit's 'bloodiness' symbolises the physiology of an underworld goddess. Ancient civilisations believed that pomegranates symbolised birth after death, as the fruit 'bleeds', and the seeds may represent children (Goldstein 2007). It is often found in tombs and on Ancient Egyptian wall paintings. It can have both positive and negative connotations; for example, within chthonic gods, particularly Earth-mothers, common representations include Side (from ancient Greek) and Hariti (from Buddhism); the sources of life and death, of health and illness, and of fertility and infertility.

Medical Applications

References to the pomegranate have been found in two different medical papyri (Ebers and Berlin) and in both the fruit was used as the cure for round worms. The active ingredient in the skin, pelletierine, is a potent medicine against worms. It paralyses the worm before the worm is passed out in the faeces (Campbell 2007).

Pomegranate is abundant in vitamins A, C, E and iron. It is also rich in folic acid, antioxidants, and polyphenols, particularly the polyphenols punicalagins which have been shown to be the responsible antioxidants in pomegranate juice for combating free radicals (Murthy et al. 2002; Schubert et al. 1999).

Pomegranate juice has been found to be effective in reducing systolic blood pressure and artherosclerosis and therefore the risk of cardiovascular diseases (Longtin 2003). Pomegranate juice is effective against prostate cancer (Malik et al. 2005), breast cancer (Kim et al. 2002), and osteoarthritis (Horowitz 2006; Minsky 2006). Different extracts are also anti-microbial (Machado et al.

2002), anti-parasitic, anti-viral and anti-cancer (Kim et al. 2002; Kawaii and Lansky 2004). The fermented juice is potently antioxidant and oil polyphenols inhibit eicosanoid enzymes cyclooxygenase and lipoxygenase (Murthy et al. 2002) and that can slow down the ageing process (Negi et al. 2003). An extract of the flowers lowers blood sugar in rodents (Jafri et al. 2000). The fresh juice inhibits low density lipoprotein oxidation and atheromatous plaque formation in rodents and humans (Kim et al. 2002).

Side effects of the fruit or its interactions with common medications are not widely known by the public (Hidaka et al. 2005, Sorokin et al. 2006). Pomegranate products are capable of inhibiting enzymes responsible for drug metabolism and/or increasing drug intake into the circulation if used with medication. The pelletierine tannate found in the root of pomegranates might be a good remedy for tapeworms. High doses, however, can paralyse the lungs (Campbell 2007; Cheeke 1989, 89).

Research has shown that methanol is best for extracting the active ingredient from the plant. Ancient Egyptians used beer or water for extraction (Campbell 2007). The ethanol in beer is not as potent in extraction as methanol is. However, the former is capable of extracting a therapeutic amount of pelletierine and the latter is poisonous and therefore unsuitable for consumption (Singh et al. 2002).

Pomegranate Phylogeny

Archaeological findings of ancient seeds tell us much about ancient civilisations and, in particular, about the stages through which the domestication of crop plants took place.

The gene chosen for phylogenetic study was the chloroplast gene, ribulose-1,5-bisphosphate carboxylase (*rbcL*). It is the gene responsible for encoding the large subunit of the *rbcL* protein. It has proved to be phylogenetically informative and has emerged as the preferred gene for examining higher-level phylogenetic relationships (Conti et al. 1993; Gustafsson et al. 1996; Bousquet et al. 1992; Soltis et al. 1990; Bradley et al. 2007; Huang and Shi 2002; La Du et al. 2002; Wikstrom and Kenrick 2000).

The author attempted DNA extraction with seeds and rind. A polymerase chain reaction was used to isolate and amplify the target region. The lengths of primers were varied from 20 to 28 base-pairs and were selected from different literature (Bradley et al. 2007, 2; Huang and Shi 2002, 220; La Du et al. 2002, 244; Savolainen et al. 2000, 259; Kress et al. 2005, 8370) as well as self-designed using information obtained from Genbank.

Fresh pomegranate samples were bought from local supermarkets and grocers and their origins investigated. They were then put into a 40°C oven for drying for a week. Information about the samples is summarised in Table 1.

Sample	Origin	Part of fruit used	Country of origin	Amount used in extraction (mg)	Year of Harvest
1	Tesco	Seeds	India	70	2008
2	Marks and Spencer's (ready to eat)	Seeds	Various	100	2008
3	Rusholme grocers 1	Rind	India	100	2008
4	Rusholme grocers 2	Rind	India	100	2008
5	Sainsbury's (whole fruit)	Rind	India	100	2008
6	Sainsbury's (ready to eat)	Seeds	Egypt	70	2008
7	Sainsbury's (whole fruit)	Seeds	India	60	2008
8	Rusholme grocers 2	Seeds	India	60	2008
9	Rusholme grocers 1	Seeds	India	70	2008
10	Leverhulme Collection 1	Seeds	South Sinai	50	2007
11	Leverhulme collection 2	Seeds	South Sinai	80	2007
12	Leverhulme collection 3	Seeds	Unknown	40	2005

Table 1: Sample number, the parts of the fruit used, the country origin and the amount used. Unless otherwise stated, the whole fruit was obtained. 2 and 5 - it is unknown how the fruit was treated after the removal of peripulp. 10 - obtained from a wild tree on desert flood plain in S. Sinai. The fruit was opened at harvest and the pulp was eaten by wasps, only 3 seeds were available. 11 – obtained from the same tree as 10, whole fruit was obtained. 12 – small fruit with thick pericarp from a 450yr old tree in Chelsea Physic Garden, London. No special storage conditions were arranged. 10, 11 and 12 were stored in plastic bags in a store cupboard after harvest.

DNA was successfully extracted and amplified from all of the seeds apart from the oldest sample (Figure 1).

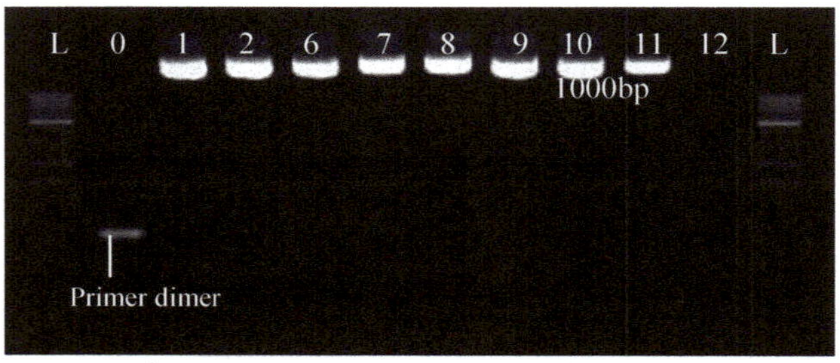

Figure 1: DNA gel of different samples of PCR reaction, where 1000bp of the rbcL gene was isolated. Lane L represents the DNA ladder (MiniSizer 50bp), ranging from 25 to 650bp; and Lane 0 represents the negative control, where water was used instead of DNA template. DNA is not present in Lane 12. The other numbers correspond to the sample number. A minute amount of primer dimers were formed. The fragments of amplified DNA are 1000bp.

This investigation concluded that all the Indian samples have the same genetic makeup in the *rbcL* region as the South Sinai samples. The quality of 'one year old' DNA (sample 10 and 11) did not seem to differ from 'fresh' DNA. However, no DNA was amplified from the oldest sample (12).

Conclusion

This study investigated the history and origin, medical applications and the phylogeny of different pomegranates. Further studies should be constructed to investigate why DNA was not obtained from the '3 year old seeds' as the nature of seeds is to protect their host DNA and to pass on their genetic information when the plants are under stress. Genetic material from archaeological samples should also be compared and related to its phenotypic differences, together with the climatic/environmental changes through the centuries.

Acknowledgements

The author would like to thank Dr. Angélique Corthals for advice and assistance in the laboratory; Dr. Jacqueline Campbell for sourcing research materials and advice on Egyptian medicine; Dr. Leander Wolstenholme for the different materials available at the University of Manchester Museum for research.

Bibliography

Agha-Jaffar, T. (2002) *Demeter and Persephone: Lessons from a Myth.* McFarland and Co.

Bajaj, Y.P.S. (1991) *Tree:III (Biotechnology in Agriculture and Forestry).* Springer-Verlag.

Anesini, C. and Perez, C. (1993) 'Screening of plants used in Argentine folk medicine for antimicrobial activity'. *Journal of Ethnopharmacology* 39, pp. 119-128.

Bousquet, J., Strauss, S.H., Doerksen, A.H. and Price, R.A. (1992). Extensive variation in evolutionary rate of rbcL gene sequences among seed plants. *Proceedings of the National Academy of Sciences* 89, pp. 7844-7848.

Bradley, B.J., Stiller, M., Doran-Sheehy, D.M., Harris, T., Chapman, C.A., Vigilant, L. and Poinar, H. (2007). Plant DNA sequences from feces: Potential means for assessing diets of wild primates. *American Journal of Primatology* 69, pp. 1-7.

Campbell, J. (2007) *Lecture in MSc Biomedical and Forensic Studies in Egyptology.* The University of Manchester.

Cheeke, P.R. (1989) *Toxicants of Plant Origin: Alkaloids. Volume I.* CRC Press.

Conti, E., Fischbach, A. and Sytsma, K.J. (1993) Tribal relationships in Onagraceae: Implications from rbcL sequence data. *Annals of the Missouri Botanical Garden.* 80 (3), pp. 672-685.

Goldstein, A. (2007) *Pomegranates and the New School Years.* [Online]. Available from: http://www.npls.eclipse.co.uk/Sermons/New/Pomegranates%20and%20New%20School%20Years.html [Accessed 24 August 2008] .

Gustafsson, M.H.G., Backlund, A. and Bremer, B. (1996). Phylogeny of the Asterales sensu lato based on rbc sequences with particular reference to the Goodeniaceae. *Plant Systematics and Evolution* 199, pp. 217-242.

Hidaka, M., Okumura, M., Fujita, K., Ogikubo, T., Yamasaki, K., Iwakiri, T., Setoguchi, N. and Arimori, K. (2005). Effects of Pomegranate juice on human cytochrome P450 3A (CYP3A) and carbamazepine pharmacokinetics in rats. *Drug Metabolism and Deposition* 33 (5), pp. 644-648.

Horowitz, S. (2006). The Power of Pomegranate: Biblical Fruit with Medicinal Properties. *Alternative and Complementary Therapies* 12 (3), pp. 121-126.

Huang, Y. and Shi, S. (2002). Phylogenetics of Lythraceae Sensu Lato: A preliminary analysis based on chloroplast rbcL gene, psaA-ycf3 spacer, and nuclear RDNAinternal transcribed spacer (ITS) sequences. *International Journal of Plant Sciences.* 163 (2), pp. 215-225.

Jafri, M.A., Aslam, M., Javed, K. and Singh, S. (2000) Effect of Punica granatum Linn. (flowers) on blood glucose level in normal and alloxan-induced diabetic rats. *Journal of Ethnopharmacology* 70, pp. 309-314.

Kawaii, S. and Lansky, E.P. (2004) Differentiation-promoting activity of pomegranate (*Punica granatum*) fruit extracts in HL-60 promyelocytic leukemia cells. *Journal of Medicinal Food.* 7 (1), pp. 13-18.

Kim, N.D., Mehta, R., Yu, W., Neeman, I., Livney, T., Amichay, A. Poirier, D., Nicholls, P., Kirby, A., Jiang, W., Mansel, R., Ramachandran, C., Rabi, T., Kaplan, B. and Lansky, E. (2002) Chemopreventive and adjuvant therapeutic potential of pomegranate (*Punica granatum*) for human breast cancer. *Breast Cancer and Treatment* 71, pp. 203-217.

Kress, W.J., Wurdack, K.J., Zimmer, E.A., Weigt, L.A. and Janzen, D.H. (2005). Use of DNA barcodes to identify flowering plants. *Proceedings of the National Academy of Sciences* 102 (23), pp. 8369-8374.

Krymow, V. (2002) *Healing Plants of the Bible: History, Lore and Meditations.* Wild Goose Publications.

La Du, J., Erdner, D., Dyhrman, S. and Andeson, D. (2002). Molecular approaches to understanding population dynamics of the toxic Dinoflagellate Alexandrium fundyense. *Biological Bulletin* 203, pp. 244-245.

Longtin, R. (2003) The Pomegranate: Nature's Power Fruit? *Journal of the National Cancer Institute* 95 (5), pp. 346-348.

Machado, T.B., Leal, I.C.R., Amaral, A.C.F., dos-Santos, K.R.N., da-Silva, M.G. and Kuster, R.M. (2002) Antimicrobial ellagitannin of Punica granatum fruits. *Journal of the Brazilian Chemical Society* 13 (5), pp. 606-610.

Malik, A., Afaq, F., Sarfaraz, S., Adhami, V.M., Syed, D.N. and Mukhtar, H. (2005) Pomegranate Fruit juice for Chemoprevention and Chemotherapy of Prostate Cancer. *Proceedings of the National Academy of Sciences* 102 (41), pp. 14813-14818.

Manniche, L (1989) *An Ancient Egyptian Herbal.* British Museum Press.

Minsky, B.C. (2006) *Super Foods*. [Online]. Available from:
http://www.nutritionalconcepts.com/Articles/Super%20Foods%204-24-06.pdf
[Accessed 24 August 2008].

Murthy, K.N.C., Jayaprakasha, G.K. and Singh, R.P. (2002). Studies on antioxidant activity of Pomegranate (*Punica granatum*) peel extract using in vivo models. *Journal of Agricultural and Food Chemistry* 50, pp. 4791-4795.

Negi, P.S., Jayaprakasha, G.K. and Jena, B.S. (2003) Antioxidant and antimutagenic activities of pomegranate peel extracts *Food Chemistry* 80 (3), pp. 393-397.

Pliny The Elder (1991) *Natural History: A selection.* Translated by Healy, J. F. Penguin Books Ltd.

Savolainen, V., Fay, M.F., Albach, D.C., Backlund, A., van-der-Bank, M., Cameron, K.M., Johnson, S.A., Lleda, M.D., Pintaud, J., Powell, M., Sheahan, M.C., Soltis, D.E., Soltis, P.S., Weston, P., Whitten, W.M., Wurdack, K.J. and Chase, M.W. (2000). Phylogeny of the Eudicots: a nearly complete familial analysis based on rbcL. *Kew Bulletin* 55 (2), pp. 257-309.

Schubert, S.Y., Lansky, E.P. and Neeman, I. (1999) Antioxidant and Eisosanoid enzyme inhibition properties of pomegranate seed oil and fermented juice flavonoids. *Journal of Ethnopharmacology* 66, pp. 11-17.

Seeram, N.P., Schulman, R.N. and Heber, D. (2006) *Pomegranates: Ancient Roots to Modern Medicine.* CRC Press.

Singh, R.P., Murthy, K.N.C. and Jayaprakasha, G.K. (2002). Studies on the antioxidant activity of pomegranate (*Punica granatum*) peel and seed extracts using in vitro models. *Journal of Agricultural Food Chemistry* 50, pp. 81-86.

Soltis, D.E., Soltis, P.S., Clegg, M.T. and Durbin, M. (1990). rbcL seuence divergence and phylogenetic relationships in Saxifragacea Sensu Lato. *Proceedings of the National Academy of Sciences* 87 (12), pp. 4640-4644.

Sorokin, A.V., Duncan, B., Panetta, R. and Thompson, P.D. (2006). Rhabdomyolysis associated with Pomegranate juice consumption. *The American Journal of Cardiology* 98 (5), pp. 705-706.

Wikstrom, N. and Kenrick, P. (2000). Relationships of Lycopodium and Lycopodiella based on combined plastid rbcL gene and trnL intron sequence data. *Systematic Botany* 25 (3), pp. 495-510.

THE MAN WHO KNOWS BULLS – VETERINARY PRACTICE IN ANCIENT EGYPT

C. Lord

KNH Centre for Biomedical Egyptology, The University of Manchester, UK

Abstract: *The advancement of knowledge regarding human disease in ancient Egypt, and the treatment thereof, is evident from the numerous current studies on this subject. What has not been explored is the health and disease of the animals from this time and in turn, the possibility of veterinary intervention. This field of veterinary medicine especially is a little researched area of the ancient Egyptian medical knowledge. The reasons for this are easy to understand as the only compelling evidence for the concept comes from the Veterinary Papyrus of Kahun, which has largely been ignored by Egyptologists, probably due to the extreme fragmentation of the original document. All that remains comprehensible is one main segment outlining three treatments for ailing bovines.*

Supporting the Veterinary Papyrus is such circumstantial evidence as inscriptions that hint at a connection between the wab priests of Sekhmet with some area of animal care as well as the depictions and literature that attest to the ancient Egyptians' well developed knowledge of animal husbandry. There can be no doubt that animals were of paramount importance to the ancient Egyptian people in both the secular and sacred arena and a study into their care, health and disease, with the evidence available, can only advance the overall knowledge of ancient Egyptian society. As with many aspects of ancient Egyptian scholarship, there are no definite answers available; however, a look at the evidence collectively supports the hypothesis that veterinary intervention did exist in Pharaonic Egypt, while the exact form and how widespread this type of intervention was, remains, for now, unknown.

Key words: Egyptian art, animal husbandry, animal disease, veterinary intervention, Veterinary Papyrus.

Animals in Ancient Egypt

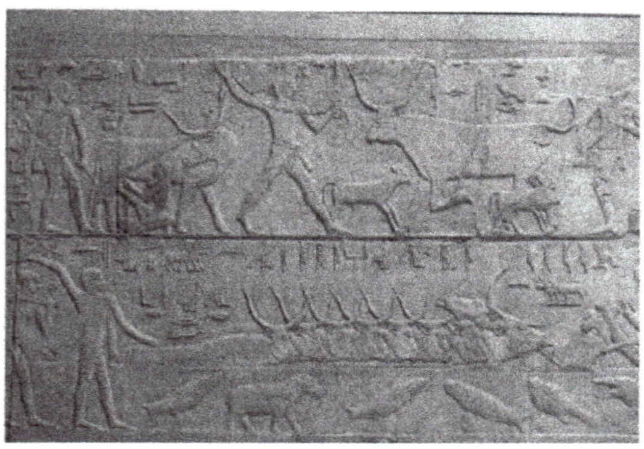

Figure 1: Cattle fording river (Tomb of Kagemni, Dynasty 6) – (Donovan and McCorquodale, 2004: plate 3.2)

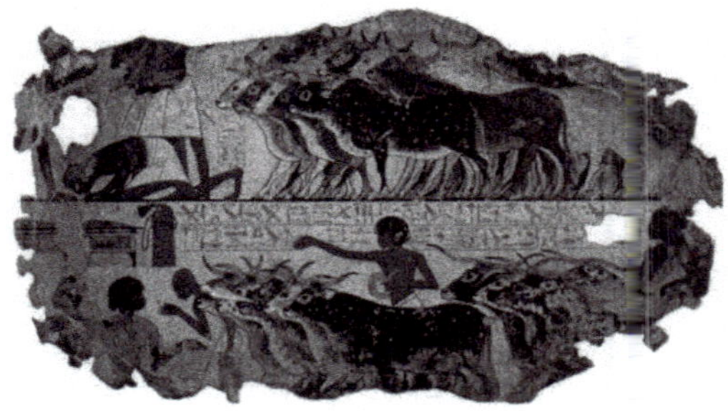

Figure 2: Cattle counting in the tomb of Nebamun Dynasty 18 (Parkinson 2008, 93)

Looking at the images above, it is easy to see the skill of the ancient Egyptian artists who decorated the tomb walls of the nobles and officials of the country. These wall paintings reflect the everyday life of the people, the natural elements that surrounded them, their religion and the influence of king and state (Donovan and McCorquodale 2004, 1). The rich relationship between the animal kingdom and the ancient Egyptian people can be seen throughout these artistic representations; animals were valued, interacted with and sometimes feared. The depiction of animals in these tomb scenes occurs in various different themes such as agricultural, butchery, offering formulae, branding, and cattle and geese counting for the purpose of calculating tax. The tomb scenes are one source that enables a reconstruction of ancient Egyptian agricultural and pastoral practices and an insight into their knowledge of animal husbandry and the genuine affection that the ancient Egyptians had for many of their animal charges (Scanlan 2004, 85). However, the depiction of sick animals and their care is completely lacking, although it must be kept in mind that it is also extremely rare for depictions of human illness.

Animals had three very important roles in the lives of the ancient Egyptian people. Firstly, the religious relationship; the many gods of Egypt were often depicted in animal form and could have connections to certain individual animals or whole species of animals. Secondly, animals had the practical function of providing meat, milk, bone, horn, skin, hide and/or wool, all necessary for a more comfortable existence. Finally, although it may be a case of superimposing modern sentiment onto an ancient civilisation, it would appear the ancient Egyptians had various species of animals as favoured pets.

The significance of cattle is a wonderful example of the ancient Egyptian culture where the secular and sacred aspects of life were often fundamentally linked. As an agricultural people, the Egyptians understood the value of an animal that could provide meat, milk, fat and horn and be used as a reliable beast of burden for ploughing and therefore, domestic cattle were of paramount economic importance (Houlihan 1996, 10).

Cattle, however, also covered another important aspect of Egyptian life: that of the sacred. The deification of animals in ancient Egypt existed even before the unification of the country around 3100 BC (Shaw and Nicholson 1995, 310). Various animals were worshipped in different nomes and among the most important animal cults were the bull cults. The powerful bull was believed to embody the personality of the king. The bull's characteristics of great strength and virility were seen as necessary qualities for the pharaoh of Egypt (Wilkinson, 2003, 57). These two aspects, the domestic and the sacred, ensured that cattle in ancient Egypt would be of utmost value to king and peasant alike.

Evidence for Animal Husbandry in Ancient Egypt

The majority of cattle were herded and range fed and considerable herds of cattle were attached to temples and personal estates. In the Tomb of Khnumhotep at Beni Hasan, cattle and other animals are shown being fed by hand.

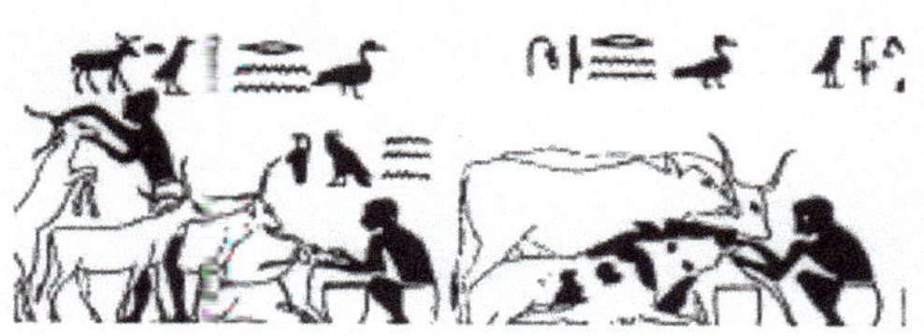

Figure 3: Animals being hand fed (Tomb of Khnumhotep, Middle Kingdom) (Scanlon 2004, 94).

These cattle were often tethered on short ropes so they could not stand and hand fed, resulting in obesity so they would be, as in other ancient cultures, the best specimens for sacrifice and offerings to the deceased or as part of the daily temple ritual offerings (Scanlan, 2004, 86). Specific joints of meat had significance when offered to the gods or the deceased; for example, the foreleg was presented as a symbol of strength and rejuvenation. The majority of slaughtering scenes from tombs concentrate on beef cattle so the prosperous Egyptians could feast on beef forever (Donovan and McCorquodale 2004, 101).

Today, the care of animals, especially cattle and other herd animals, is divided into two areas of responsibility. Firstly, for everyday treatment and care of field animals, experienced herdsmen have responsibility. Only if an animal is very ill, is a 'vet' called in. This concept transfers well to ancient Egypt. In agriculturally based societies, a close association between people and animals can develop and these herdsmen would have known their animals extremely well and, through experience, would be able to deal with many animal husbandry issues. Tomb reliefs give evidence of this with many images depicting herdsmen assisting with cows giving birth, branding of cattle and the force-feeding of animals. There is, however, no evidence of veterinary surgeons caring for these herds of animals. While it is obvious from archaeological remains and tomb reliefs that animals were indispensable for the function of ancient Egyptian agriculture, it is likely that the experienced herdsmen carried out most animal needs. As these herdsmen would have mostly been illiterate, any skills and knowledge would not have been written down in a form such as the Veterinary Papyrus but was passed down orally or learnt by trial and error.

In many scenes involving herdsmen and their charges, the men can be seen making magical gestures of protection toward the animals. Dialogue attached to these scenes includes simple charms aimed at protecting both the animals and the people on the land. There have been suggestions that these herdsmen may have been part-time priests who obtained their knowledge of protection charms from the temple books (Ghalioungui 1983, 13; Schwabe 1978, 160). However, the herdsmen are depicted in such a way that indicates that these men were not of a high enough status to belong to any sector of the priesthood. Like the practical knowledge of animal husbandry, the basic magic involved in the protection spells would have been passed down orally from generation to generation (Pinch 1994; 59).

The second area of animal care in ancient Egypt may have come in the form of veterinary surgeons who would have only been called in to practise if the herdsmen were unable to manage. Ghalioungui (1983, 12) believes that the absence of priestly or medical qualification in scenes of calving and other animal husbandry representations is evidence against a widespread veterinary field. While it may ultimately be true that veterinary procedures were not common practice in ancient Egypt, this particular pictorial absence is not the evidence to prove this assumption. In today's agricultural community cows' calving would be handled by the farmer; only if the cow is in distress or having difficulty is a vet called in to assist. Ancient Egypt had experienced and skilled herdsmen, as evidenced from tomb models, wall paintings and literary texts, and there is no reason to believe they would have required any veterinary assistance in a straightforward calving.

The Veterinary Papyrus of Kahun

In the late 1880s, the renowned archaeologist W. M. Flinders Petrie excavated a necropolis and town site, which he called Kahun, located at the eastern edge of the Fayum (a large fertile depression covering 12,000 sq kms in the Libyan Desert). The Fayum region flourished in the Middle Kingdom when the Egyptian capital was moved to Itjtawy (unlocated but north of Kahun, close to el Lisht). Kahun, in the Middle Kingdom, was originally developed to house the pyramid builders and officials for the royal funerary monuments of Sesostris II (Shaw and Nicholson 2002, 156). Here, Petrie discovered a large number of papyri dating to the late Middle Kingdom, their contents ranging from religious and medical documents to personal communications. One of the more unique discoveries was the Veterinary Papyrus of Kahun, as it is now known. It is the only papyrus that has been found relating to the medical treatment of animals. Even so, Egyptologists have largely ignored it, probably due to the severe fragmentation of the original document. All that remains is a main fragment outlining 3 case studies concerning the treatment of ailing bulls, and some smaller fragments for which their positioning in the overall papyrus is unknown. Griffith (1898, 12), the original translator, believes that the complete papyrus was probably of great length.

The papyrus script is that of cursive hieroglyphs, reading in columns from right to left in the illustration. Interestingly, this form of hieroglyphs is usually reserved for religious documents; of the twelve medical papyri, only one (Ramasseum V) is written in cursive hieroglyphs. The main fragment is 25 inches long and 5 ½ inches wide with 48 columns and 3 horizontal headings (Walker 1964; 199).

Figure 4: The Veterinary Papyrus (Copyright of the Petrie Museum of Egyptian Archaeology, UCL, UC32036).

Of the known medical papyri from ancient Egypt, the Edwin Smith Surgical Papyrus is probably the most comparable to the Veterinary Papyrus of Kahun. Both have a logical approach and, rather than being a collection of remedies, appear to concentrate on case studies. The approach and content of both these papyri testify to their practical use rather than simply as objects of historical curiosity.

The few scholars that have analysed the Veterinary Papyrus (Griffith 1898; Walker 1964; Bardinet 1995; Lord 2005) have had difficulty naming the three diseases described in the case studies, mainly due to the generality of the symptoms, as well as the language challenges.

It can be speculated as to what diseases would have inflicted the animal world of ancient Egypt; the well watered fertile land along the banks of the Nile and its Delta branches attracted a heavy concentration of livestock, which would have rendered it susceptible to re-occurring plagues of environmental origin (e.g. anthrax). Animals brought into Egypt as tribute or from invasion origin could have transmitted respiratory and enteric diseases such as Rinderpest, said to be one of the ten plagues of Egypt of the Bible (Walker 1964, 198; Dunlop and Williams 1996, 73). The high concentration would have also encouraged a high level of parasitic disease and the frequent droughts and sand storms would have, most likely, resulted in an elevated incidence of animal eye disease as it did for humans (Dunlop and Williams 1996, 73).

The first case study has invoked the most wide-ranging diagnoses. It has been suggested that it is a description of the deadly Rinderpest, German meaning 'cattle plague', although the positive outlook for the patient 'you will recognise that he will be well when...' (Walker 1964, 198) is contrary to its extremely high (95-100%) mortality rate in cattle (www.agric.nsw.gov.au/reader/an-health/a0933.htm). An alternate diagnosis of an external infestation of the still prevalent, but much less lethal, screwworm fly has been suggested (Lord 2005, 64).

The second case study has elicited more agreement with the symptoms being synonymous with those of Bovine Malignant Catarrh (BMC) (Walker 1964, 199; Lord 2005, 68; Dunlop and Williams 1996, 68). The bull is suffering the common BMC symptoms of pyrexia, swollen lymph glands in the head and neck, reddened gums and depression.

The third case study appears to concentrate on an eye complaint identifiable with an animal suffering photosensitisation (Lord 2005, 73), a common complaint worldwide still, where skin and eyes become abnormally sensitive to bright sunlight after stock have eaten certain toxic plants: (www.agric.nsw.gov.au/reader/an-health/a0933.htm).

Other Evidence for Veterinary Knowledge in Ancient Egypt

The only firm evidence for veterinary intervention in ancient Egypt is the Veterinary Papyrus of Kahun and this text is unable to assist with any firm identification of the diseases being treated. Everything else regarding the care of sick animals is circumstantial. This includes a hieratic graffito from the Twelfth Dynasty from the alabaster quarries of Hatnub (near Tell el-Amarna).

This graffito contains the biographical detail of two men. The main figure is called Hery-shef-nakht who claims to be chief of the king's physicians and a wab priest of Sekhmet. Next to his graffito, and of a much inferior size, is the information regarding one of Hery-shef-nakht's colleagues, Aha-nakht, wab priest of Sekhmet. Aha-nakht claims to be 'rekh kau' or one who knows oxen (Nunn 2003, 129). Very early in the history of ancient Egypt, the priests of Sekhmet were associated with the medical profession. Sekhmet was the lion-headed goddess who could inflict death and disease. Her priests were charged with the responsibility to intervene in the favour of those whom she punished (Nunn 2003, 101). From the Old Kingdom, three Sekhmet priests are also pictured on tomb walls supervising the sacrificial butchery of offering cattle. One such scene is of Wenen-nefer, in the tomb of Ptahhotep, who was both a wab priest of Sekhmet and an inspector of physicians. Ghalioungui (1983, 13) believes this suggests that the wab priests of Sekhmet were probably the ones charged with veterinary responsibilities

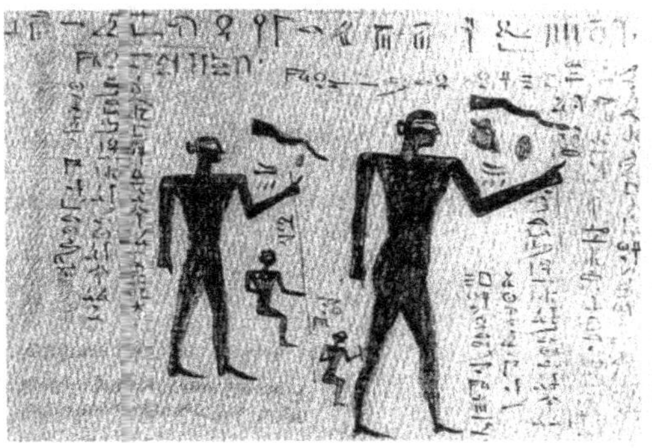

Figure 5 - Hatnub graffito. The smaller of the two main figures, Aha-nakht, claims to be one who knows oxen (Nunn 2003, 129).

Alongside the Hatnub graffito, there is one other inscription that could support the idea of the existence of veterinary surgeons, as well as the suggestion of Ghalioungui that the wab priests were involved in veterinary practice. This comes from the Tomb of Petosiris at Tuna el-Gebel (Ptolemaic Period – 332-30 BC) where there is a text in which Petosiris' daughter says:

> *Your herds are numerous in the stable,*
> *thanks to the science of the priest of*
> *Sekhmet*
>
> (Ghalioungui 1983, 12).

The evidence discussed above should be positioned beside that of the Veterinary Papyrus itself, attestation of animal husbandry practices and the undisputed importance of animals, both sacred and domestic, in the lives of the ancient Egyptians. Only then is a more complete picture of the care of animals during the pharaonic period accessible.

Summary

Although the Veterinary Papyrus of Kahun is the only concrete evidence for veterinary practice in dynastic Egypt, it offers no insight into the diseases that would have plagued the ancient Egyptian farmers and should not be looked at in isolation. Beside this limited proof must be placed all the circumstantial, or suggestive, evidence. This includes all the tomb and temple scenes, literary texts and tomb models showing the rich and compassionate relationship between people and animals. The scenes of daily life show that experienced and skilled herdsmen, with a genuine affection for their charges, existed in ancient Egypt.

There is also evidence from the discovery of the medical papyri which show the scientific knowledge and skill of the ancient Egyptians was capable of assisting many human ailments and therefore, why not animals? Disease was present and debilitating for the ancient Egyptian population, and it can be assumed that animal disease was a problem for the economy and also had ramifications for the health of the human population. Diseases such as bovine tuberculosis and anthrax can be transferred to the human population from both close contact with an infected animal or through drinking the contaminated milk (Mays 2002, 127). The ancient Egyptians were an agricultural people; close contact with animals and a reliance on their products was part of everyday life.

There can be no doubt that animals in ancient Egypt were exceedingly important; they were necessary for survival and also were a component of the sacred world. Bulls and cows were especially significant and the sacred bull cults existed through Egyptian history. These individual animals were worshipped in their own right but also had connections with certain gods and with the pharaoh. The bulls were cared for as befitting their sacred status, given the best food, shelter and attention. Despite the lack of evidence, it is difficult to believe that if one of these precious animals fell ill, it was not given some form of veterinary care from its priestly careers.

The identification of animal disease and the possibility of veterinary care for animal disease in ancient Egypt is yet another fascinating aspect of a sophisticated and intriguing ancient people and worthy of investigation.

References

Bardinet, T. (1995). *Les Papyrus médicaux de l'Égypte pharaonique*. Fayard.

Donovan, L. and McCorquodale, K. (2004). *Egyptian Art – Principles and Themes in Wall Scenes.* MU Press.

Dunlop, R. and Williams, D. (1996). *Veterinary Medicine.* Mosby.

Ghalioungui, P. (1983). *The Physicians of Pharaonic Egypt.* Al-Ahram Center for Scientific Translations.

Griffith, F.L. (1898). *The Hieratic Papyri of Kahun and Gurob*. University College.

Houlihan, P. (1996). *The Animal World of the Pharaohs.* Thames and Hudson.

Lord, C. (2005) *How now sick cow*? Unpublished Masters Dissertation, The University of Manchester.

Mays, S. (2005). Tuberculosis as a zoonotic disease in antiquity. In Davies, J. and Fabis, M. (eds) *Diet and Health in past animal populations.* Oxbow Books.

Moens, M. and Wetterstrom, W. (1988). The agricultural economy of an Old Kingdom town in Egypt's west delta. *Journal of Near Eastern Studies* 47 (3), pp. 159-173.

Nunn, J. (2003 reprint). *Ancient Egyptian Medicine.* British Museum Press.

Pinch, G. (1994). *Magic in ancient Egypt.* British Museum Press.

Quirke, S. and Collier, M. (2004). *The UCL Lahum Papyri: Religious, Literary, Legal, Mathematical and Medical.* BAR Publishing.

Scanlan, B. (2004). Animals: The Hunted and The Domestic, In Donovan, L. and McCorquodale, K. (eds). *Egyptian Art – Principles and Themes in Wall Scenes.* MU Press, pp. 83-90.

Schwabe, C.A. (1978). *Cattle, Priests and Progress in Medicine.* University of Minnesota Press.

Shaw, I. and Nicholson, P. (eds) (1995). *The British Museum Dictionary of Ancient Egypt.* The British Museum Press.

Walker, R.E. (1964). The Veterinary Papyrus of Kahun. *The Veterinary Record* 76, pp. 199-200.

Wilkinson, R. (2003 reprint). *Reading Egyptian Art.* Thames and Hudson.

Animal Health and Disease:
www.agric.nsw.gov.au/reader/an-health/a0933.htm
[Accessed 01/07/08]

A PRIMACY IN HISTORY: THE DOCTORS OF THE PHARAOHS

S. Malgora

Curator of the 'Ur Sunu Project' and the Egyptian section of Buonconsiglio Castle, Trento.

Abstract: *'Ur Sunu. Great Doctors of Ancient Egypt. Diseases and Cures in the Land of the Pharaohs' is the title of a new exhibition about ancient Egyptian medicine which has provided a chance to review current knowledge about this topic, which has never been the focus of an exhibition before.*

Key words: Medicine, doctors, specialisation, hierarchy, Egypt

Introduction

An exhibition of more than 150 objects from important national and international museums took place from 27th September 2007 to 10th of January 2008 in the historical building of the Sannazzaro Palace (middle of XVIII century) in Casale Monferrato (north-west Italy). The exhibition came from the desire of the Brotherhood of Misericordia, the exhibition organisers, to promote historical and scientific events, linked to medicine and surgery and their development over the centuries. The Misericordia are a brotherhood founded in 1527 by the influential members of the town of Casale, the capital of Monferrato. The principal aim of the association is to give free medical assistance to the people during difficult periods, like the Black Death of the 1600s.

In the 500th anniversary of its foundation, the Misericordia wish to investigate the roots of the history of medicine with an international exhibition of findings from the Nile Valley. Ur Sunu (www.ursunu.org.) is now a project for studying the history of the medicine and for moving the exhibition to foreign countries. The exhibition provides a good view of an uncommon side of the ancient Egyptian civilisation which, nevertheless, has afforded us with an insight into past medical traditions.

The ancient Egyptians were, as evidenced by the highly interesting and numerous findings of the exposition, very skilled doctors with advanced specialisms and cures. Their reputation as such in the ancient world appears to be justified. The testimony of the Greek historian Herodotus about this fact is therefore supported by the archaeological evidence.

The success and professional reputation of Egyptian doctors was such that pharaoh's doctors were a reference for all Mediterranean countries. Homer (Odyssey IV, 229-232) said:

> *'There, every man is a doctor, every man knows better than all the others how to treat all manner of disease.'*

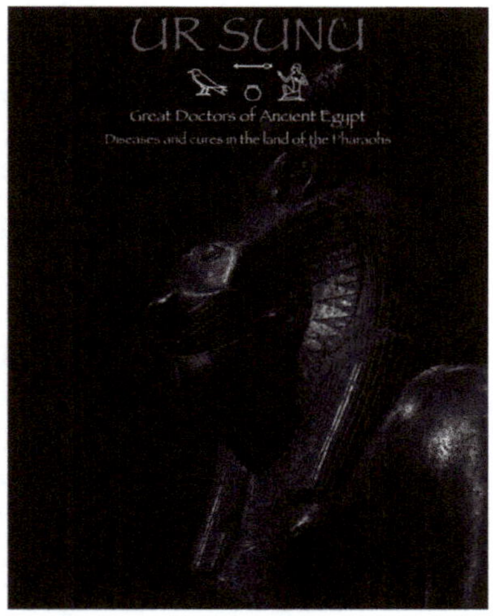

Figure 1: The poster of the exhibition

We can observe the Egyptian culture and society from many different points, but certainly medicine is one of the best, with information coming from architecture, images, sculpture, papyrology and anthropology. In this way, it is possible to understand the figure of the doctor with his hierarchy and specialisations during the long history of ancient Egypt.

We know the names of 150 doctors, 21 of which are specialized, mainly teeth and eye doctors. The word to define the doctor and the translation of the Greek *iatros* is *swnw*. The first doctor ever attested is Hesyra (reign of Djoser, 2667-2648 BCE). He was *wr swnw*, chief of doctors and *wr ibhy*, chiefs of dentists. Hesyra was buried in a mastaba at Saqqara (Malgora 2008, nota 2-3). The meaning of *swnw* is confirmed several times by the medical papyri such as the Ebers, Chester Beatty, Berlin and Leiden papyri, where the word is related to the cure of diseases, and in the Coptic word for doctor '*SAEIN*', which comes from *swnw*.

The Hierarchies

The medical profession was integrated into the elaborate scheme of Egyptian hierarchy; the stelae and funerary inscriptions of doctors show a large assortment of titles and qualifications, starting from the Old Kingdom. The first level includes the generic medical profession, called '*swnw*'. Doctors were subjected to the authority of a 'chief of doctors', *wr swnw*, like Gua and Seni, XI-XII dynasty, 2125-1773 BCE (BM 30840; BM 30842; Willems 1988, cat no. B1L, cat no B3L). This is the most frequent title found and it is found during the entire pharaonic period. It was held by Wedja-hor-resnet, XXVII dynasty, 404-399 BCE, represented in a basalt naophorus statue, with many other titles: royal sealbearer, sole companion to the king, administrator of the palace and commander of the royal navy (Nunn 1996, 129; Vatican Museum inv. n. 22690).

Resuming the hierarchy, there is *kherep swnw*, 'administrator of doctors' only attested by Medunefer, Old Kingdom, who was also an ophthalmologist of the doctors of the royal palace. Then there is *hery swnw*, 'one with the authority over doctors', mainly attested during the New Kingdom, *imy-r swnw,* an 'overseer'and *sehedj swnw,* an 'inspector', attested only during the Old Kingdom. To these titles should be added that of *semesu swnw,* 'doyen of the doctors', a courtesy title, as attested by the inscription on the sarcophagus of Neferi, who died at an advanced age (Leca 2002, 87).

An intriguing figure is the *wr swnw* Iuty, XVIII-XIX dynasty, 1550-1186 BCE; he holds the prestigious position of *wr swnw n neb taui,* 'chief of doctors of the Lord of the Two Lands'. Then there is *imy-r swnwt,* 'overseer of the female doctors' attested only by Peseshet, V-VI dynasty, 2494-2345 BCE (Nunn 1996, 124; Malgora 2008, 38). Peculiar is the title *imy-r gesuy depet swnw per aa*, overseer of the two sides of the boat of doctors of the palace.

In spite of definitions, the hierarchical range is not certain, as the details of the competences, duties, roles and the authorities are unclear. The administrative authority of the doctors set territorial restrictions: *wr swnw* of Upper and Lower Egypt, or of a village, or as one of the necropolis, Pura, New Kingdom, XIX-XX dynasty, 1295-1069 BCE, *wr swnw* of the Place of Truth.

A centre of medical activities is the royal palace. *Swnw per âa* is the 'doctor of the Great House', the doctor of the royal palace. Serving the court is the duty of a team of doctors, who follow the king, his family and those living and working at the court. For example, Ni-ankh-sekhmet, IV dynasty, reign of Snefru, 2613-2589 BCE, is *wr swnw per âa*, chief of the doctors of the palace, and also chief of the dentists of the palace. The top position is taken by the king's personal doctor, *wr swnw mehu shena,* 'chief of the doctors of the North and the South', whose authority covers all of the court, as well as all Upper and Lower Egypt (Nunn 1996, 117-119; Malgora 2008, 39-41).

The Specialisations

> *'The practice of medicine is so divided amongst them that each physician treats one disease and no more. There are plenty of physicians everywhere. Some are eye doctors, some deal with the head, others with the teeth or the belly, and some with hidden maladies ...'*
>
> Herodotus (II, 84)

Possibly Herodotus, a famous visitor to Egypt in 450 BCE, went too far, but even if the documentation is not complete and homogeneous, the tendency towards specialization among the ordinary physicians long after the pharaonic era is clear.

Dentist: *ibhy*, the one who cures teeths, and *iry ibh*, a person who deals with teeth. During the Old Kingdom: Neferiretes, Menkauraankh and the famous Hesyra, who was also an *wr ibhy* or chief of dentists. During the XXVI dynasty in the reign of Amhose II (570-526 BCE) Psammetekseneb was 'chief of the dentists of the palace' and 'chief of doctors of Upper and Lower Egypt' (Malgora 2008, 43)

The anatomical finds reflect modern problems. Over the course of time, a richer diet including meat and cooked food increased tooth decay. Moreover, the teeth are certainly worn from minerals contained in bread (Leek 1972; Peluso 1980). They drained abcesses, extracted teeth and cured them, as in the Ebers Papyrus (Eb.) paragraph 739 states, 'Beginning of the cures in order to strengthen a tooth: spelt wheat 1, ochre 1, honey 1. Make a poultice and fill the tooth with it' (Bardinet 1995, 354).

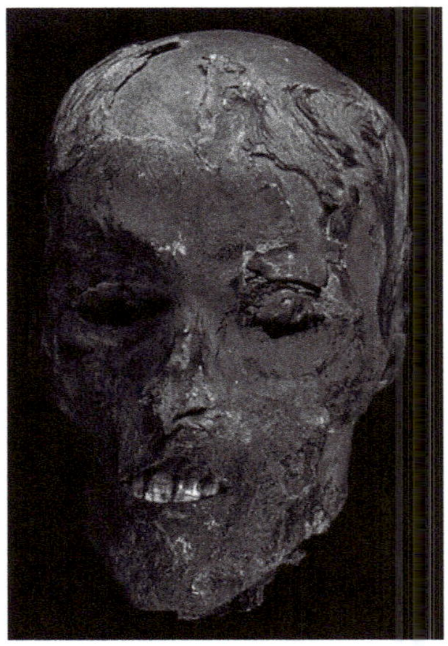

Figure 2: The mummified head showing signs of dental disease. The teeth have clear stripes visible on their surface, which can be recognised as hypoplasia of the enamel. This illness can be congenital or caused by poor nutrition.VI-XI dynasty, 2345-2055 BCE. From the necropolis of Gebelein or Assiut (inv. N. M6/911). Courtesy of Museum of Ethnography and Anthropology of Turin

Ophthalmologist: *swnw irty*, 'doctor of the two eyes' or *swnw irt*, 'doctor of the eye', or *swnw seneb irty*, 'doctor who cures the eyes'. The ophthalmologists are particularly well represented and their skill is not confined to the Egypt only: Cyrus, king of Persia, asks Ahmose II for the services of the best oculist in Egypt to cure his ocular disease, as Pliny the Elder records (*Naturalis Historia,* 26.3). During the Old Kingdom, the work of Wai, IV-V dynasty, 2613-2345 BCE, is attested by his tomb at Giza (Lepsius 1849-1859, II, 93, a) and also Nefertjes, connected with the royal palace (Hassan 1936, 179-201, pls. 74-76). During the First Intermediate Period, 2160-2055 BCE, Irenakhti is *swnw irty per aa.*

During the New Kingdom, Hui is administrator and chief of the ophthalmologists of the palace; during the Late Period there is Padi, during the XXVI dynasty, 664-525 BCE, and Wai, 'gastro-enterologist and ophthalmologist', *swnw khet irty* (Malgora 2008, 43).

The ocular ailments, especially the *nehat*, 'Egyptian ophthalmia' are frequent in the figurative arts; blind persons are represented, especially harpists, and a significant part of the Ebers papyrus is dedicated to these diseases. For example, in case of conjunctivitis it suggests (Eb. 384):

> '*Another remedy to remove the blood from the eyes: two bowls of clay, one of spelt flour and milk of a woman who gave birth to a male child, and the other with vaccine milk. Let it settle for the night to the dew. You should fill your eyes in the morning with this compound. After, clean your eyes with the rest of the milk four times a day*'
>
> (Bardinet 1995, 308).

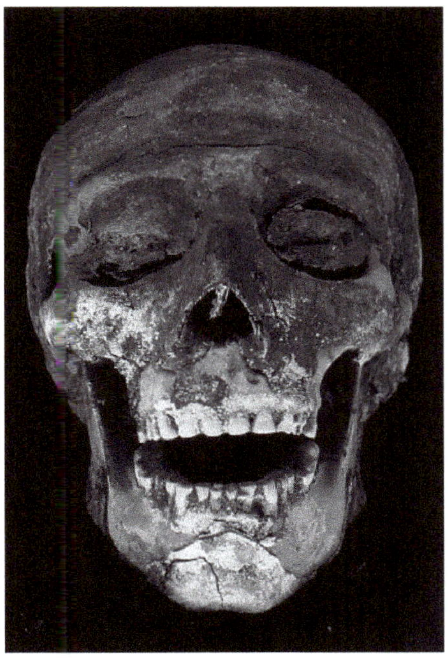

Figure 3: The dental arches show a uniform degree of occlusal wear, due probably to hard lateral bite and antero-posterior motion with probable biting use of the dentition. VI-XI dynasty, 2345-2055 BCE From the necropolis of Gebelein or Assiut (inv.n.M27/V). Courtesy of Museum of Ethnography and Anthropology of Turin

Proctologist: *Neru pehut*, 'guardian of the anus' is the doctor who prescribes and administers the medicine via the rectum. Herodotus (*Historiae*, II, 77) deals with the care of the rectum, saying that the Egyptians 'follow this model behaviour. Every month, for three days they purge the body taking care of the health with emetics and clysters, thinking that all kind of disease come from the food…' Four hundred years later, Diodorus Siculus (*Bibli. St.* 1.82) states 'in order to prevent sickness they look after the health of their bodies by means of drenches, fastings and emetics'. The use of clysters was wide spread, being used several times a month as prevention, as confirmed in many papyrus writings. The primary source devoted to the colorectal diseases is the Chester Beatty VI papyrus. For example, 'what is necessary to eliminate the anal inflammation by means of a refreshing enema: hemp 1/4; colocynth 1/32; stir water 1/16+1/64 to inject through anus for four days' (Ch. B., 7,8-9; Bardinet 1995, 456). Proctologists include Khui, VI dynasty, reign of Teti and Pepi I, 2345-2287 BCE, who is also a dentist and *swnw per aa*, and also *wr swnw mehu shema*, and *semesu swnw per aa*, as his stele from Saqqara attests. The *neru pehut* could be the doctor's assistant, who can be identified with the Greek *iatroklystes* (Malgora 2008). Great attention is given to curing this part of the body where the decay begins, a phenomenon so opposed by a people who must preserve the body for their afterlife.

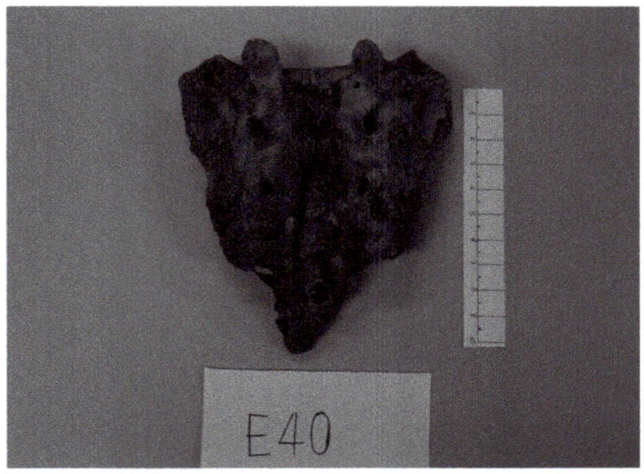

Figure 4: Sacrum with *spina bifida occulta*, VI-XI dynasty, 2345-2055 BCE. From the necropolis of Gebelein or Assiut (inv. n. E40). Courtesy of Museum of Ethnography and Anthropology of Turin

'One who knows the organs of the human body that are hidden from sight and interpreter of the liquids in the *netnetet*'. The former is a specialist of internal organs, the latter an expert in urinary disorders. As *netnetet* is in fact a membrane or an organ with the form of a sac, it could perhaps be the bladder. Khui has two specialisations, like his successor, the plurally titled Irenakhty, who was doctor and inspector of the royal doctors, proctologist, ophthalmologist and priest of Serqet.

Doctor of the belly: *swnw khet* could be a gastro-enterologist and a gynaecologist, because of the double meaning of the word *khet*. Wai is *swnw khet*, but also an ophthalmologist (Malgora 2008, 44).

Community doctor: Although the sources give little information, Metjen (IV dynasty, reign of Snefru) was attested as *swnw meret*, 'doctor of the workers' (For the title see Jonckheere 1958, 37; Leca 1986, 90; *swnw gereget,* doctor of settlers; Nunn 1996, 211; Daglio 1998, 41. For the documents: Maspero 1890, 113-246).

During the Middle Kingdom, Renefseneb (reign of Amenemhat III, 1831-1786 BCE) was *wr swnw* for the workers of a quarry at Serabit el-Khadim in Sinai. In the alabaster quarry of Hatnub, Herishefnakht, *wr swnw n nesu*, 'chief of the doctors of the king', XII dynasty, was probably there only for a visit, being too important to be settled in that place. There is also a chief of doctors in the Theban necropolis - Pura, XIX dynasty, 1295-1186 BCE, *wr swnw* of the Place of Truth. Neferhor, XIX dynasty, is maybe the doctor of the funerary temple.

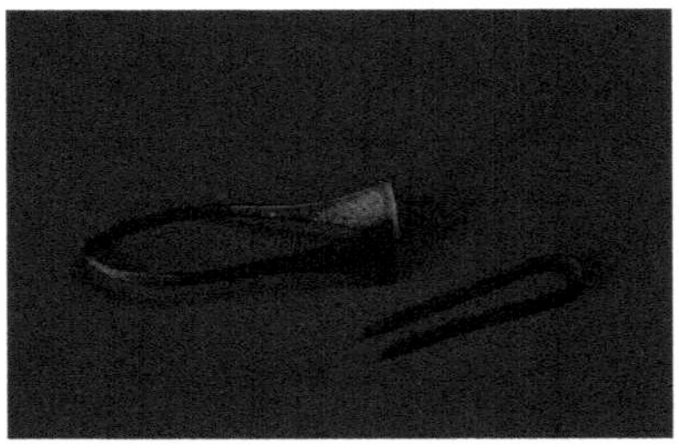

Figure 5: Bronze tweezers. Date unknown, from the necropolis of Thebes (inv. N.n. 6863, 3186). Courtesy of Egyptian Museum of Florence

Surgeon: In the papyri and funerary texts there are no clear indications and therefore it is not possible to understand if surgery was a branch of medicine. In the Ebers Papyrus, in the prescriptions, there are instructions for minor surgery, e.g. 8.57-8.77 referring to tumours, the *sa hemen*, the men of cauterization, could be surgeons. In the Edwin Smith papyrus, the 'surgical' one, alongside the swnw, is cited the *uab* of Sekhmet, who could be recognized as the surgeon (Malgora 2008, 45).

The Pharmacist: The sources unfortunately do not allow us to outline this profession and it is especially difficult to understand if this task was undertaken by the doctor himself or if it did exist as a separate profession. On the contrary, we have plenty of information about the ancient Egyptian pharmacopoeia; about 400 names of drugs are mentioned in the Ebers Papyrus (Malgora 2008).

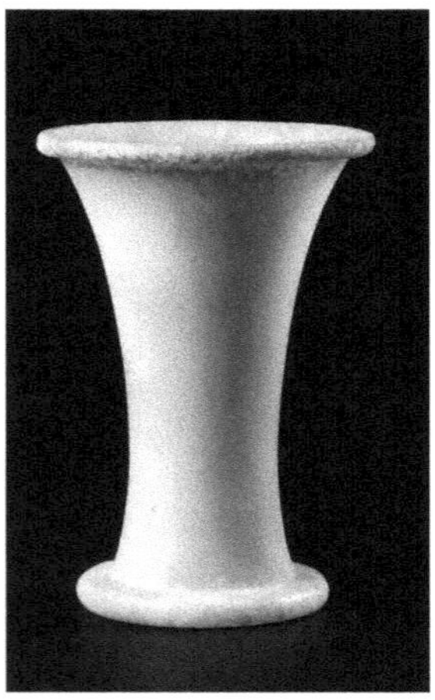

Figure 6: Ointment alabaster vase. V-VI dynasty. (inv. n. 3335) Courtesy of the Egyptian Museum of Florence

Remuneration

As with every other professional activity, the physician too is assured of remuneration for his work. The use of money was only introduced just before the XXX dynasty, 380-343 BCE, so the doctors were paid by barter, controlled by the government. Some documents found in the settlement village of the workers, Deir el Medina, supply details about remunerations: the lowest monthly salary is rations of the main products of the diet: wheat, barley, bread and beer. An *ostrakon*, XX dynasty, 1186-1069 BCE, states that the doctor receives an additional payment in comparison with the other workers - a quarter of a *khar* of wheat and a *khar* of barley, in addition to four *khars* of each cereal (Jansen 1975, 460). A fragment of the Vatican papyrus, XIX dynasty, confirms that doctors could receive honoraria in the form of copper and natron, in addition to their monthly salary.

Remuneration is largely affected by the wealth of the patient. The decorations in tombs show remuneration scenes, such as the example in the tomb of the doctor Nebamon, XVIII dynasty, reign of Amenhotep II, 1427-1400 BCE, at Dra Abu el Naga, where he receives a lavish remuneration from a Syrian prince and his wife: slaves, livestock, copper and natron. In the scene in the funerary chapel of his tomb, Pentju, chief of doctors of the palace, XVIII dynasty, reign of Akhenaton, 1352-1336 BCE, is honoured by the king for his services with the gift of gold collars. The doctors of the palace who regularly get a monthly salary could be also honoured with a gift of symbolic value that overcomes the material one, such as a funeral chamber, the funerary equipment for the life after death, or a commemorative stele.

Doctors with Priests' Titles and Others with Magical Aspects

In the Ebers papyrus (Eb.854a), in the 'Treatise of the Heart' and in a gloss of the Smith papyrus, three exponents of the medical profession are mentioned: 'if every *swnw,* every *wab* of Sekhmet or every *saw* (of Serqet) puts his two hands or his fingers on the head, on the head back, on the hands, on the heart place...' (Bardinet 1995, 239).

In the text therefore we have three figures - the doctor, the priest of the 'powerful one', an enchanter, and a real magician. To understand that role differentiation, one should make reference to the concept of illness in ancient Egypt. The suffering in a person can be caused even by a negative power, or by a divinity or by a demon. The doctor's role was also that of fighting and beating the invisible power, which was upsetting the patient, by reciting magical formulae and religious spells.

The *Hekay* are an example of these experts, a sort of 'shaman', the only ones who, in these special cases, were able to win - with a real exorcism - against the 'dark side'. The *Hekay* were linked to Heka, a natural yet divine force but also a component of the human being which, after death, becomes a circumpolar star, of the type that never fades. Religion and the divine rite also played an important role in curing illnesses, as the deities had protective faculties. Therefore, it is not unusual that lots of doctors held priestly titles. (Malgora 2008, 45-46; Rosati 2008; Guzzon 2008)

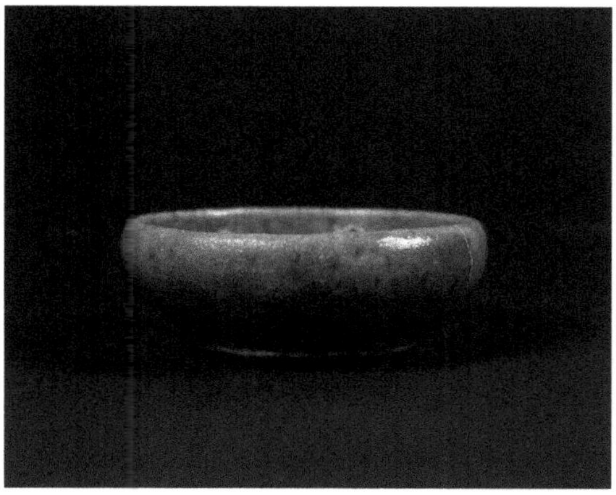

Figure 7: Faïence bowl. Late Period, 664-332 BCE (inv. 3531) Courtesy of the Egyptian Museum of Florence

Medical Practice

The primary sources, especially the Ebers and Edwin Smith papyri, allow us to understand some aspects of medical practice and of the approach to the patient. In front of an ill person, the doctor conducts a medical investigation in a rather modern approach based on three different stages to deliver a diagnosis, a prognosis, the prescription of the medicaments to take and the care to follow.

In the first stage, the doctor asks for information on the psycho-physical condition of the patient, to learn the problem and which part of the body hurts. Then he inspects the face, the expectoration, the urine, the excrement, and then he pays attention to the body, evaluating wounds, haematoma, other deformations of the skin, looking for interesting elements, like trembling, stiffening, paralysis. No aspect is forgotten, because every detail is important and helpful. The sight, the smell and the touch all work in synergy. Palpation has also a symbolic importance, because it requires contact between doctor and patient, and in some cases is intended to circumscribe and to extirpate the illness (Halioua and Ziskind 2005, 25). After the investigation, the doctor points out and marks the symptoms. In the Edwin Smith papyrus, unfortunately not complete, there are 48 cases to which the doctor can refer 'if you examine a man having'.

Then come the solemn moments of the diagnosis and of the prognosis characterized by the following statements: 'you will say what is the matter with him: a patient suffers from....' The patient is not abandoned, even in the case of a negative prognosis. Not in every case does a right diagnosis follow a good understanding of the symptoms. The doctors are not free to treat the patient as they like, but they had to follow the ancient texts. These texts are considered sacred and immutable, of divine inspiration. With reference to this aspect of medicine, Diodorus Siculus says that the doctors respect these texts with scrupulousness, because if what is suggested from the books does not lead to the recovery, nothing will be ascribed to his work; on the contrary, if he acts according to his opinion and without following the holy texts, most probably he will be accused and sentenced to death (I, 82). This may appear to be too rigid, but this represents the birth of the first medical procedures, forerunners of modern guidelines and of diagnostic and therapeutic procedures. (Halioua and Ziskind 2005, 27; Daglio 1998, 46).

The practice of medicine also included magic, since illness is seen as the result of the intervention of an entity that must be fought in order to obtain the recovery of the patient. By means of magic, one can look for the cause of a problem, putting it on a divine level; for the gods, the recovery of the patient is a way to re-establish the world order.

References

Bardinet, T. (1995) *Les papyrus médicaux de L'Égypte pharaonique*. Fayard.

Daglio, C. (1998) *La medicina dei faraoni. Malattie, ricette e superstizioni della farmacopea egizia*. Ananke.

Diodorus Siculus, *The Library of History*, (ed.) Oldfather, C.H., Sherman, C.L., Welles, C.B., Geer, R.M., Walton F.R., (1933-1967), Loeb Classical Library 12 vols.

Guzzon, E. (2008) Magia e medicina nell'antico Egitto. In Malgora, S. (ed) *Ur Sunu. Great doctor of ancient Egypt. Diseases and cures in the land of pharaohs*. Saviolo Vercelli.

Jansen, C. (1975) *Commodity prices from the Ramessid Period: an economic study of the village of necropolis workmen at Thebes*. Brill.

Jonckheere, F. (1958) *Les médecins de l'Égypte Pharaonique*. Fondation Égyptologique Reine Élisabeth.

Halioua, B. and Ziskind, B. (2005) *Medicine in the days of the Pharaohs*. Harvard University Press.

Hassan, S. (1936) *Excavation at Giza II*. Cairo Government Press.

Homer, *Odyssey*, (ed.) Murray, A.T., revised by Dimock, G.E. (1998), Loeb Classical Library, 2 vols. Harvard University Press.

Leca, A.P. (1986) *La medicina egizia*. SBM Scientific Book Market.

Leek, F.F. (1972) Bite, attrition and associated oral conditions as seen in ancient Egyptian skulls. *Journal of Human Evolution* 1 (3), pp. 289-295

Lepsius, C.R. (1849-1859) *Denkmäler aus Äegypten und Äthiopien*. I-IV, Berlin.

Malgora, S. (2008) I medici della terra dei faraoni. In Malgora, S. (ed) *Ur Sunu. Great doctor of ancient Egypt.*

Diseases and cures in the land of the pharaohs. Saviolo Vercelli.

Maspero, G. (1890) *L'Égypte au temps de Ramsès* II, 1 vol. Paris.

Nunn, J.F. (1996) *Ancient Egyptian Medicine*. British Museum Press.

Peluso, A. (1980) Patologia orale in una antica popolazione egiziana. *Antropologia Contemporane* 3 (1), pp. 57-60

Pliny the Elder, *Natural History*, (ed) Jones, W.H.S. and Andrews, A.C. (1956) Loeb Classical Library, 10 vols. Harvard University Press.

Rosati, G. (1998) il sacerdote *wab* di Sekhmet. In Malgora, S. (ed) *Ur Sunu. Great doctor of ancient Egypt. Diseases and cures in the land of the pharaohs*. Saviolo Vercelli.

Willems, H. (1988) *Chests of life: a study of the typology and conceptual development of Middle Kingdom standard class coffins*. Ex Oriente Lux.

A CURE FOR BALDNESS: ANCIENT EGYPTIAN PHARMACOLOGICAL REMEDIES FOR THE HAIR AND SCALP

N.C. McCreesh[1], A.P. Gize[2] and A.R David[1]

[1]The KNH Centre for Biomedical Egyptology, The University of Manchester, UK
[2]School of Earth Atmospheric Environmental Sciences, The University of Manchester, UK

Abstract: *The majority of pharmacological knowledge comes from ancient Egyptian documents, specifically the Ebers papyrus. This document lists a wide range of pharmacological prescriptions including those to be applied to the hair and scalp, not only for the treatment of ailments but also for vanity, such as cures for baldness and grey hair. Hair is an ideal archaeological resource to study due to the fact that it remains well preserved, and can be analysed for evidence of medical defects or treatments applied to the hair.*

This communication will discuss hair as an archaeological resource and give examples of the information to be gained from cuticle diagnostics, in comparison with analyses of the remedies listed in the Ebers papyrus and their efficacy to known disorders of the hair and scalp. The possibilities of finding physical evidence of such prescriptions on human remains will be discussed. Insight will also be given regarding the perception of vanity in ancient Egypt when the often unusual extents to cure hair loss and loss of hair colour are discussed.

Key words: Mummy, mummification, hair, scalp, pharmacy

Features of the Hair

Human hair is extremely stable and resistant to decomposition and enzymatic digestion. It is therefore often the least degraded part of human and animal remains. With the scarcity of archaeological remains, taking a sample of hair is much less intrusive or destructive than more frequently studied samples such as skin and bone. From a single strand a wealth of information may be gained. Cuticle diagnostics can be used to develop medical diagnoses (Dawber 1997), indicating specific hair or scalp defects and other diseases affecting the hair; and states of nutrition and climate (Wilson 2005). Though hair is very strong it can become damaged, the causes of which may be grouped into two main factors: environmental factors, such as weather and climate; for example heat, sun, and wind can all have damaging effects on hair; mechanical factors include artificial manipulation of the hair, such as brushing or curling.

Environmental damage is not usually a main cause of hair damage, as the hair is naturally resistant to daily wear. It is mainly mechanical trauma which causes damage to the hair (Grey and Dawber 1999, 70). Most damage to the hair is caused by practices which place stress on the hair, such as mechanical trauma from combing wet hair and using heated appliances; and chemical stress such as permanent waving or bleaching. The hair is damaged when such activities disrupt the cuticle and cortex, as this can involve loss and lifting of the cuticle scales, exposing the cortical fibres which can then become frayed (Grey and Dawber 1999).

The hair may also be affected due to medical conditions. This can include scalp disorders such as dandruff and psoriasis, extraneous matter such as fungi and lice, and also disorders which damage the hair shaft and cause hair loss (Dawber 1997). Some irregularities of the hair shaft caused by environmental and chemical damage can exhibit similar features to those from a medical origin such as Trichorrhexis nodosa. This condition is generally caused by cosmetic procedures; however, it can also be caused by an inherent weakness of the hair shaft such as sulphur deficiency (Grey and Dawber 1999).

Archaeological Hair

Modern scientific techniques and medical knowledge can be used to study ancient hair. Generally, ancient Egyptian hair is well preserved due not only to the natural stability of hair, but also to a protective layer of embalming material often found coating the hair. The embalming material is formed from a hard resinous material which would have been hot and fluid when applied. When the coating is removed a negative cast of the hair is left in the coating. This is vitally important as the cast preserves the hair in the condition it would have been in at the time of death. In one example, the embalming material coating was not evenly applied over the head. This resulted in parts of the hair being free of the coating, and thus the hair was damaged with cuticle lifting and peeling. This is an important finding as it implies that the state of the hair as it is today is not necessarily indicative of its condition when the person was living (McCreesh et al. *In press*).

Environmental / Mechanical

Most ancient Egyptian hair samples show healthy hair with little damage. Many of the hair samples studied by the authors show evidence of mechanical treatments such as cutting and styling, indicating that the hair was well looked after. Many mummies are also found with long hair, contrary to the belief that all ancient Egyptians shaved their hair and wore wigs (Elliot Smith 2000).

Medical

Though there are many known medical defects of the hair today, evidence for ancient Egyptian examples are rare, possibly due to the limited studies on the hair and scalp rather than a lack of occurrence. Hair lice and eggs, however, have been found in ancient Egyptian hair (Fletcher 1995; Leslie and Levell 2006) and also on combs (Palma 1991), so we know that the ancient Egyptians suffered with them. Damaged hair has been found, mainly consisting of cuticle peeling and lifting, but this is likely to be the result of post-mortem damage (McCreesh et al. *In press*).

A likely case of eczematous etiology was identified on a female mummy from the Predynastic period. The cause of the condition was suggested to be seborrheic eczema, or possibly contact dermatitis associated with hair dyes such as henna (Leslie and Levell 2006, 618). Although it has been frequently suggested that henna was used, there is no unequivocal evidence for the use of the dye in ancient Egypt.

Treatment

Along with physical assessment of the hair for medical defects, there is also evidence of ailments from prescribed treatments. The treatments are listed in medical papyri such as the Ebers and Hearst papyri, and can be assessed for efficacy or comparison with modern prescriptions and remedies.

'Swelling in the hair, hemispherical and soft, and its contents are growing' (Ebbell 1937, 125) to be treated with 'the knife treatment' (Nunn 1996, 167). This prescription is the only mention of an actual defect - the 'swelling of the hair' to be treated. It is most likely referring to a swelling of the scalp beneath the hair, rather than a swelling of the actual hair shaft. In this case, it is likely to refer to a type of cyst, which would be lanced off; cysts often contain hair (Nunn 1996, 167).

Though there is evidence that the ancient Egyptians suffered from head lice, there does not appear to be any direct remedy in the medical papyri. There are however treatments for other ailments which could have been used to treat the head lice. The treatments, which involved making a mixture of oils made into a paste to be applied to the head as an unguent, would have been effective in treating head lice, as such a paste would suffocate the lice, and the lice and eggs could then be removed through combing the hair with a fine toothed comb. Lice have been treated throughout history by simple methods such as this, and fine toothed combs have been found to contain lice eggs (Palma 1991).

The Ebers papyrus has an entire section for ailments of the hair, which can be divided into 3 types: those prescribed for a medical nature such as to treat exanthema of the scalp and dandruff; those for vanity such as expelling grey hair and to make hair grow, and those for revenge - 'to cause the hair to fall out', if applied to the head of a hated woman!

The efficacy of prescriptions listed in the Ebers papyrus has been evaluated and compared to modern counterparts (Campbell 2007). To treat discharging exanthema of the scalp 14 prescriptions are listed, for example: seed of ricinus, grease, balanites oil [moringa] (Campbell 2007, 105), mixed together and anointed daily (Ebbell 1937, 77). This prescription may have had some soothing effect as castor oil is used as an emollient for skin complaints (Campbell 2007, 105). Another includes honey, date wine and silphium (along with some unidentifiable ingredients), to be rubbed into the condition (Ebbell 1937, 77). Mercury, analogous with silphium, was used to treat skin eruptions during the 20th century (Campbell 2007, 105). Again, for the same ailment, red ochre, fresh 'carob pod / colocynth' oil (Campbell 2007, 106) are mixed and used to anoint the ailment (Ebbell 1937, 78). Oil and carob are soothing, whilst ochre is mildly astringent (Campbell 2007, 106).

Ostrich fat, fish gall, *kmw*, sory [resin] (Campbell 2007, 106) turpentine [pine tar] (Campbell 2007, 105) and frankincense are mixed and the ailment is anointed for four days. This is an unusual remedy as turpentine would be more likely to cause eczema (Campbell 2007), as shown by its high frequency in painters, who are regularly exposed to turpentine. Alternatively, the ingredient may have been pine oil which, in strong quantities, could possibly cause dermatological conditions. In small doses, however, the antibacterial properties may have aided a skin complaint such as eczema by preventing the wounds from becoming infected. Pine oil is found in small doses in remedies available for the treatment of eczema today.

There is one remedy to expel dandruff which lists a mixture of roasted barley, roasted *amni* [emmer] (Campbell 2007, 109) and grease to be anointed, followed the next day by anointing with fish oil and hippopotamus fat. This is followed on the third day by anointing with laudanum and finally, on the fourth day, the crown is anointed with sour wheat bread. It is suggested here that this remedy may have lessened the condition by helping to condition and moisturize the scalp which lessens flakes caused by dry skin.

There are 20 prescriptions to expel baldness and promote hair growth, for example:

> '*Remedy to expel spotted baldness: prickles of hedgehog, are burnt, immersed in oil and applied to it*'
>
> (Ebbell 1937, 107).

This prescription does not have any known efficacy, but perhaps the quills may have been used as a stimulus or form of acupuncture; how the quills are to be used is not stated. The main benefit from these types of treatment would be that rubbing in an unguent may have provided some stimulus to the scalp to promote hair growth. One remedy includes red ochre and beer (Ebbell 1937, 107). The beer may have provided some results as it is often used even today to rinse the hair, giving shine and body. The inclusion of coloured products with a staining action such as the red ochre and ink powder (Ebers translated Ebbell 1937, 107), may have given some form of tint to the hair like a dye, allowing a notable, visual difference to the appearance of the hair.

The remedies for expelling greying of the hair are very interesting. None of the ingredients are efficient in a pharmacological manner. Yet they all contain black (or very dark brown-black) coloured ingredients; for example, blood of black calf, shell of tortoise, backbone of raven, ravens egg, blood from the horn of a black ox, brain of synodontis fish, tadpole, burnt hoof of an ass, fat of a black snake (Ebbell 1937, 78-79). It is possible that this was the use of sympathetic magic; by using things with a black colour they would project this property onto the hair. It is also possible, however, that this may have been an attempt to dye the hair. It is presumed that most native ancient Egyptians would have had black or very dark brown hair, and thus covering any grey with a dark stain may have helped to disguise the grey.

Conclusion

Through the combined study of traditional Egyptology and modern science it is possible to build up a wide understanding of hair care in ancient Egypt. It is well known that the ancient Egyptians practised forms of hair dressing, but not much is known about their reaction to conditions affecting the hair and scalp. The medical papyri provide extensive prescriptions for treating ailments such as balding and greying of the hair, but treatments are also provided for medical complaints such as dandruff and exanthema of the scalp. Through detailed studies of mummified remains, the hair and scalp can be studied, to understand more fully the medical complaints suffered in ancient Egypt and the methods of dealing with them.

References

Campbell, J.M. (2007) *An assessment of the pharmaceutical and therapeutic merit of remedies within the Kahun, Edwin Smith, Ebers and Chester Beatty ancient Egyptian medical papyri.* Unpublished PhD Thesis. Manchester: The University of Manchester.

Dawber, R. (1997) *Diseases of the Hair and Scalp.* 3rd Ed. Blackwell Science Ltd.

Ebbell, B. (1937) *The papyrus Ebers: the greatest Egyptian medical document / translated by B. Ebbell.* Oxford University Press.

Elliot Smith, G. (2000) *The Royal Mummies* 2nd Ed. Duckworth.

Fletcher, A.J. (1995) *Ancient Egyptian hair: a study in style, form and function.* Unpublished PhD Thesis. Manchester: The University of Manchester.

Grey, J. and Dawber, R. (1999) *Hair and Scalp Disorders. An illustrated Guide.* Blackwell Science.

Leslie, K.S. and Levell, N.J. (2006) Cutaneous findings in mummies from the British Museum. *The International Journal of Dermatology* 45, pp. 618-621.

McCreesh, N.C., Gize. A.P. and David, A.R. (In Press) Hair: an untapped forensic resource. *Proceedings of the International Symposium on Archaeometry,* Siena 2008. Springer e-Book.

Nunn, J.F. (1996) *Ancient Egyptian Medicine.* British Museum Press.

Palma, R.L. (1991) Ancient head lice on a wooden comb from Antinoë, Egypt. *Journal of Egyptian Archaeology* 77, pp. 194.

Wilson, A.S. (2005) Hair as a Bioresource in Archaeological Study. In Tobin, D.J. (ed). *Hair in toxicology – an important bio-monitor.* The Royal Society of Chemistry.

GOOD FOR WHAT ALES YOU – A PROSPECTIVE STUDY INTO THE ROLE OF BEER IN ANCIENT EGYPTIAN MEDICINE

R.J. Metcalfe

KNH Centre for Biomedical Egyptology, The University of Manchester, UK

Abstract: *The medical papyri make it clear that beer was extensively used in ancient Egyptian pharmacy. However, the question of whether it was used simply as a diluent or whether it played a more important and active role has not yet been answered.*

There are good reasons to suspect the latter. The fermentation process would help to limit the amount of viable bacteria in the water used for brewing, making it a more suitable carrier for someone with a suppressed or strained immune system. Providing that the mixture was not heated sufficiently to vaporise the alcohol, the beer would add a slight soporific and euphoric effect.

Previous research into brewing has established that, in contrast to previously held beliefs, the methods used in ancient Egypt were quite sophisticated. A number of putative methods determined using different techniques are available, and several possible variants have been identified that would alter the character of the beer significantly. We aim to use these recipes to study the potential for different types of beer to act as a carrier for pharmaceutically active substances derived from plants and resins as well as their bactericidal effects.

Key words: Brewing, beer, pharmaceutical remedies, traditional medicine.

Ancient Egyptian Beer and Brewing

It is well known that beer formed a staple part of the ancient Egyptians' diet (Kemp 1989, 126). Originally, this was thought to be a fairly primitive process, based on lightly baked, heavily yeasted bread mixed with water and allowed to ferment (Curtis 2001, 106). Confirming or refuting this assumption using preserved tomb scenes and models was difficult, as these were not meant to be informative and instructional, but merely indicative. The close association in many such scenes between images of brewing and of baking appear to reinforce the suggestion that the two were intimately linked, but as production of both required large amounts of grain and yeast, could it not be that it was simply more efficient logistically to have them near to each other?

Rather than relying on artistic interpretations of the process, Samuel analysed residues of the beer itself using electron microscopy (Samuel 2000). This revealed the process to be more sophisticated than previously thought. Both malted and non-malted grain was used, with some cooked to gelatinise the starch. Mixing this with uncooked grain allowed enzymes to convert the starch to sugars, which were then fermented.

Other methods were devised by Ishida based on analysis of tomb scenes (Ishida 2005). Reproductions of these methods produced residues that were similar to those studied by Samuels, though as they were based on a modern interpretation of an ancient artistic representation, they may not be entirely accurate. It is, however, extremely unlikely that the Egyptians had only a small number of recipes for brewing, given that several different brews are given specific names in the literature, and that they were brewing on a large scale from the Predynastic period onwards.

Pharmaceutical Preparations

As well as forming a major part of the diet, beer is mentioned in many of the remedies mentioned in the surviving pharmaceutical papyri (Ghalioungui 1987). Whether it is being used simply to dissolve and aid mixing of the other ingredients is not known, neither can we say if it was being used as a gentle soporific or euphoric to make the patient feel better.

There is good reason to suspect that it was included in the pharmaceutical corpus for more important reasons, however. Both lactic acid bacteria and yeast are thought to have been used for fermentation of beer. These produce lactic acid and ethanol respectively, which limit the growth of other organisms without affecting the viability of the other (except at higher concentrations) (Rowen et al 1998) forming what has been referred to as a 'fermentation wall' (Ishida 2005). Using fermentation to clean the drinking water would have obvious benefits to those with weakened immune systems.

The ethanol content provides another potential reason for using beer rather than water. It is possible that including such a solvent improved the dissolution of pharmaceutically active compounds. If this is the case, then the different alcohol content of different beers may have provided a way of controlling the amount of substance in the final remedy, and thereby controlling the dose. The opposite is also a potential function for beer, i.e. using the alcohol to remove or reduce the concentration of harmful substances by washing or soaking before use.

Not Just a Vehicle

It is possible that beer had a function beyond a dose mediator and vehicle for the drug, and actually had a function of its own. Perhaps the most immediately obvious possibility to an Egyptological audience would be tetracycline, an antibiotic thought to be present in stored grain that has been infected with Streptomycetes (Bassett et al. 1980), and the emetic power of beer may be attested by anyone who has witnessed the Dionysian fury of a University Fresher's week.

Beer is also known to contain B vitamins (Denke 2000 and references therein), for example, though excessive consumption of alcohol may also prevent the uptake of vitamins and minerals (Tomasulo et al. 1968). Phenolic acids found in the beer may help to protect the body against oxidative stress, which is related to neurodegenerative disorders and cardiovascular disease (Ghiselli et al 2000). However, these are perhaps better seen as being long-term, nutritional benefits rather than pharmacologically useful properties *per se*, and so could not be taken as having a directly observable effect that would influence their continued use as an ingredient in remedies.

An Egyptian Template

Though a number of other medical traditions use beer in their remedies (see, for example, Powell 1993; Cano and Volpato 2004), perhaps the most thoroughly understood of the ancient examples is that of the Egyptians. A great deal of work has been carried out not only to translate the surviving medical papyri but to understand their pharmaceutical efficacy. This, combined with the above mentioned research into their brewing practices, therefore represents the ideal starting point for research into the use of beer in traditional medicine. It is hoped that chemical analysis will allow the various beneficial and detrimental properties of ancient Egyptian style beers to be illustrated. This would then provide a stepping-stone for research into the use of other alcoholic beverages, such as wine, and into other medical traditions, such as that of Mesopotamia.

Acknowledgements

The author would like to thank The Leverhulme Trust who funded this research.

References

Bassett, E.J. Keith, M.S., Armelagos, G.J., Martin, D.L. and Villanueva, A.R. (1980). Tetracycline-Labelled Human Bone from Ancient Sudanese Nubia (A.D 350). *Science* 209, pp. 1532-1534

Cano, J.H. and Volpate, G. (2004). Herbal Mixtures in the Traditional Medicine of Eastern Cuba. *Journal of Ethnopharmacology* 90, pp. 293-316

Curtis, R.I. (2001). *Ancient Food Technology*. Brill.

Denke, M.A. (2000). Nutritional and Health Benefits of Beer. *The American Journal of the Medical Sciences* 320, pp. 320-326

Ghalioungui, P. 1987. *The Ebers Papyrus*. Academy of Scientific Research and Technology.

Ghiselli, A., Natella, F., Guidi, A., Montanari, L., Fantozzi, P. and Scaccini, C. (2000). Beer Increases Plasma Antioxidant Capacity in Humans. *The Journal of Nutritional Biochemistry* 11, pp. 76-80

Ishida, H. (2005). Two Different Brewing Processes Revealed from Two Ancient Egyptian Mural Paintings. *The Master Brewers Association of America Technical Quarterly* 42, pp. 273-282.

Kemp, B. (1989). *Ancient Egypt: Anatomy of a Civilization*. Routledge.

Powell, M.A. (1993). Drugs and Pharmaceuticals in Ancient Mesopotamia. In Jacob, I. and Jacob, W. (eds). *The Healing Past*. Brill, pp. 47-67

Rowen, N.J., Anderson, J.G. and Smith J.E. (1998). Potential Infective and Toxic Microbiological Hazards Associated with the Consumption of Fermented Foods. In: Wood, B.J.B. (ed). *Microbiology of Fermented Foods*. Blackie Academic and Professional, pp. 812-837

Samuels, D. (2000). Brewing and Baking. In Nicholson, P.T. and Shaw, I. (eds). *Ancient Egyptian Materials and Technology*. Cambridge University Press, pp. 537-576.

Tomasulo, P.A., Kater, R.M.H. and Iber, F.L. (1968). Impairment of Thiamine Absorption in Alcoholism. *American Journal of Clinical Nutrition* 21, pp. 1341-1344.

MOLECULAR METHODS FOR THE STUDY OF ANCIENT PHARMACY

R.J. Metcalfe

KNH Centre for Biomedical Egyptology, The University of Manchester, UK

Abstract: *The application of DNA analysis to ancient pharmaceutical research promises to provide a range of useful data. Perhaps most importantly it is hoped that identifying the remains of plants, with complementary evidence from the literature, pharmacognitive research and palaeobotany, will help with the firmer identification of plants from preserved medical texts. Given that the Middle East and North Africa are centres of endemism, it is also hoped that it will be possible to identify the sources of pharmaceutically useful plants used in ancient Egypt, thereby potentially indicating the source of the remedies that used those plants.*

Given the difficulties associated with ancient DNA research and the irreplaceable nature of ancient samples, it was considered appropriate to conduct numerous tests on models before performing destructive analytical techniques. Therefore, models mimicking preservation by charring in a variety of environments were designed to determine which protocols are best able to produce extracts suitable for analysis via PCR. A model for the application of a topical remedy was also prepared to assist in sample selection to maximise the potential for success in future experiments.

The data from these models will be presented not only to share the data with people to whom it may be of interest, but also in the hope of demonstrating the potential of experimental models in archaeological science to help refine techniques and reduce the requirements for ancient, irreplaceable samples.

Key words: Ancient DNA, plants, experimental models.

Introduction

The heavy reliance placed by the ancient Egyptians on plants to supply their pharmaceutical requirements opens up possible areas of research into their origins and uses that may otherwise not be available. The potential for ancient DNA techniques to identify plant residues and remains should not be ignored, as it may supply additional information to that obtained from textual or pictorial sources, palaeobotany, and that interpreted using pharmacognitive methods. The positive identification of plants from preserved pot residues, for example, in a mixture corresponding directly to a prescription included in one of the medical papyri would obviously be of great interest. More modest findings, such as the identification of a medicinally useful plant imported from another country, should not be overlooked as they could also provide insights into the origins of ancient Egyptian medicine.

The prospects for this type of research are improved thanks to the high level of endemism found in North Africa and the Middle East. The level varies widely, from as high as 31.8% in Socotra to 0% in Qatar (Boulos 1997). Although variation over time should also be expected as environments and agricultural practices etc. change, this high level of endemic species raises the spectre of being able to pinpoint the origin of imported plants with some accuracy. Achieving this does, of course, rely on having suitable genetic sequences for the various plant species from the area to compare to ancient samples, and on finding intact DNA of a suitable size and quality in the archaeological specimens.

Preserved ancient specimens are rare and, by definition, irreplaceable, and aDNA techniques difficult and expensive, thus using experimental models to test theories and refine techniques can help prevent wastage of this valuable material. Charring represents not only a common method of preserving plant remains (Murray 2000), but is also a damaging process that can help to test the abilities of various experimental methods to extract clean and usable DNA from the sample. By varying the reaction conditions, it is possible to use the model to determine which samples stand the best chance of success. For example, restricting access to the material by oxygen (which is known to damage DNA in a variety of ways (Lindahl 1993)) would be expected to reduce the degradation of the sample and would therefore indicate that ancient specimens recovered from sealed containers should be better subjects for analysis (O'Donoghue et al. 1996). Testing this using models will establish whether this is the case or not, as sealing out air will also prevent water, which also damages DNA extensively (Lindahl 1993), from escaping as vapour during heating. Which of these factors, restricting oxygen or allowing water to be removed, has the most effect is something that models can show unequivocally.

Another way in which experimental archaeology can assist in the choice of samples for pharmaceutical research is by reproducing remedies preserved in the medical papyri to determine how their preparation affects the survival of DNA from the plants and other constituents. Several of these remedies require extensive or potentially damaging formulation such as prolonged soaking (e.g. Ebers remedy 48 (Ghalioungui 1987)) or boiling, either to heat or to reduce the volume (e.g. Ebers remedies 18 and 23 respectively (Ghalioungui 1987)). This will show whether the genetic investigation of preserved residues would be worth pursuing with today's technologies. Alternatively, as many of the remedies were designed for external application, it is possible that residues adhering to the body would be a useful source of information.

Materials and Methods

Two models were prepared, one to test the effects of charring on DNA preservation and the other to determine the possibility of a poultice leaving sufficient DNA on the skin after application for identification of its constituents.

Charring Model: Grapes were used in this model as they are mentioned in medical papyri (e.g. Ebers remedy 223 (Ghalioungui 1987, 76), are easily obtained commercially, and have been well studied genetically. Whole grapes and naked seeds were heated in a furnace at 250°C and 300°C, either sealed in foil packages to create an anoxic environment or in open trays. Whole fruit were heated for 90 minutes to allow complete charring of the exposed samples, and naked seeds were heated for 30 minutes.

PCR was used to determine how well preserved the samples were by targeting a long (631 base pair (bp)) and a short sequence (229bp). PCR amplicon length is inversely proportional to the amount of damage inflicted to the DNA molecule, as missing or damaged bases retard or stop the polymerase enzyme (Hofreiter et al. 2001).

Poultice Model: This model was based on the reproduction of remedy 129 from the Ebers papyrus. The original recipe is as follows:

> *Another, to break pain-matter: Wheat flour 1; barley flour 1; flour of emmer 1; myrtle 1; honey 1; bandaged therewith.*
>
> (Ghalioungui 1987, 41)

Some slight alterations were made to the experimental poultice. Neither myrtle nor emmer wheat was easily available, and so myrtle was omitted and spelt substituted for emmer. Equal quantities of the grains were ground by hand and mixed with honey to form a thick paste. This was then spread over pieces of pig skin obtained from a butcher, which were subsequently dried in a synthetic 'natron' made up from laboratory chemicals in proportions indicated to provide a high degree of preservation (60% anhydrous sodium carbonate, 20% sodium bicarbonate, 20% sodium chloride) (Garner 1979). The samples were split into several different groups so that a number of parameters, such as length of exposure to the poultice, the presence of a wound in the skin, and the effects of washing the poultice from the skin before mummification, could be tested for their effects on preservation.

Results and Discussion

Grape Model: The fruit samples showed very low levels of reproducibility, with some extracts showing high levels of preservation, and others showing little or none. This suggests that the size of the fruit allows differential preservation throughout its volume. The environment surrounding the fruit is likely to be responsible for this, especially in the samples sealed to prevent oxidation. In these samples, the juice evaporated significantly more slowly than in the open samples, instead forming a layer on the bottom that the fruit sat in, exposing them to boiling juice throughout the length of the experiment. It is feasible, therefore, that the parts of the fruit most exposed to this liquid were more damaged than those above it, which dried more quickly and so were exposed only to heat, rather than heat and water.

Naked seeds showed a wide range of preservation, with those heated at 250°C without oxygen showing amplification of both the 229bp and the 631bp products. All the other samples only showed positive results for the 229bp product, with the 300°C without oxygen samples being marginally better than the open samples. As the seeds have much less free water than the fruit, the potential degradation pathways are limited to heat and oxidation. Conversely, the heat damage to the fruit samples would be limited as the water would have to be evaporated before the internal temperature would rise above the boiling point of the juice.

Seeds taken from the fruit samples showed an extremely high level of preservation. All the samples showed positive amplification of both 229bp and 631bp fragments. The pattern of preservation differed from that of the naked seeds in that those samples heated with oxygen were better preserved. However, those heated at 250°C were still better than those heated at 300°C. This is most probably caused by the same conditions encountered with the fruit samples. The anoxic samples had the seeds bathed in boiling juice throughout a significant portion of the experiment, which had a deleterious effect on preservation. However, it does appear that the presence of fruit around the seed has a protective effect, as the level of preservation seen in these samples is greater than seeds heated directly.

Poultice Model: The results from this model indicated that traces of DNA from a poultice can remain detectable on skin after mummification. 'Wounded' samples showed slightly larger quantities of PCR products, indicating the presence of slightly more DNA, though the difference was slight. Samples that had the poultice left on for 24 hours at 4°C were marginally more positive than those exposed for 1 hour at room temperature, again indicating that slightly more barley DNA had been transferred. Washing the poultice from the samples before mummification had a strong deleterious effect on the detectability of barley DNA on the samples, as should be expected, but there was still a very slight positive result.

These results show that there is definite transfer of detectable amounts of DNA from a poultice to the skin, which can be detected after mummification. However, the amounts are small, especially after the poultice has been rinsed off under water. A more thorough or vigorous washing, or one that includes a cleaning or scouring agent, would almost certainly reduce the amount surviving even further. Additionally, as these traces would be on the exposed surfaces of the body, they may be more susceptible to degradative processes.

The combination of these factors appears to make the detection of the constituents of poultices unlikely on Egyptian mummies. The 'classic' method of mummification described by Herodotus (De Selincourt 1996, 115) includes several washing steps, some of which use palm wine. The comparatively long period since their production, when compared to those of other cultures such as Incan mummies, will have exposed any surviving traces to greater degradation.

Instead of investigating wound sites for the presence of DNA from a poultice, it would be better to look at the remedy itself. Though the thorough ritual cleaning of the body seen in Egypt would make it unusual to find such a thing, it may be possible in other mummies. The body of Maria d'Aragona, for example, was found with a poultice still in position on her arm (Fornaciari et al. 1989).

Conclusions

From these results, it appears that the possibility of finding identifiable DNA residues from a topical remedy on an Egyptian mummy is unlikely as the washing stages in mummification would almost certainly remove the larger deposits that would provide the most realistic chance of success. The trace amounts of genetic material transferred to the body itself by the poultice appear to be so small that they would probably degrade over the intervening centuries. However, this could be an avenue of investigation worth pursuing in mummies from other cultures, or where the material is still in place.

Fruit seeds appear to be more highly resistant to degradation as a result of charring than expected, with high molecular weight PCR amplicons retrievable from samples heated to 300°C. The presence of fruit around the seed appears to improve its preservation, especially in samples exposed to oxygen during the heating. Rapid removal of juice from the fruit appears to be key to this, as having the seeds exposed to liquid at high temperature, as seen in the sealed samples where vapour could not escape, increased their degradation. These results may be useful in guiding future research by influencing sample choice to provide the best chance of success and limiting the use, and therefore wastage, of samples that are unlikely to provide results.

Acknowledgements

The author would like to thank The Leverhulme Trust who funded this research.

References

Boulos, L. (1997) Endemic flora of the Middle East and North Africa. In Barakat, H.N. and Hegazy, A.K. (eds.) *Reviews in ecology: Desert conservation and development*. Metropole, pp. 229-260.

De Selincourt, A. (1996) *Herodotus: The Histories*, Penguin.

Fornaciari, G., Castagna, M., Tognetti, A., Tornaboni, D. and Bruno, J. (1989) Syphilis in a Renaissance Italian mummy. *The Lancet* 614, pp. 8663.

Garner, R. (1979) Experimental Mummification. In David, A.R. (ed). *The Manchester Museum Mummy Project*. Manchester University Press, pp. 19-24.

Ghalioungui, P. (1987) *The Ebers papyrus. A new English translation, commentaries and glossaries.* Academy of Scientific Research and Technology

Hofreiter M., Serre, D., Poinar, H.N., Koch, M. and Pääbo, S. (2001) Ancient DNA, *Nature Reviews Genetics* 2, pp. 353-359).

Lindahl, T. (1993) Instability and decay of the primary structure of DNA. *Nature* 362, pp. 709-715.

Murray, M.A. (2000) Cereal production and processing. In Nicholson, P.T. and Shaw, I. (eds.) *Ancient Egyptian materials and technology*. Cambridge University Press, pp. 505-536.

O'Donoghue, K. et al. (1996) Remarkable preservation of biomolecules in ancient radish seeds. *Proceedings: Biological Sciences* 263 (1370), pp. 541-547

PALAEOPATHOLOGICAL - RADIOLOGICAL EVIDENCE FOR CEREBRAL PALSY IN AN ANCIENT EGYPTIAN FEMALE MUMMY FROM A 13TH DYNASTY TOMB

A.G. Nerlich[1], S.Panzer[2], E. Hower-Tilmann[1] and S. Lösch[1]

[1]Institute of Pathology, Academic Hospital Munich-Bogenhausen, Munich, Germany
[2]Dept. of Radiology, Trauma Clinic Murnau, Germany

Abstract: *The palaeopathological investigation of mummified human remains is an important and direct approach to reconstructing living conditions and diseases in past populations. Besides typical osseous pathologies in rare cases complex disorders may also be identified. The present report describes such an example.*

The palaeopathologic examination of the human remains from a 13th dynasty tomb (c. 2000 BC) of the necropolis of Dra-Abu-el-Naga, Thebes-West, Upper Egypt, revealed the partly skeletonized, partly mummified remains of a mature female individual of 50 – 60 years of age which was found – although disrupted by tomb robberies – adjacent to a very well-decorated sarcophagus of a high ranked female of the pharaonic court named 'Geheset'. An extensive anthropological and palaeopathological analysis showed severe dental attrition affecting the left-sided teeth more severely than those of the right side, along with severe left temporo-mandibular arthritis. Additionally, the right hand was deformed and partly wrapped in linen bindings. Radiologically, the hand showed extensive flexion in the radiocarpal joint and hyperextension in the phalangeo-interphalangeal (PIP) joints. Reconstruction of the hand position in intact burials precludes postmortal malformation. There is no evidence for osseous destruction; the well-preserved tendon apparatus is shortened. In consequence, the hand malformation is highly suggestive of a long-standing disturbance of the hand innervation. Post-traumatic cerebral ischemia is unlikely as this produces flexion deformities in all hand joints. In summary, the hand malformation is most likely the result of a chronic cerebral paresis such as seen in uni- or bilateral infantile cerebral palsy (M. Little).

Introduction

The palaeopathological analysis of human remains may provide considerable insight into living conditions and diseases in individuals of historic populations. The amount of available information is dependent on the type of preserved material and its conservation conditions. Since in the majority of cases bone tissue is the only preserved biomaterial, analysis is usually limited to those diseases that manifest in bone. However, occasionally important observations have been made in soft tissue residues as well (Aufderheide 2000). In rare cases, the palaeopathologic pattern of disease may provide a distinct diagnosis of a complex syndrome. In the present report, we describe the complex pattern of a severe neurological disease in a fragmented and significantly skeletonized female mummy describing the, as yet, oldest case of cerebral palsy (possibly of the congenital type) in the palaeopathological literature.

Material

The individual was found during an excavation of the German Archaeological Institute Cairo (under the heading of Prof. Dr. D. Polz) in the necropolis of Dra Abu-el-Naga, Thebes-West where a 13th dynasty tomb had been discovered with a very elaborate sarcophagus (for details of the burial see Polz (2007)). The sarcophagus inscriptions identify that the owner was a female named 'Geheset'. Although still unclear, it has been speculated that she was the wife (or another relative) of a royal official named 'Imeni', suggesting a higher social burial dating back to the Middle Kingdom period (i.e. between c. 1950 – 1750 BC). During the excavation, the partly skeletonized residues of the mummy were found in front of the opened sarcophagus with signs of extensive grave robbery.

The human remains were subjected to a detailed anthropological and palaeopathological examination, including a radiological analysis of body parts. In order to investigate the potential role of burial practice, the observed pathological findings were compared to the evidence depicted in the royal mummy catalogue (Smith 1912).

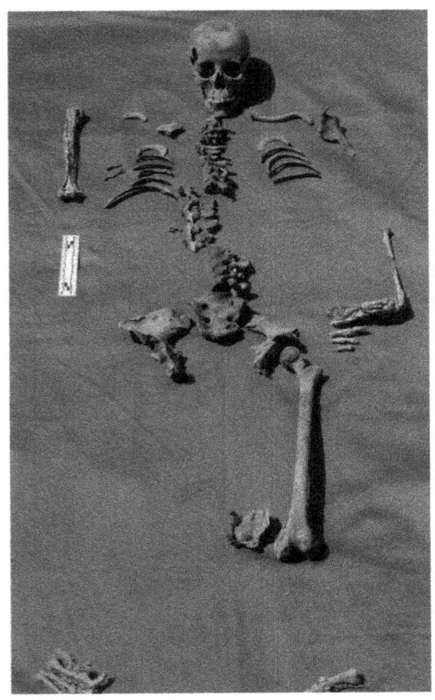

Figure 1: The skeletal residues of the mummy after reconstruction of the severely damaged mummy.

Observations

The skeleton belongs to a mature female with well preserved bones of the skull, upper and lower vertebra, several rib fragments, both clavicles, part of the left scapula, right humerus, left forearm, part of both pelvis, left femur and patella and isolated bones of both fore feet (Fig. 1). Most remarkable was the left fore arm/hand which presented as the only preserved, almost intact piece with mummified skin and soft tissues, hand and finger bones and the still attached distal radius and ulna covered by some linen bindings.

The detailed inspection of the skull sutures and the pelvic symphyses suggests an age at death of more than 50 years and a body height of approx. 1.53 m (determined from the length of the right humerus and left femur according to Bach (1965) and Szilvassy (1988)).

The skull revealed a significant prognathism so that Nubian ancestry was taken into consideration, although no other metric or non-metric evidence for such an assumption was available. The teeth showed extensive abrasion of the enamel which, however, was unevenly distributed. Accordingly, the left labial teeth were significantly more affected than the right sided ones. Furthermore, the buccal aspect of the left teeth was also less severely affected than the labial side. In addition, the left temporo-mandibular joint was severely deformed, its surface was extensively pitted and the joint cavity was strongly eroded while the right-sided contralateral joint cavity presented with a smooth and regular surface and without deformation (Fig. 2).

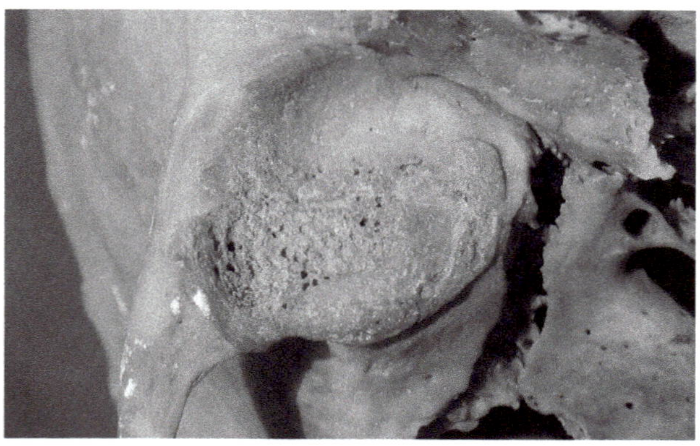

Figure 2: Severe deformation of the left temporo-mandibular joint with deformation and superficial erosion of the joint cavity.

Most remarkable was the almost intact left hand which presented as strongly flexed in the radio-carpal joint, along with hyperextension in the phalangeo-interphalangeal joints of all digits and extension of the thumb with inward rotation (adduction) (Fig. 3). The soft tissue and skin appeared intact. On radiographs these findings were confirmed along with some evidence for sclerosis of the ossa metacarpalia joints, the os scaphoideum was slightly deviated to the palmar side. There was some evidence for contracture of the soft tissue mantle along with intact tendons and ligaments.

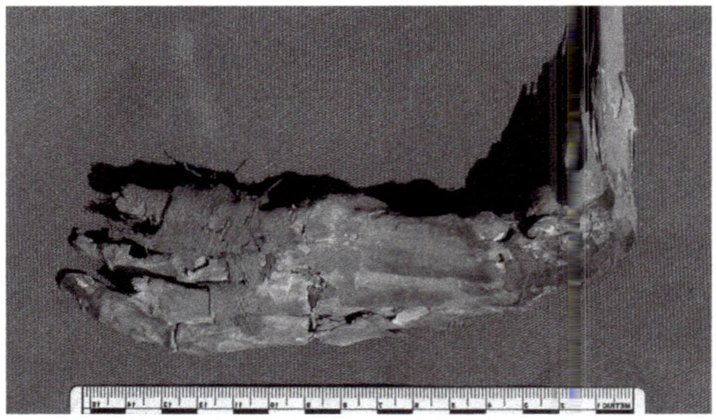

Figure 3: The mummy´s left hand shows strong flexion in the radio-carpal joint and hyperextension in the metacarpo-phalangeal joints suggesting a neuromuscular disorder.

Discussion

We investigated here an extensively skeletonized and fragmented mummy of an ancient Egyptian female individual dating back to the Middle Kingdom. Due to the archaeological findings these human remains could be attributed to a socially high-ranked female named 'Geheset' (which means 'gazelle') whose remains had been contained in a very well decorated sarcophagus (Polz 2007). The anthropological investigation confirmed the individual´s sex, thereby providing a further independent confirmation of some of the archaeological findings. In summary, the burial strongly suggests a high class burial presumably from the entourage of a ruler of ancient Egypt during the Middle Kingdom. Archaeological findings by Polz (2007) identified that the necropolis of Dra Abu-el-Naga/Thebes-West, Upper Egypt served at that time as the main necropolis for the pharaohs of the Middle Kingdom. At that time, Thebes was the capital of the ancient Egyptian empire. However, we do not have enough archaeological data to identify the specific role of 'Geheset' in ancient Egyptian history, nor is there enough data that identifies aspects of her personal biography. In consequence, some anthropological features, such as that of significant prognathism suggesting a probable Nubian ethnicity, remain uncertain.

The detailed and careful anthropological and palaeopathological investigation showed a mature, slender female individual of approx. 1.53 m body height of more than 50 years of age. The palaeopathological analysis identified a very unusual pattern of osseous (and soft tissue) pathology. Most remarkably, the left sided teeth and the left temporo-mandibular joint showed severe abrasion (at least when compared to the contralateral right side) along with degenerative changes. This suggests a significantly stronger 'use' of the left side during mastication providing some evidence for reduced function of the right-side masticatory muscles.

In turn, the left hand showed severe malposition with extensive flexion in the proximal and hyperextension in the middle and distal hand joints along with extension and adduction of the thumb. The focal sclerosis of the subchondral zone of several ossa metacarpalia indicates a 'chronic' status indicating long-standing 'malposition' of the hand bones. For this deviation we suggest the following differential diagnosis:

- abnormal position of the hand due to postmortal deviation (e.g. during the embalming process);
- sequels of (direct or indirect, e.g. cerebral) trauma;
- sequels of a muscular or (non-traumatic) neurological disease.

A comparison of the hand position of numerous female mummies, mainly those shown in the Catalogue of the Royal Mummies now housed in the Egyptian Museum at Cairo (Smith 1912), revealed hand positions that were all different from our case. There, the hands were positioned either along the body side or slightly crossed over the pelvis, but there was no instance of the strong deviation seen in our mummy. A virtual superimposition of the mummy's hand with the royal female mummies showed an incompatible feature fairly ruling out that the hand position was the effect of postmortal deviation during the embalming process.

During this comparative analysis we had detected the abnormal position of both hands of the Pharaoh Seqenen-Ra, an imperial ruler during the time period of reconciliation of the ancient Egyptian empire after severe warfare with the Hyksos (17th dynasty). His hands show a malposition partly similar to the findings with Geheset. However, the mummy of the pharaoh additionally reveals several premortal osseous skull defects, most probably as the result of blunt force trauma by a sharp weapon. Bockenheimer et al. (1978) and Metzel (1981) previously have suggested that the wounds on the pharaoh's skull had produced intracerebral bleeding resulting in a secondary neurologic defect with post-traumatic hand paresis. However, the skull of Geheset did not provide evidence of direct trauma or residual trauma, so that this cause also was ruled out.

Finally, we considered the possibility of a severe neuro-muscular disease. It is significantly important that the left side of the teeth was used more than the right side and that the left temporo-mandibular joint was more severely eroded than that of the right fossa temporo-mandibularis. These observations strongly suggest a hypofunction of the right-sided masticatory muscles, indicating hemiparesis of the right side of the face. Taking the pathological hand position and hemiparesis of the face into account, we may conclude a severe neurological disorder of Geheset. Since we have no evidence for direct or indirect post-traumatic disease, the pattern of alterations is most compatible with cerebral palsy (*M. Little*, named after the English surgeon William John Little in 1843) which may present as hemiparesis of either one side or paresis of opposite body parts (uni- or bilateral paresis) as seen in the remains of this mummy.

In consequence, we may speculate both on the physical, but also the social consequences of this severe disease. Individuals affected by *M. Little* are frequently (but not necessarily) struck by dyskinesia (strange movements) and ataxia. In most instances, cerebral palsy affects newborns with an estimated frequency of one in 1,000 babies. The risk is highest in premature and underweight babies and the disease seems to result from a hypoxic status either within the uterus or during a prolonged birth period. Although cerebral palsy is often a congenital (present at birth) syndrome, it is not genetically inherited. It is characterised by slow, writhing movements, usually in the limbs, but it may also affect facial muscles, including the tongue. This can lead to drooling, strange facial expressions, and an inability to form some words or sounds. Usually, the mental and intellectual development of affected individuals is normal. Ataxia is a rare additional symptom showing poor coordination and depth perception which makes people with ataxic cerebral palsy unsteady walkers, with a wide-based gait. They may suffer from intention tremor, in which the arm or hand trembles when reaching for an object and the trembling gets worse the closer the hand gets to the target. Symptoms do not generally get worse over time, as the underlying disease is not progressive. Atrophy, however, can worsen muscular symptoms and, in children, prevent proper growth. Since there is no evidence for disease progression with age, life expectancy seems not to be reduced and it is certainly not considered a fatal condition.

Geheset may in consequence have presented as a very 'unusual' person. Since we know that persons with particular personal presentation sometimes had a high position at the pharaoh's court (likewise it is well known that dwarfs occupied high positions in the pharaoh's entourage (Dasen 1983)), we may speculate that the clinical features of Geheset may have made out of her a person with a 'divine' presentation and that this may have been the reason for her high social status manifested by the well crafted sarcophagus (and the burial in the imperial necropolis next to the pharaoh's tomb). This study provides good evidence that palaeopathology may uncover socially relevant information.

References

Aufderheide, A. (2000) Progress in soft tissue paleopathology. *JAMA* 284, pp. 2571-2573

Bach, H. (1965) Zur Berechnung der Körperhöhe aus den langen Gliedmaßenknochen weiblicher Skelette. *Anthropologischer Anzeiger* 29, pp. 12-21.

Bockenheimer, S., Eickhoff, U., Metzel, E. and Voigt, K. (1978) Radiological densitometric examinations of the skull injuries of pharaoh Seqenenre. *Röntgenforschung* 128, pp. 691-694

Dasen, V. (1993) *Dwarfs in ancient Egypt and Greece.* Oxford Mongraphs on Classical Archaeology. Clarendon Press.

Metzel, E. (1981) Neurotraumatology in ancient Eygpt. *Neurochirurgia* 33, pp. 78-80.

Polz, D. (2007) *Für die Ewigkeit geschaffen. Die Särge des Imeni und der Geheset.* Philipp von Zabern Mainz.

Smith, G.E. (1912) *Catalogue général des antiquités égyptiennes du Musée du Caire. The Royal Mummies.* Institut Français d'Archéologie Orientale.

Szilvassy, J. (1988). Altersdiagnose am Skelett. In Knußmann, R. (ed). *Anthropologie. Handbuch der vergleichenden Biologie des Menschen.* Gustav Fischer Verlag, pp. 421-435.

SURGERY IN ANCIENT EGYPT – PALAEOPATHOLOGICAL EVIDENCE FOR SUCCESSFUL MEDICAL TREATMENT BY SURGERY

A.G. Nerlich[1], S.Panzer[2] and S. Lösch[1]

[1]Institute of Pathology, Academic Hospital Munich-Bogenhausen, Munich, Germany
[2]Dept. of Radiology, Trauma Clinic Murnau, Germany

Abstract: *Surgery is an important branch of modern medical treatment. Until recently, there existed only indirect evidence that the ancient Egyptians practised surgery, and therefore there is no palaeopathological evidence. The present report describes the palaeopathological findings in the remains of three ancient Egyptian mummies, confirming the ancient Egyptians (successfully) performed surgery.*

During our palaeopathological survey of the human remains found in several 'Tombs of the Nobles' of the necropolis of Thebes-West, dating to the New Kingdom and subsequent periods (approx. 1550 – 700 BC), we identified two cases of intravital surgery: one almost complete female mummy and an isolated disarticulated foot that clearly showed intravital amputation of either the big toe or the complete fore foot, respectively. The female mummy was found in tomb TT95 and archaeological findings suggest that she dates back to the 21st dynasty (ca. 1070-850 BC). The isolated foot was found in tomb TT183, a Ramesside tomb on the hill of El-Khokha (20th dynasty, approx. 1300-1000 BC). Both amputation sites were covered by intact layers of soft tissue and skin indicating intravital amputation a long time before death. In addition, the amputated big toe had been replaced by a carefully crafted wooden prosthesis. A third case with evidence for intravital surgery comes from our own mummy collection where the head of a Theban male mummy revealed signs of operative removal of bone fragments at a severe trauma site of the left parietal bone.

With these cases, we provide clear evidence for intravital (successful) surgery in ancient Egypt.

Introduction

Extensive literary evidence indicates that the ancient Egyptians practised medicine at a high level. Likewise, Homer (IV, 229-232) describes in his 'Odyssey' that:

> *'Here (i.e. in Egypt) everyone is a medical doctor outnumbering the medical experience of any other people'.*

Furthermore, Herodotus (II, 84) indicates a significant sub-specialisation of doctors with those responsible for the treatment of eyes, ears, teeth, the stomach and the rectum. However, this list does not contain mention of surgeons. Up to now, there exists an open debate as to whether the ancient Egyptians practised surgery or not. Indirect evidence has been deduced from written sources, but until now no palaeopathological findings confirm surgical treatment. Likewise, the medical papyri, e.g. the Papyrus Edwin Smith, describe the treatment of traumatic lesions, but do not indicate surgical treatment directly (Kolta 1992). In addition, there exists up until now no proof from palaeopathological findings that surgical treatment was indeed performed in ancient Egypt, although the description of externally treated fractures of the forearm by wooden splints (Smith and Dawson 1924) or a IXth dynasty bone finding (c. 2500 BC) of a (presumably post-traumatic) amputation of the forearm with subsequent distal synostotic fusion of radius and ulna (Brothwell et al. 1963) are very suggestive of this. Very recently, Dupras et al. (2008) described three skeletons from Deir el-Bersheh Upper Egypt, which presented with amputations of the feet and signs of healing. However, the authors suggest that these conditions resulted from traumatic amputation.

Further, though 'indirect', evidence for surgery comes from Old Kingdom tomb wall paintings showing circumcision, this may not represent surgery, but a religious practice. The depiction of surgical instruments on the temple wall of Kom Ombo, Upper Egypt date to the Roman period and might therefore already represent the Graeco-Roman influence on Egyptian medicine in the final period of ancient Egypt.

The present report describes three cases where the palaeopathological findings indicate the successful practice of surgical treatment, including amputation, in ancient Egypt. Thereby, we observed one case of ancient 'neurosurgery' and two cases of amputation of a toe and the forefoot respectively. Furthermore, in one of those two cases of amputation, the amputated limb – the big toe – was replaced by a carefully crafted wooden prosthesis which was not only manufactured for the afterlife, but provides clear evidence for intravital use (Nerlich et al. 2000). Therefore this is the, as yet, oldest known prosthesis used for medical treatment.

Description of the Findings

During the last several years we have performed an extensive palaeopathological survey on the human remains from ancient Egypt coming from various sources: a major part of our work is related to excavation campaigns of the German Archaeological Institute, Cairo (in close collaboration with the Supreme Council of Antiquities of Egypt), and further work has been done on the mummified human remains from various collections in Europe. The excavation material analysis covers numerous tombs and tomb complexes from Abydos (Pre- / Early Dynastic), Dahshur (Old Kingdom) and Thebes-West (Middle Kingdom, New Kingdom until Late Period and Coptic Period). This global approach has provided us up to now with paleopathological data on more than 1,500 individuals amongst which we examined the following three cases.

Case 1

This particular case was that of a mummified complete skull with intact external soft tissues which was at least in the major part covered by linen bindings (Fig. 1A). The skull belongs to an adult male individual of c. 40 – 60 years of age and archaeologically, it most likely dates from IIIrd Intermediate Period until Late Period (i.e. 1070 – 300 BC). The skull had been found in the necropolis of Thebes-West. Unfortunately, no further information is available on the postcranial part of the mummy or on the archaeological context that might give a hint as to the socio-economic living conditions of that individual.

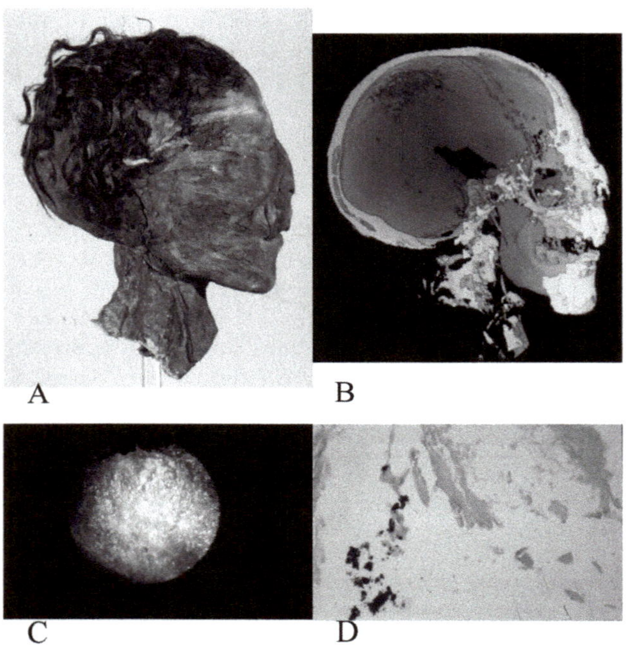

Figure 1: Macroscopic, radiologic, endoscopic and histological findings in Case 1 presenting with a defect of the left parietal bone and missing bone fragments. The head was covered by an intact layer of soft tissue, skin and some linen bindings (A); on CT scans, however, a osseous defect is visible (B), while the endocranial endoscopy reveals an intact brown layer at the defect zone (C) and histology shows the focal deposition of haemosiderin at the defect margin (D, Prussian blue stain, x200).

During the anthropological-palaeopathological investigation of the skull, we also conducted CT scans on the otherwise completely intact mummy head. Surprisingly, this showed an extensive osseous defect of the left parietal bone which was covered by an intact external layer of connective tissue, hair and linen bindings. The bone fragment(s) was/were completely missing (Fig. 1B). At the defect margins both bevelling of the defect edges with focal slight new bone formation as signs for osseous repair were seen. In addition, there was a fine fracture line running from the upper end of the defect into the parietal bone and there was evidence for a fracture of the petrous bone. In order to evaluate further these findings, an additional examination of the endocranial space by endoscopy was performed. Therefore, following removal of a small bitumen plug that had covered the nose, a small flexible endoscope was inserted through the open nostrils and through a small defect of the lamina cribrosa. These defects are typically seen in mummies beginning from the New Kingdom period (c. 1550 BC) until later periods. They have been made during the embalming process in order to remove the brain (Smith and Dawson 1924). On internal inspection the left middle cranial fossa was partly covered by a thin brown layer (Fig. 1C), such as residue of the dura mater. Otherwise, there was no evidence for an intracranial significant bone fragment and there was also no evidence for other residues of organic material except for a dark-brown gluey material adhering to the occipital bone, such as that seen as embalming residue in other mummies.

The further evaluation of the CT scans and an endoscopic inspection of the external and middle ear showed on the left side a complete loss of all ossicles, while the ossicle chain was present and arranged in normal position on the right side.

In order to confirm these aforementioned observations, we decided to carefully remove a small tissue sample from the defect region in order to perform a histological analysis. Following rehydration and embedding into paraffin wax, histological slides revealed regular subcutaneous structures, such as dermal connective tissue, residues of subcutaneous fat tissue with occasional hair follicles and the dense connective tissue layers of the galea and the dura mater which were separated by deposits of histochemically identified haemosiderin (Prussian blue), providing evidence for older bleeding residues in the defect zone (Fig. 1D).

In summary, this is a case showing a severe blunt trauma to the left parietal bone of the skull that has survived for at least 1-2 weeks (due to haemosiderin deposition, possibly also somewhat longer). The most interesting issue is that the bone fragment(s) is (are) missing and that both the dura mater and the galea/skin are intact so that a 'neurosurgeon' must have removed the fragment(s) from the defect zone. This makes sense since the trauma region is well known to bear the danger of epidural haematoma due to traumatic rupture of meningeal arteries which would lead to death within a few hours if untreated. Modern treatment options – such as in the ancient Egyptian case – would consist of removal of the osseous fragment(s) in order to avoid intracranial pressure. Therefore, the bone pieces might have been removed during surgical procedure.

Case 2

The disarticulated mummified foot was recovered from the necropolis of Thebes-West (El-Khoka, TT183), a tomb that had been built in the Ramesside period of the New Kingdom (c. 1300 – 1000 BC) and reused in later periods. Except for being the foot of an adult individual, unfortunately no data are available either on the respective individual or on any further pathological processes. Also, the individual´s sex is unknown.

The foot is disarticulated at the ankle and covered by an intact layer of skin and soft tissues with typically dark-brown appearance due to mummification substances. Otherwise there is no evidence for superficial defects. However, the complete fore foot is missing due to amputation (Fig. 2A). The amputation line runs through the metatarso-phalangeal line, except for the Vth digit where the metacarpus is retained. The amputation line is completely covered by skin and soft tissue and there is no evidence for any defect, major scarring, residues of stitches or surgical suture material. All these observations are confirmed on fore foot radiographs which confirm the amputation line running through the metatarso-phalangeal joints (Fig. 2B). On the radiographs there is no evidence for further pathological lesions of the bones or for soft tissue calcifications; the bones do not seem significantly demineralised.

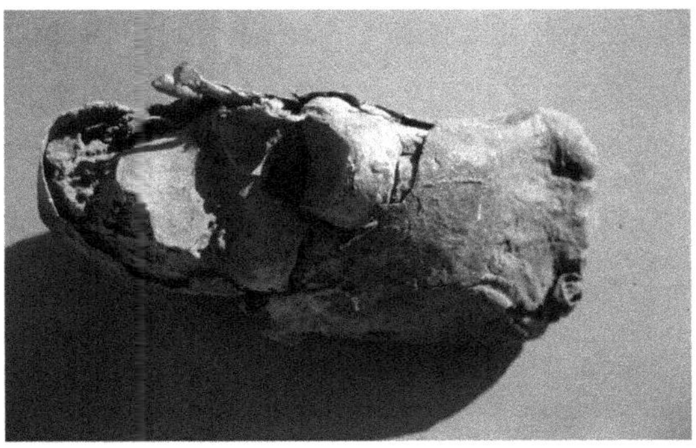

A

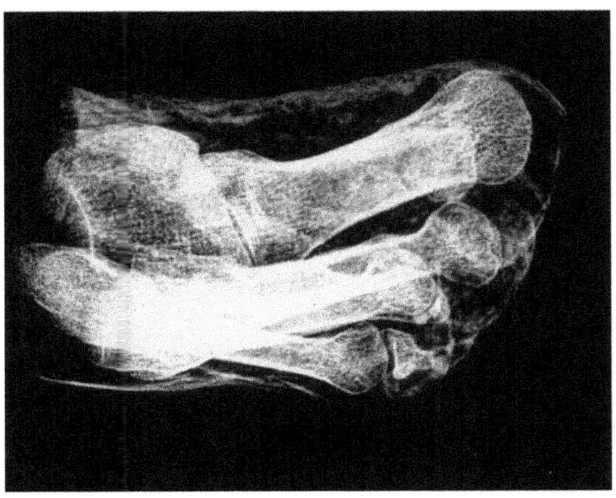

B

Figure 2: Amputation site of Case 2: Macroscopically (A) the fore foot shows an intact layer of skin and soft tissue at the amputation site; on radiological examination (B) the amputation line runs through the typical metacarpal amputation zone as in present day operations.

In conclusion, this is a case of (almost) complete and typical forefoot amputation with clear evidence for healing of the amputation line. There is no obvious cause for the amputation as the radiograms do not show the residues of any trauma in the remaining bones nor evidence for significant soft tissue calcifications, such as in peripheral arterial walls.

Case 3

This case describes the almost complete mummy of a woman with an estimated age of 50 – 55 years. A more extensive description of this case is presented in a previous publication (Nerlich et al. 2000). The mummy was found in a burial shaft of the tomb complex of the tomb TT95 which had been built in the New Kingdom. The survival of funerary objects in the respective shaft where this mummy was found indicate that this individual most likely lived in the 21st – 22nd dynasty (early IIIrd Intermediate Period, c. 1070 – 700 BC), so that the mummy most obviously dates back to this period.

The mummy was broken into several fragments which, however, could be reconstructed almost completely. Thus, only the arms and the left thigh are missing. The other body segments are wrapped in linen bindings except for the ventral thorax and abdomen which are extensively disrupted. Anthropological estimations (age at death and gender) could be performed at the skull and the pelvis; furthermore, we identified a c. 12 cm long segment of the thoracic aorta lying above the vertebral column.

The completely wrapped right foot was most remarkable, since the careful removal of superficial linen bindings showed a loss of the right big toe. Again, the amputation site was completely covered by intact skin and a tiny soft tissue layer (Fig. 3A). The other digits were normally structured and well preserved. The missing big toe was replaced by a carefully crafted wooden prosthesis which was attached to the fore foot by a textile lace, allowing firm attachment of the prosthesis (Fig. 3B). On the sole of the prosthesis, several scratch marks clearly indicated intravital use (Nerlich et al. 2000).

Radiographs and CT scans of the foot revealed an extensive exostotic bony overgrowth at the distal end of the first metatarsal along with significant demineralization of this bone in its diaphysis (Fig. 3C). The other bones were normally structured, but showed also some mild to moderate hypomineralization. Furthermore, CT scans demonstrated small arterial vessels to have thickened vessel walls with excentric calcifications indicating arteriosclerotic microangiopathy (Fig. 3D). The presence of arteriosclerotic vessel lesions was confirmed by the findings in the segment of the thoracic aorta. This aortal segment revealed extensive calcifications and an ectatic enlargement of the vessel.

In summary, this case represents a unique case of intravital amputation of the big toe, a procedure that must have been survived for at least several months and more probably several years. This is clearly indicated by the extensive bone changes in the remaining metatarsal bone which showed demineralization and distal exostosis formation. The missing toe was replaced by a finely crafted wooden prosthesis which must have been used during lifetime due to plantar erosion and scratch marks. As a cause for the amputation, we have good evidence for necrosis of the big toe (gangrene) due to macro- and microangiopathic arteriosclerosis, most probably, but as yet unproven, associated with diabetes mellitus.

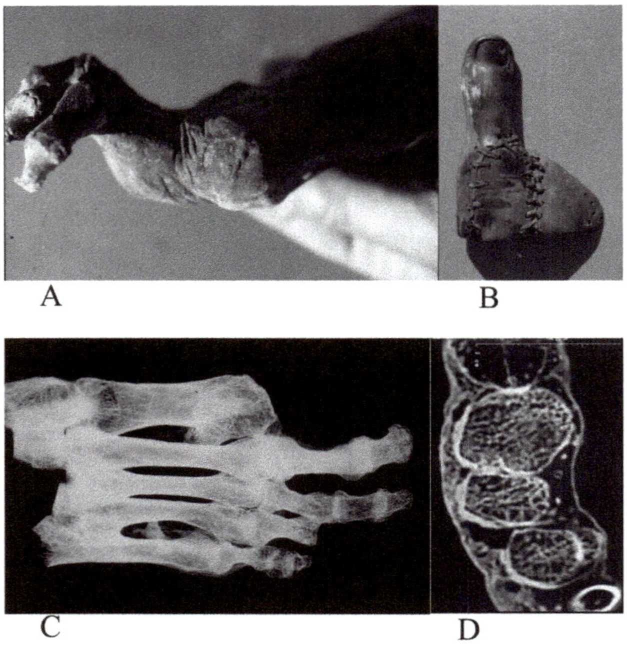

Figure 3: Amputation of the big toe and replacement of the amputation site with a wooden prosthesis: The female mummy suffered from a well-healed amputation of the big toe (A) which had been replaced by a finely crafted wooden prosthesis (B). The amputation must have been performed a considerable time before death since the distal end of the first metatarsal bone shows an exostotic bony overgrowth (C). Small arterial vessels of the fore foot reveal focal calcifications which are seen on CT scans (D).

Discussion

Until now, it has not been proven whether the ancient Egyptians practised surgical treatment or not. The only evidence therefore comes from written sources, such as the medical papyri that describe some surgical treatments, and a few skeletal findings suggesting possible medical treatment (e.g. Kolta 1992). Thus, the identification of two cases with wooden splints as treatment of broken bones (Nunn 1996) and the identification of an amputated forearm with fused ulna and radius (Brothwell et al. 1963) are suggestive of surgery, but did not present definitive proof. Very recently, Dupras et al. (2008) described the skeletons from three individuals from the site of Deir el-Bersheh with evidence of amputation. Two of these individuals (one dating to the Old Kingdom/First Intermediate period, the other Middle Kingdom period) revealed bilateral amputation of their feet through the metatarsals. They showed extensive healing and deformation of the feet. Differential diagnoses indicated that these pathologies were likely due to trauma and not disease. A third individual suffered from extensive perimortem trauma and displays cut marks on his right humeral shaft. These were placed directly over a perimortem butterfly fracture. The cut marks and the position of the right arm bones in the burial suggest that the arm was amputated before death.

In the present report, we now describe three cases originating from the necropolis of Thebes-West which present circumstantial evidence for intravital surgical operations, such as 'neurosurgical' removal of fractured bone fragment(s) and amputation of limbs. All cases can be attributed to the most advanced period of ancient Egyptian culture (New Kingdom until Late Period, i.e. between approx. 1300-700 BC) on the basis of archaeological findings. Two cases were discovered in the so-called 'Tombs of the Nobles' and it can be assumed that they belong to individuals of socially advanced classes. The type of embalming used in the third case also suggests that the affected individual lived in the socially more advanced class.

The complete covering of both amputation sites clearly indicates that both operations were survived for a considerable period of time. This fact was additionally confirmed in the second amputation case where extensive exostotic bony overgrowth indicates that this condition had persisted for long time. Therefore, we have now clear proof that the ancient Egyptians used surgery to remove limbs.

With respect to the underlying causes for the amputations, the two cases described here are different. Thus, the second case showed evidence for both arteriosclerosis of the large and small vessels (macro- and microangiopathy) (Nerlich et al. 2000) which was not seen in the first case. In this latter case, the almost complete removal of the fore foot, along with the lack of arteriosclerotic microangiopathy, suggest even more a (post-) traumatic origin. However, a definite diagnosis cannot be presented here.

As a further, very remarkable finding, the missing big toe in the third case described had been replaced by a carefully crafted wooden prosthesis (Nerlich et al. 2000). With these cases, we provide not only clear-cut evidence for intravital amputation, but also present - to the best of our knowledge - the oldest prosthesis used during lifetime to replace a missing human limb.

References

Brothwell, D.R. and Moller-Christensen, V. (1963) A possible case of amputation dated to 2300 BC. *Man* 244, pp. 192-194.

Dupras, T., Mathews, S., De Meyer, M., Peeters, C. and Vanthuyne, B. (2008) *Just cut it off: Amputation in ancient Egypt.* Paleopathol Assoc. 35th Meeting, Abstracts, pp. 6.

Kolta, K.S. (1992) Medicine in ancient Egypt – bone fractures and their treatment in the medical papyri. *Med. Forum* 26, pp. 13-20.

Nerlich, A., Zink, A., Szeimies, U. and Hagedorn, H.G. (2000) Ancient Egyptian prosthesis of the big toe. *The Lancet* 356, pp. 2176-2179.

Nerlich, A., Zink, A., Szeimies, U., Hagedorn, H. and Rösing, F.W. (2002) Skull trauma in ancient Egypt and evidence for early neurosurgical therapy. In: Arnott B et al. (ed) *Cranial Trepanation in ancient times.* Swets Publ., pp. 191-201.

Nunn, J.F. (1996) *Ancient Egyptian Medicine.* British Museum Press.

Smith, E. and Dawson, W. (1924) *Egyptian Mummies.* Allen and Unwin.

'OTHER THAN' - EGYPTOLOGY AS SCIENCE? A SELECTIVE HISTORY

P.T. Nicholson

Cardiff University

Abstract: *There has been a long established view that Egyptology is something 'other than' science. This view has not especially come from the general public (whose views are in part formed by Egyptologists themselves) but from within Egyptology and archaeology. Many archaeologists working outside Egypt have even come to regard Egyptology as 'other than' archaeology, not least because of its traditional focus on the Egyptian language (for an excellent review see Ray 1978).*

This paper seeks to look at Egyptology from a different perspective, as a part of the science of archaeology, and indeed as a pioneer in that field. It puts forward a, necessarily selective, view of the historical development of Egyptology and examines how it seemingly moved from a pioneer of archaeological science (in its broadest sense) to a language based discipline aside from the mainstream of archaeological thought. It goes on to suggest how Egyptology today is moving forward, and in some cases, leading the development of archaeology as a science whilst still maintaining its distinctive character.

Introduction

I am neither an expert in ancient pharmacy or in medical science, but rather an archaeologist working in Egypt and someone who is interested in the application of science to Egyptology. This paper attempts to review some aspects of the development of Egyptology or Egyptian archaeology and suggest that a focus on scientific method is not a diversion from the aims of the subject as some would see it but is a return to its roots. I would like to try to demonstrate that Egyptology is *not* 'other than' a science.

Beginnings

When Napoleon landed in Egypt in 1798 the country was relatively little known to the West. Arab scholars and travellers had visited over many years, and only now are their observations starting to become known to Europeans through work such as that by Okasha El-Daly (2003; 2005). Such information as was available to Europeans at the end of the 18th Century was limited and of dubious quality.

It was precisely because Egypt was virtually unknown that Napoleon determined that his expedition should be accompanied by a group of 167 scholars, the *savants*, whose job it was to record for science not only archaeological monuments but *everything* of interest which they came upon in Egypt (see Burleigh 2007; Russell 2005; Bednarski 2005). Their brief included the recording of plant and animal species; and the annual Nile flood. So far as the west was concerned then, the study of Egypt began scientifically.

Those who worked in Egypt in the two decades following Napoleon were largely collectors and/or explorers. Customarily they brought antiquities home to their patrons in Europe. Since the inscriptions which covered many of these objects could not be read the objects were studied in their own right, as artistic representations and similarities were sought between them. Attempts were made to understand them in terms familiar to Europeans of the time so, for example, the vessels used to contain mummified viscera were labelled as 'Canopic Jars' because classical writers said that they were the symbols of Canopus, the pilot of Menelaus, who was said to have died in Egypt. He was believed to have been worshipped at the site of Canopus in the form of a jar. This is not science as we would understand it today, but it was an attempt to use existing knowledge, much of it derived from the Classical world (which after all had enjoyed contacts with ancient Egypt), to inform the objects brought from Egypt. It was an attempt to work from the known to the unknown using familiar paradigms, in this case Classical mythology. The emphasis was necessarily on the 'things' and to a lesser extent on the 'places' from which they came. It is true that there was great interest in hieroglyphs but they could not be read, and so had to come second to the objects.

Decipherment

Everything changed on September 22nd, 1822. On that day Champollion's *Lettre à M. Dacier Relative à l'alphabet des Hiéroglyphes Phonétiques* was read to the Academy for Inscriptions and Belles Lettres in Paris (for a convenient English translation see Conrad 1966). This is usually regarded as the birth of Egyptology, though (for Europeans) the subject could be said to have been conceived with the Napoleonic expedition which had unearthed the Rosetta Stone on which the decipherment was built.

Decipherment changed the way in which the study of ancient Egypt was perceived. From here onward the focus was increasingly on language. Objects might be prized for their artistic merit, but valued even more if they also bore a useful text. The view was taken that everything scholars needed to know could be told to them by the Egyptians themselves. All that was needed were sufficient texts on which to work.

The following years were ones of collecting and translating texts. Sites were plundered for the sculptures and papyri they contained because they could – literally –

tell us something. The study of ancient Egypt became part of the study of language and literature which were the raw material of history. It became the study of the written word. Until very recently, for example, Egyptology has been part of the Faculty of Oriental Studies at Cambridge alongside Japanese and other oriental languages; only recently has it moved into the archaeology faculty.

It is obvious that texts in a variety of scripts and languages are of enormous importance to Egyptologists, and we can learn from them about aspects of life which would be difficult, if not impossible, to discern in other ways. Their importance cannot be diminished but at the same time they have sometimes led to a one-sided view of our subject, and one which is 'other than' scientific (if one excludes linguistic science). John Ray (1978) is one of those who has argued for a more integrated and balanced view, and within this there is scope for scientific work.

Twin Histories

After decipherment there are two histories of Egyptology: one celebrates the great discoveries, which often means the great discoveries of *inscribed* material, much of it poorly excavated. The second history applauds the great *archaeologists* and their work. Scientific archaeologists have been influential but much less numerous than the great linguists and historians in the evolution of the subject.

What I would like to do is to mention a few exceptions to the linguistic rule (in all senses!) within Egyptology before looking at where we stand today and the prospects for the future.

If one looks at a few popular histories of Egyptology, such as those by Bratton (1968) or Wortham (1971) one notes that the word 'science' does not feature in their indexes, nor generally in their contents pages. Rather we find chapters such as *'The Dawning of the Great Age: British Soldiers and Explorers in Egypt'* and *'Pyramid Explorers, Pyramidiots and some Obelisks'*. Between the two books there is just one chapter which stands out for its approach: *'Sir Flinders Petrie and the Development of Scientific Excavation'*.

This speaks volumes for the way in which our subject is perceived. Ask almost any Egyptologist to name the great scientific excavators and they will come up with two names: W.M. Flinders Petrie (1853-1942) and George Andrew Reisner (1867-1942). If asked for scientists they will come up with only one name - Alfred Lucas (1867-1945). However, the picture is a little more complicated than that, and we should not attribute all things scientific to this small, if significant, group. As we have seen, the belief in a scientific approach goes back to Napoleon's *savants*, but was essentially lost in the excitement over the decipherment of language.

Against the predominant background of looking for texts there are some notable exceptions who did much to pioneer the scientific approach to the study of Egypt. Amongst these Joseph Hekekyan (1807-1875) deserves particular mention. He was active in Egypt from 1830, but particularly from 1850 was engaged in geological work and drew stratigraphic sections at several sites in Egypt, including at Memphis where he showed one of the Colossi *in situ*. His work is still little known, but forms the subject of a new book by Jeffreys (forthcoming). Hekekyan has been a much neglected figure, and his work predates – sometimes outdoes – that of Petrie.

Flinders Petrie is, of course, one of Egyptology's best known figures and, as Wortham's (1971) chapter rightly emphasises brought a more disciplined and scientific approach to excavation. Unlike some of the great Continental scholars such as Karl Richard Lepsius (1810-1884), Petrie's background was not solely philological, nor did he concentrate only on Egypt. He had a long background of survey work in Britain, and had made an accurate survey of Stonehenge between 1874 and 1877 (Drower 1985, 22-24), as well as of other sites. His skill as a surveyor made him the ideal person to survey the Giza pyramids in 1880-82, a survey made in order to test a fantastical interpretation of the Great Pyramid published by Charles Piazzi Smyth (1819-1900) (Smyth 1864). In other words, Petrie's first work in Egypt had a scientific purpose – it was a hypothesis test, based on the collection of raw data unrelated to Egyptian language.

He went on to undertake numerous excavations in Egypt, but what marks him out from other excavators of the time is the *way* in which he worked. Attention was paid to the objects in graves, and to their relationship to one another and to the body. His tomb cards from the excavations at Abadiyeh and Hu allowed him to develop his sequence dating method, what we would today call seriation (Petrie 1901). He is in fact regarded by statisticians – who know relatively little of his archaeological work – as a pioneer in their field. He also observed carefully, and made careful notes. His contribution to *How to Observe in Archaeology* (British Museum 1929) makes it clear that the positions of archaeological features should be determined by 'bearings to mapped points' (British Museum 1929, 20) and that plans, sketches and photographs are all of importance to the accurate recording of sites. He was also acutely aware of the need to observe detail, and it is perhaps this as much as his other contributions which have set his work apart.

At Amarna, for example, whilst he was looking for historical clues, he realised that he might also be able to reconstruct the glassmaking process (Petrie 1894, 25-7) and he attempted to do so. He was able to do this because he had a wide knowledge of industrial processes and had read well outside the realms of Egyptian history and language. Few of his contemporaries would have been able to make such steps, and still fewer would have been interested to do so – since they took the view that all that was worth knowing had been written down by the Egyptians. It is worth noting that even today we have still not discovered any *written* evidence for the manufacture of glass in Egypt. A scientific, forensic, approach is the only one to offer results in this and many other areas.

Petrie, as someone well aware of scientific developments outside Egyptology, was quick to have analyses made of some of his finds. Some of his glassmaking materials from Amarna were analysed by Dr. William James Russell, F.R.S. (1830-1909) then Lecturer in Chemistry, Medical School, St Bartholomew's Hospital, London (Petrie 1894, 25). It may also have been from Russell that he learned of the potential of x-rays.

The first use of x-rays on Egyptian material seems to have been by Carl Koenig (1859-1936) in 1896 (Böni *et al.* 2004, 203-4). He examined the knee of the mummy of a child and also the mummy of a cat. The same year Thurstan Holland (1863-1941), working in Liverpool, took an x-ray of a bird mummy and it may be that his work was the inspiration for Petrie's x-ray. Boni et al. (2004) comment that Petrie said nothing about the potential of the technique for the study of mummies. However, that may simply be because it was not his purpose to do so and what he wished to do was to illustrate the remains. At one level the fact that he uses the technique, essentially without comment, may imply that he simply recognised this as a tool suitable for use in Egyptology. There was no need to trumpet the fact that it was taken from 'science' because for him Egyptian archaeology *was* part of science, not something separate – something 'other than'.

Petrie is rightly praised for his prompt publication of his work. However, this prompt publication sometimes meant that he did not spend time extensively researching areas of his data. Although he undertook some controlled examinations of mummies (1909, 1911) his work in this area is less prominent than that of others, such as the anatomists Grafton Elliot Smith (1871-1937) and Warren Dawson (1888-1968). However, one of Petrie's pupils made a very significant step toward unifying traditional Egyptology and medical science.

Dr. Margaret Murray (1863-1963) trained with Petrie (see Murray 1963), and not only was she one of the first professional female Egyptologists but she was quick to see the benefit of careful laboratory examination of mummies and worked alongside those with medical training. It was she who examined the mummies of the 'Two Brothers' in Manchester in 1908. This may be regarded as the first time that a trained Egyptologist fully participated in such an autopsy and can be regarded as the first step in the chain of collaborative development which has led up to the establishment of centres such as The KNH Centre for Biomedical Egyptology and to fully collaborative meetings between Egyptologists and scientists such as that at which this paper was presented. Such meetings would have been almost unimaginable even 30 years ago.

Reisner was mentioned above as another, arguably *the* other, well known name in scientific excavation. Like Petrie he was a great observer of his material and made detailed studies of architecture and finds. However, he was generally less interested in laboratory science and one might wonder why so many gifted Egyptologists confined themselves to linguistic studies and the historical narratives which they derived from them. It seems that one reason for this was the view of science held by Egyptologists for much of the late 19th and early 20th centuries, a somewhat different view to that which we take today.

So far as many Egyptologists were concerned, 'science' within Egyptology largely seems to have meant *medical* science, and as we have seen that was dominated by figures such as Smith and Dawson, and later by Armand Ruffer (1859-1917). Beyond medical science, other 'scientific' questions were regarded as having been adequately covered by Petrie and more especially by Lucas.

Alfred Lucas (1867-1945) worked as chemist for the Egyptian government from 1897 to 1945 (Dawson et al. 1995, 263-4). From 1923 to 1932 he was chemist to the Antiquities Service, a role he continued in a consulting capacity until his death. It was Lucas who carried out numerous analyses of Egyptian materials, including mummies, and his book *Ancient Egyptian Materials and Industries* (Lucas 1926) remains a classic work. It first appeared in 1926 and its last revision with an updated bibliography appeared in 1962. It remained as '*the* book on science' other than medical science, in Egyptology until the end of the 20th century and is still in print. It was only in 2000 that a new version with 35 contributors instead of a single author appeared (Nicholson and Shaw 2000).

Many Egyptologists, including myself, greatly admire Lucas's work. However, there can be no better example of the view that 'science is other than' Egyptology than the fact that his book remained in service for so long and that it had no rival. For most Egyptologists the science had been *done* by Lucas and he had provided all that it was necessary to know. Scientific analyses were but an interesting aside to the real business of learning from texts. Whilst Egyptologists would be quick to update their own work as new linguistic discoveries were made, the science was considered to have been done, it was a static field.

The last twenty five years has done much to change that view. Egyptologists such as Barry Kemp began to ask questions which could not be answered by traditional techniques, and which started to involve archaeologists who had not trained in Egyptology, as well as scientists from other disciplines. Rosalie David revived and expanded the pioneering work begun by Murray and in 1986 produced her highly influential book *Science in Egyptology* (David 1986), probably the first time that the words 'Science' and 'Egyptology' had appeared together in a book title. That the book was mainly concerned with medical science in Egyptology, and that within this it contained a great diversity of papers is a testimony to the regeneration of the subject in Britain and beyond. However, it also included a number of papers on aspects of science beyond the medical, on pottery and metalwork for example. Such studies were common in archaeology, but much less so in Egyptology. *Science in Egyptology* could fairly be said to mark the beginning of a new era and a new approach; it was a statement that it was acceptable to be explicitly scientific, and that it did not prevent one from being considered an Egyptologist.

From the work of the many distinguished contributors to that volume has come the development of the research group which now forms Manchester's KNH Centre. That new generation of Egyptologists have also made new links. The West has at last realised what the East knew all along – namely that there is a huge and untapped potential amongst the people of Egypt and the Near East, that the Bedouin of Sinai and the farmers of the Nile Valley know the properties of the plants in their environment, and that by working with these groups and through the collaboration between Egyptian and foreign scientists, there is the potential to develop a much greater understanding of ancient Egyptian pharmacy and medicine.

There have, of course, been significant studies in the flora and fauna of Egypt, but until recently they have not been conducted by or alongside archaeologists. The work of individuals such as Mary Anne Murray and Wilma Wettestrom, trained in archaeology *and* botany has been a great step forward. Similarly Professor Rene Cappers, a botanist, is the co-director (with Willeke Wendrich) of a major archaeological project in the Fayum.

I recently read Jacqueline Campbell's thesis (2007) which provided an excellent example of the use of an interdisciplinary approach. The potential of Egyptologists with a science background working alongside the Egyptian Bedouin and in collaboration with Egyptian scholars cannot fail to yield good results. The use of traditional Egyptological approaches, the study of the language in the terms used for different plants, along with knowledge of the plants and of their pharmaceutical properties offers new insights into all manner of questions. To review the list of contributors to this volume is to see that Egyptology is ceasing to be 'other than' science, and that it is returning to its scientific roots. That is long overdue. It is time that Egyptology resumed its place at the forefront of archaeological science.

Acknowledgements

I am grateful to Professor Rosalie David and Jenefer Cockitt for the invitation to speak at the *Medicine and Pharmacy in Ancient Egypt* meeting. I am also indebted to Janine Bourriau who was kind enough to comment on a draft of this paper.

References

Bednarski, A. (2005) *Holding Egypt: tracing the reception of the Déscription de l'Égypte in nineteenth-century Great Britain.* Golden House Publications.

Böni, T., Rühli, F.J. and Rethy, K. (2004) History of paleoradiology: early published literature, 1896-1921. *Canadian Association of Radiologists Journal* 55 (4), pp. 203-210.

Bratton, F.G. (1968) *A History of Egyptology.* Apollo.

British Museum (1929) *How to Observe in Archaeology.* British Museum (2nd Edn.).

Burleigh, N. (2007) *Mirage: Napoleon's Scientists and the Unveiling of Egypt.* Harper.

Campbell, J.M. (2007) *An Assessment of the Pharmaceutical and Therapeutic Merit of Remedies within the Kahun, Edwin Smith, Ebers and Chester Beatty Ancient Egyptian Medical papyri.* Unpublished PhD thesis. The University of Manchester.

Conrad, V.M. (Trans) Champollion deciphers the hieroglyphs In Ceram, C.W. (ed). *The World of Archaeology.* Thames and Hudson, pp. 162-170.

David, A.R. (ed.) (1986) *Science in Egyptology.* Manchester University Press.

Dawson, W., Uphill, E.P. and Bierbrier, M. (1995) *Who Was Who in Egyptology.* E.E.S.

Drower, M. (1985) *Flinders Petrie: A life in Archaeology.* Gollancz.

El-Daly, O. (2003) Ancient Egypt in Medieval Arabic writings. In Ucko, P. and Champion, T. (eds.) *The Wisdom of Egypt.* UCL Press, pp. 39-63.

El-Daly, O. (2005) *Egyptology: The Missing Millennium: Ancient Egypt in Medieval Arabic Writings.* UCL.

Jeffreys, D. (Forthcoming) *The Survey of Memphis IV: Sources.* E.E.S.

Lucas, A. (1926) *Ancient Egyptian Materials and Industries.* Longman Green and Co.

Murray, M. (1963) *My First Hundred Years.* Kimber.

Nicholson, P.T. and Shaw, I. (2000) *Ancient Egyptian Materials and Technology.* Cambridge University Press.

Petrie, W.M.F. (1894) *Tell el-Amarna.* Methuen.

Petrie, W.M.F. (1901) *Diospolis Parva: The Cemeteries of Abadiyeh and Hu 1898-9.* E.E.F.

Petrie, W.M.F. (1909) *Qurneh.* B.S.A.E.

Petrie, W.M.F. (1911) *Roman Portraits and Memphis IV.* London: B.S.A.E.

Ray, J.D. (1978) The world of North Saqqara. *World Archaeology* 10 (2), pp. 149-157.

Russell, T. (2005) *The Discovery of Egypt: Vivant Denon's Travels with Napoleon's Army.* History Press.

Smyth, C.P. (1864) *Our Inheritance in the Great Pyramid.*

Wortham, J.D. (1971) *British Egyptology 1549-1906.* David and Charles.

ANCIENT EGYPTIAN HEADACHES: *ICHTHYO* - OR *ELECTRO*THERAPY?

R. Park

Independent Scholar

Abstract: *There are several remedies in the medical papyri which refer to the use of 'Nar' fish – the Egyptian catfish. The place of fish and in particular the Nile electric catfish, in art and iconography will be discussed. The diagnosis and treatment of headache as an example – both in the Egyptian and the subsequent Greek and Latin literature - is explored. The tantalising question of whether some unique forms of ichthyotherapy might actually have constituted an early form of electrotherapy is speculated upon.*

Key words: Fried, electric catfish, *Nar*-fish, Torpedo ray-fish

Introduction

It is a nice conjunction that the start of the Christian Era, often known as the 'Age of Pisces', brought to light in Graeco-Roman medical annals a few curious fishy treatments. The ones this paper explores are quite remarkable due to the electrical properties of the fish.

Setting the scene

Almost on a par with the 1,500 recipes in the *Hippocratic Corpus*, the early Egyptian medical papyri could impressively claim some 1,350 general prescriptions (see Estes 1989). However, only 38 treatments call for the use of Nile fish, or parts thereof. In the ancient Egyptian language, 50 names of fish are recorded but sadly 30 words are fish specimen words still to be identified by us. The few species that we can identify in the medical recipes include the mullet, tilapia, Nile perch and catfish.

The first thing to understand about Egyptian medical remedies is that words in the texts may hide an alternate meaning. A Late Roman papyrus [PGM 12.408-444] written in Greek offers the information that the medical ingredient 'Crocodile dung' is a synonym for 'Ethiopian clay'! Since the first English translation of the Ebers papyrus by Ebbell in 1937 gave rise to 'sewage pharmacology', it has been bandied about by medical historians as recently as 2004, that widespread *coprotherapy* was practised in Ancient Egypt (Parkins 2005). Laskaris' work (2005) shows that crocodile excrement is only one of the many listed code names used by Egyptian healer-priests to throw the untrained off the scent.

It is difficult to say at what stage disguised ingredients such as the euphemistic 'tears of the sacred baboon' rather than the actual component 'dill juice' were introduced into the nomenclature of ancient Egyptian medical-magical papyri. Many specialist words for diseases and treatments perplexed the New Kingdom scribes writing up replacement papyri from earlier periods, and required from them the insertion of glossed words with sometimes a great deal of explanation. Suffice to say that we, as well as those New Kingdom scribes copying earlier papyri, do experience many translating difficulties especially when unique words, phrases or concepts could have been codified to preserve the secrecy of the physician's knowledge.

King Narmer's fish

Taxonomy played an important part in depictions of aquatic scenes with 23 different forms of fish, some having subtle distinguishing features that are not obvious to present day Nile fishermen. Catfish belong to 32 families, 7 of which are known in Africa (Burgess 1989). Catfish *per se* are generally called 'nar fish', and five *genera* of Nile river catfish are clearly differentiated by skilled Old Kingdom tomb artists (see Brewer and Friedman 1989).

The earliest representation of catfish which also names the species is the famous record on the slate palette of Narmer - the conquering king who unified Egypt in 3100 BC. The heraldic animal adopted as his totem and used as a spelling rebus for 'Narmer' is uppermost in the *serekh*-frame of both sides of the slate palette. What made the catfish so awesome that the ruthless Narmer chose it over all the Nile predators as his particular emblem of power?

Known in Africa today as the 'Vundu' fish, it was identified as the *Heterobranchus* by Gamer-Wallert (1970, 10). Modern fish breeders describe the heterobranchus as a greedy and voracious predator, capable of growing in captivity to 1 metre in length. The heterobranchus is known to produce a mild electric current, and to an observer above water looking down on it swimming in the water, it is hard to distinguish from its more powerful cousin, the electric catfish *malapterurus electricus* (Figure 1). The electric catfish can grow up to 120 cm in length and weigh over 20 kg and, when attacked, will discharge between 100-450 volts. The electric catfish is nocturnal with a voracious appetite, being most active in feeding 4 to 5 hours after sunset. These features would have been highly significant in Egyptian religious thought – i.e. the passage through the hours of darkness of Osiris who had his phallus eaten by a fish, and even allegorically in the 'Tale of the Two Brothers' where the young brother castrates himself and throws his member to the catfish in the river.

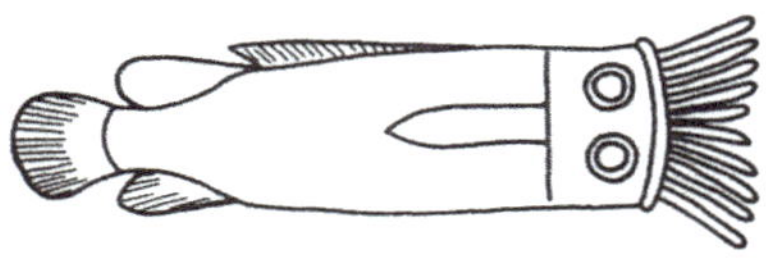

Heterobranchus as depicted on the Narmer Palette

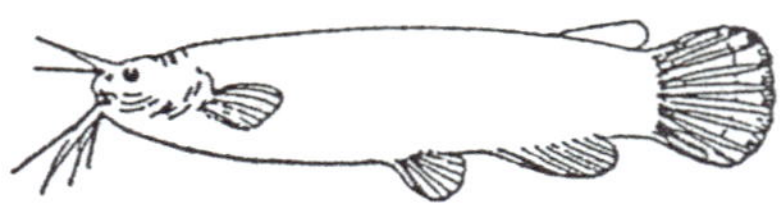

Malapterurus electricus - Nile electric catfish

Figure 1. Line drawings of Heterobranchus and Malapterurus electricus Nile River catfish.

Visual sources can provide a valuable complement to written sources and could modify or add another dimension to what has been left to us in the hieroglyphic accounts. As to the archaeology, Old Kingdom catfish remains have been recovered and recent scholarship (Mysliwiec 2000) claims that the catfish was one of the sacred animals of the feared god Seth, which may account for it not appearing in traditional fish scenes after the Old Kingdom. Likewise, the eel mysteriously disappeared from the visual record in 2000 BC. Herodotus claiming the eel to be the most sacred fish to the Egyptians may be right after all since, in bronze effigies on rare coffins of eels *circa* 25th Dynasty, an association with the god Atum has been made by Mysliwiec (2000, 99). Possibly the art-work 'speaks' of a changing politico-religious situation: in the often published (see Steindorf's 1907 Plate illustration) witty scene from the Saqqara Old Kingdom tomb of Ti, for instance, a mischievously behaved Narmer catfish (capable of living out of water for many hours) is about to die from a smiting blow from a lowly fisherman. The paradox could surely be, that, 700 years after Narmer's conquest, his totem-fish about to expire, still has capable cunning and compulsion to toss his tentacle-barbel onto the boat and steal a loaf of bread.

By the Late Period, the apparent taboo or ban on 'nar'-fish, seems to have lifted. Catfish have been found to be included in votive fish mummies. Strange anthropomorphic catfish deities in the ritual of 'stretching the cord' appear on some 26th Dynasty coffins of the Saite Period (664-525 BC) which brings us to the early Hellenistic period in Egypt. This period of scientific 'consciousness' rediscovered interest in all natural phenomena including electric fish. The 'Greek Enlightenment' and the birth of Hippocratic medicine around 650 BC seems to have resonance or foundation with a bygone age in the Nile valley which I hope to demonstrate further.

The 'nar-ke' fish of Greece

Athenaeus of Naucratis (2nd-3rd century AD) wrote a list of 16 fish he remembered in the Nile. The first fish he named was the Torpedo ray-fish – the 'Narke' (Ghalioungui 1977, 363). Now the ancient Greek name for the electric ray is NA'PKH (νάρκή) and, according to D'A. Thompson (1947, 172), it is a non-Greek word of unknown origin.

The phenomenon of electricity from a fish fascinated many Greek and Latin writers including Plato, Aristotle, Erasmus, Oppian and Pliny – for a fuller list see Sharples (1995). The physician Galen made at least six references to the Torpedo electric ray-fish (*torpedo/nobiliana /marmorata*). Aristotle (384-322 BC) studied the Mediterranean ray-fish and observed that its stun defence mechanism ejected a kind of 'poison or elixir, yet being neither' (*Hist.An620b19-20).* His pupil Theophrastus did describe how the hands of fishermen were numbed when in contact with the fish, and he remembers how the shocks even travelled through the clubs, spearing irons and fishing nets. This recalls the Nile electric-catfish being called *Abu Raash*, the 'Releaser', as the transmitted shock to fishermen makes them release their catch back into the river (Seton-Williams, 1985, 137). To briefly mention a few other citations, let me run through several references:
Plato wittily compared Socrates to 'the flat torpedo fish who *torpifies* those who come near him';
Plutarch in *Moralia* describes the electricity discharge as 'effluvium of its nature'; while Pliny used the descriptive word 'exhalations'.
The 2nd century poet Oppian of Corycus remarked that the electric ray-fish 'on a sudden would eject poisoned charm'.
Dioscorides in his *De material medica* [Book II, 15] says that the electric ray-fish assuages the intensity of chronic pains when 'plastered' (translated by Beck, 2005, 98) around the head.
His contemporary Pliny (*Book XXXII*, 94) discusses the medical and especially gynaecological *prolepsus* (*ib.105 [ch.Diosc.ii.15]*) of and in relation to electric fish treatments. It is Pliny who apparently was the first to differentiate between the two unconnected electric fish – that is, the Mediterranean torpedo-fish and the Nile catfish.
Thompson (*ibid*., 171) assumed in his commentary on Pliny's knowledge of electric fish that:

> *'As the marine Torpedo would be awkward to manage and difficult to keep alive, one may imagine that Pliny was referring, in part at least, to the Egyptian fish*'.

The Right Word

It can be seen from the above, that the Greek philosophers and Roman doctors had a problem finding the quintessential word to describe the electric organ discharge belonging to their curious Mediterranean fish. We can only make guesses as to how the Egyptians viewed the concept of Nature's electricity, and, if they came up with an appropriate word, what it might have been.

It should be borne in mind that fishermen may tend to cling to very ancient words. The Arabic name *ra'ad* by which Nile fishermen even today identify the electric catfish literally translates as 'thunder' (this brings to mind: a 'thunderbolt' or 'lightning'). According to Brewer and Friedman (*ibid.*), the word implies a 'sense of quivering' experienced by those who touch the creature.

The medical doctor Engelbert Kaempfer, who did scientific research in the Persian Gulf in 1712, said the Torpedo fish there was similarly called *ra'ad* (Carrubba, 1996, 9).

In hieroglyphs, the word 'to tremble' *snwr* uses a fish determinative. The word in our medical recipe for 'fried' uses a fire determinative, but more of this later on. One word *h3t* (pronounced 'kat'), seemingly linked in concept, has several meanings either the fish we call 'the elephant-snout or sharp-nosed fish', or other meanings e.g. 'corpse' or 'cadaver', as well as 'marshy swamp' and a 'quarry or mine' (see Schumann-Antelme and Rossini 2002, 122).

It is interesting that this elephant-snout fish is another type of electrically charged Nile fish (*Gymnarchus* of the *Mormyriformes* family) with an organ discharge between 196-326 Hz. It is the sacred emblem of the Oxyrhynchus Nome and this 'Oxyrhynchus' hieroglyph is used by the Ancient Egyptians as a repeating word *h3h3ty* to mean 'thunderstorm' (Gardiner 1957, 586).

There may not be any surviving written evidence of the morbid capabilities of the electric Nar-fish, but a 6th Dynasty Dahshur tomb scene (unpublished item 1784, Cairo Museum) shows the electrocution of a decoy calf in a variation of one of those typical cattle-crossing river scenes with a lurking crocodile below.

Ebers 250

As this discussion must be brief, let us dive into the semantics of the medical prescription of Ebers 250 – and review a unique type of headache and its suggested cure. The translation of Ghalioungui (1987) is herewith shown in hieroglyphs and transliteration (Figure 2):
Kt nt mrwt m gs tp dnnt n<r snwh hr mrht gs tp im r hrw 4

> '*Another for disease in one half of the head: skull of catfish fried in oil/fat; the 'half-head' (? condition) is anointed therewith on 4 days*'.

Breaking this down a bit, and I am grateful to John Nunn's comments here (personal communication October 1993):
Mrht is 'oil' or 'grease' but Westendorf gives an alternative meaning of 'ointment' (or 'unguent').

The second *gs* at the end of the sentence – not to be confused with the *gs tp* (= 'half head' meaning 'migraine') at the beginning of the sentence – means 'anoint' or 'smear'.

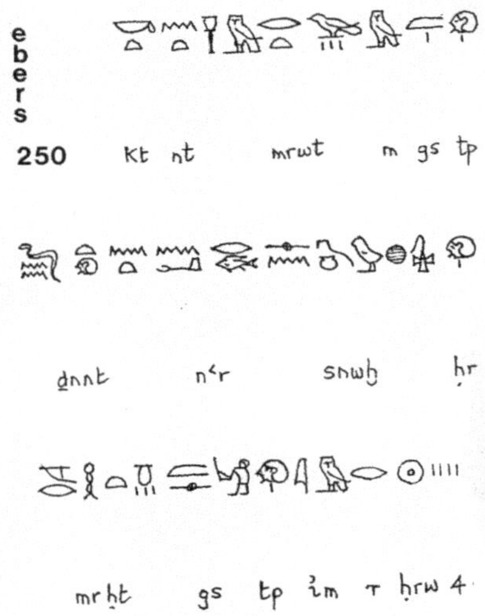

Figure 2. Ebers 250 in hieroglyphs and transliteration.

Snwh is a very troublesome word which Westendorf translates as 'overcooked' after a three-page long discussion, in German; whereas Faulkner translates the word as 'boil'; Nunn agreed 'fried' was by far the better word.

In her Chapter contribution 'Rationality versus Irrationality in Egyptian Medicine in the Pharaonic and Graeco-Roman Periods' David (2004, 141) gives a simpler translation of Ebers 250 as:

> '*Another [remedy] for suffering in the head. The skull of a catfish fried in oil*'.

Ebers 250 French translation by Bardinet (1995, 289) fries up the head of a European catfish:

> '*crane de silure (Silurus glanis), frit dans la graisse/huile. Enduire la tête avec (cels), quatre jours de suite*'.

With the patient having a severe migraine attack, why would the Egyptian healer want to take time out to fry up in an oil medium the head of a dead fish which is already naturally oily anyway? In this instance, linguists are translating a word with a determinative sign for 'fire' from a medical corpus. It might very well have a more technical meaning akin to 'diatherme' for example, rather than debating which culinary method best suits cooking the head of the catfish. My suggestion is that the Egyptian word for 'fried', rather than denoting a mode of cooking, is the frying capability of the fish – the best-fit technical word the Egyptians could come up with for the related concepts of 'electrophysiology'. The prescription perhaps becomes more lucid as a topical application or counter-irritant if it is reworded:

'head of the frying-Narfish (or the fish which causes 'to fry') applied to the migraine sufferer's head (once every) 4 days'.

Egyptian Catfish Remedy

Apart from the electric catfish remedy, the 'upside down' catfish *Synodontis* with its poisonous spine features in several recipes; and in the Ramesses V medical papyrus there is even the provocative use of the blood of the sacred Oxyrhynchus fish. Notwithstanding the Heterobranchus or the Malapterurus variety – both with electric charges - the Nar-fish occurs in only five prescriptions of the Ebers papyrus (128, 250, 639, 656 and 730). Ebers 128 duplicates in Hearst 203, and Ebers 656 is copied in the Ramesses V papyrus.

Worthy of mention is the use of the Nar-fish for a toe affliction in the Hearst papyrus (H. XIII, 10) dated to the reign of Tuthmosis III (1479-1425 BC). Elsewhere I have argued (Park 2006) that the Egyptian word *sfw-t* is the most likely word for gout, and where the recommended application is of Narfish, plus honey - the honey would seemingly serve as a barrier to skin burning. Alternatively, this could have been used as a conductive 'jelly' to the anticipated 100-350 volts from a tormented Nile electric catfish! The electric fish which Scribonius Largus would have used does not have quite the same ferocity of up to 200 volts, but the charge of the Torpedo fish is better conducted in salt-water.

Scribonius Largus (1-50 AD) in *Compositiones* advised therapeutic shocks from the Torpedo ray-fish in the management of both headache (*XI*) and gout (*CLXII*) – the latter being the celebrated case of his patient, a freedman from Tiberius, who undertook to stand on the shore and have repeated shocks from the ray-fish beneath his feet, and this apparently numbed the gout pain. For a torturous cure for chronic and unbearable head pain, Nero's physician Largus recommended the application of two or three live torpedo fish to the head.

That great advocate of traditional 'Hippocratic medicine', Galen (129-216 AD) researched the medical texts in Alexandria at his disposal, many of them obviously being quite ambiguous. In his experiments of wanting to know if dead electrical fish might be useful in the treatment of headache, and possibly hysteria, he found negative results. But then, from '*On the temperaments and Properties of Simple Drugs (XI.48==XII)*, he writes:

> *'It is often reported that the whole sea animal – the Torpedo fish – applied to the head can cure a headache, or check a disturbed womb (cf. Pliny's prolapsus?), but I tried it and found it did not work. Then I thought, perhaps one should apply it to the head while it was still alive, and found it acted like other things which can dull sensation. I believe that the first man to use this treatment started from this sort of reasoning'.*
>
> (Nutton, personal communication 1995)

Head-pain in Egypt

When ill, the Egyptians called in either a priest or a doctor who consulted his written manuals for traditional treatment. But when such specialists were not available, such as in the case (reported in Davies and Friedman, 1998, 176) of a 19th Dynasty village healer at Deir el-Medina, the problem of the 'head pain demon' was dealt with by cursing him and making a talisman to ward him away. In the more learned medical texts, notably the Ebers, Hearst and Berlin papyri, many different types of headache are described. These include 'excess fluid' headache and 'women's' headache amongst a list of 9 headaches in the Ebers papyrus alone. Remedies for bothersome head pain are also catered for in the medico-magical prescriptions of the Leiden and Budapest papyri written very late in Egyptian history, when all known medical knowledge of the Egyptians, Hebrews, Greeks and Romans had amalgamated at Alexandria.

Let us be reminded that the mention of migraine in Egyptian is called by Nunn (1996, 93): 'One of the most celebrated passages in the medical papyri'. Goodwin recognised the 'half-head' - the Egyptian word *ges tep* - as the origin of the Greek word for migraine as long ago as 1873; and, as philologist Sir Alan Gardiner said in 1935: 'There could be no more eloquent testimony to the dependence of Greek upon Egyptian medicine'. The written record for *ges tep* appears in Egyptian records in three known instances: around 1500BC in Ebers 250 (47.14-15) which we have just discussed, followed 3 centuries later in Chester Beatty V papyrus (verso 4, 1-19); and finally in the Leiden (1,348 [8]) thought to date to 250 AD – a time span of 1,750 years.

As to the Nar-fish, it is probably a safe assumption that the strange fish capable of air-breathing on land, having no scales but whisker-like barbels, will always remain as a 'cat'-fish to early Egyptians and modern lexicographers alike. We do not know how the secret cult of Sekhmet healer-priests treated headache. Sekhmet, the big Cat deity herself, often described as a 'burning and scorching' (link to 'fry'?) goddess, could have had those easy to rear fish looking like cats reared in the ponds of her temple precinct for the purpose of shock-cures, alongside the prerequisite catfish bred for votive mummy offerings. As every simple fisherman knows, when mis-handling the electric catfish, 400 volts will zap away a pre-existing headache or, alternately, cause one. It would be best to kill the Nar-fish first as can be witnessed in the Luxor fish market today – for there you will find live catfish in the 'catch of the day' except for *malapterurus electricus* who has a stun-gun bullet hole in its head.

Conclusion

One and a half thousand years before the birth of Hippocrates and those who followed in his tradition, the ancient Egyptians recorded in the Ebers papyrus the Nile 'nar' fish for the treatment of that most difficult to manage headache *viz.* migraine, and a toe-swelling ailment (most probably gout). In the first and second centuries AD Graeco-Roman medical writers described the use of the Mediterranean 'nar-key' fish for headache and gout, which I find to be too much of a coincidence. Modern scholars presume *the* therapeutic catfish indicated in the Ebers papyrus to have been dead. But, like Galen, I suspect King Narmer's fiery fish worked better on intractable medical conditions whilst it was still alive.

Acknowledgement

The author wishes to thank Professor Vivian Nutton for his help in the Galen translation.

Bibliography

Bardinet, T. (1995) *Les papyrus Médicaux de l'Égypte Pharaonique.* Fayard.

Beck, L. (2005). *Pendanius Dioscorides of Anarzabus translation of 'De material medica'.* Olms-Weidmann.

Brewer, D. and Friedman, R. (1989). *Fish and Fishing in Ancient Egypt.* Aris and Phillips.

Burgess, W. (1989). *An Atlas of Freshwater and Marine Catfishes.* T.F.H. Publications.

Carrubba, R. (1996) translation of *Engelbert Kaempfer [1712] 'Exotic Pleasures'.* Southern Illinois University Press.

David, R. (2004). Rationality versus Irrationality in Egyptian Medicine in the Pharaonic and Graeco-Roman Periods. In Horstmanshoff, H. and Stol, M. (eds.), *Magic and Rationality in Ancient Near Eastern and Graeco-Roman Medicine.* Studies in Ancient Medicine 27. Brill.

Davies, V. and Friedman, R. (1998). *Egypt Uncovered.* British Museum Press.

Estes, J. (1989). *The Medical Skills of Ancient Egypt.* Canton.

Gammer-Wallert, I. (1970). *Fische und Fischkulture in alten Ägypten.* Weisbaden; Ägyptologische Abhandlingen 21.

Gardiner, A. (1957). *Egyptian Grammar.* Griffith Institute.

Ghalioungui, P. (1977). *Food: The Gift of Osiris – Volume II.* Academic Press Inc.

Ghalioungui, P. (1987). *The Ebers Papyrus. A New English Translation, Commentaries and Glossaries.* Cairo.

Laskaris, J. (2005). *Drug Synonyms and the Transmission of Pharmaceutical Knowledge* (in press). Paper read at Approaches to Ancient Medicine Conference, Newcastle, August 2005

Mysliwiec, K. (2000). *New Riddles in West Saqqara – Discoveries and Conservation work of the Polish-Egyptian Mission in Autumn 2000.*

Mysliwiec, K. (2000). *The Twilight of Ancient Egypt.* Cornell University Press.

Nunn, J. (1996). *Ancient Egyptian Medicine.* British Museum Press.

Park, R. (2006). *Gout in Ancient Egypt.* Paper read at History of Ancient Medicine Conference, Reading University, August 2006.

Parkins, M. (2005). Pharmacological Practices of Ancient Egypt. In Whitelaw, W. (ed.) *History of Medicine Days 2004.* Calgary.

Seton-Williams, V. and Stocks, P. (1985). *Blue Egypt Guide, 3rd edition.* Black.

Thompson, D'Arcy (1947). *A Glossary of Greek Fishes.* Oxford University Press.

Sharples, R. (1995). *Theophrastus of Eresus: Sources for his Life, Writings, Thought and Influence, Commentary volume 5, Sources on Biology.* Brill.

HEALING MEASURES: *dja* AND *oipe* IN ANCIENT EGYPTIAN PHARMACY AND MEDICINE

T. Pommerening

Institute for Egyptology and Ancient Near Eastern Studies Johannes Gutenberg University Mainz

Abstract: *At the dawn of the New Kingdom (ca. 1550 BC) an innovation in Egyptian medicine emerged: prescriptions suddenly began to indicate precise measurements for each ingredient in a preparation, particularly those remedies prescribed for internal administration. This metrological information was expressed in two systems of dyadic fractions, but without any specification of their base units of measurement. Hence, the absolute quantity of each substance used in a given remedy remains unknown. To establish the efficacy of ancient Egyptian medicines and ascertain the dosage form, it is necessary to know the exact units of measurement used in these recipes. The aim of this paper is to summarize my works on the units dja and oipe which I recovered as the main units in a healing context.*

Key words: Horus Eye; medicinal papyri; measuring cups; fractions; metrology

Introduction

Approximately 2000 ancient Egyptian formulae are known at the present time, a quarter of which contain metrological information consisting of one or two fractional numbers following an ingredient.

Studying these numbers in the extant formulae, two sequences of dyadic fractional numbers emerge (Fig. 1). The two columns on the left show the so-called Horus Eye numerals in hieratic script and hieroglyphic transcription. When combined together, the hieroglyphic signs constitute the Eye of Horus (Fig. 2).

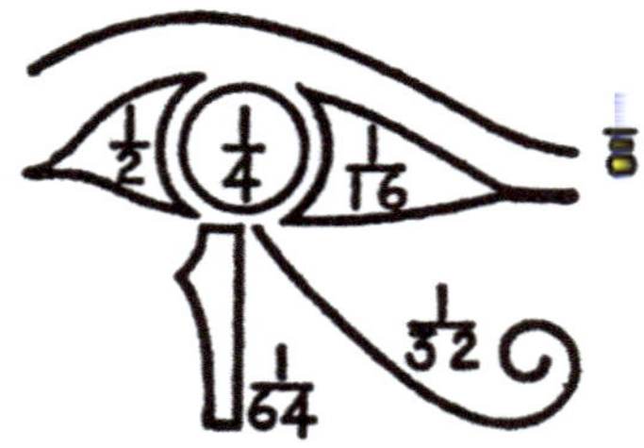

Figure 2: Eye of Horus

It is common editorial practice to transliterate hieratic papyri into hieroglyphic characters. Although no palaeographical records of the hieroglyphic Horus Eye fractions have survived from the period before the 19th dynasty, these hieroglyphic fractions are nevertheless used in modern editions of papyri from earlier periods. In my opinion this correlation between the hieratic and the Horus Eye is admissible from the moment when the ancient Egyptians began to indicate exact measurements in their medicinal texts, because medicinally and mythologically there are strong connections between the Horus Eye and the measuring vessels used for medical purposes, as I will presently demonstrate. Furthermore, this endeavour to interpret the hieratic signs as parts of the Horus Eye also enables us to distinguish linguistically between the two systems of numerals for fractions found in the medical papyri. The 'normal' one is shown in the two columns on the right.

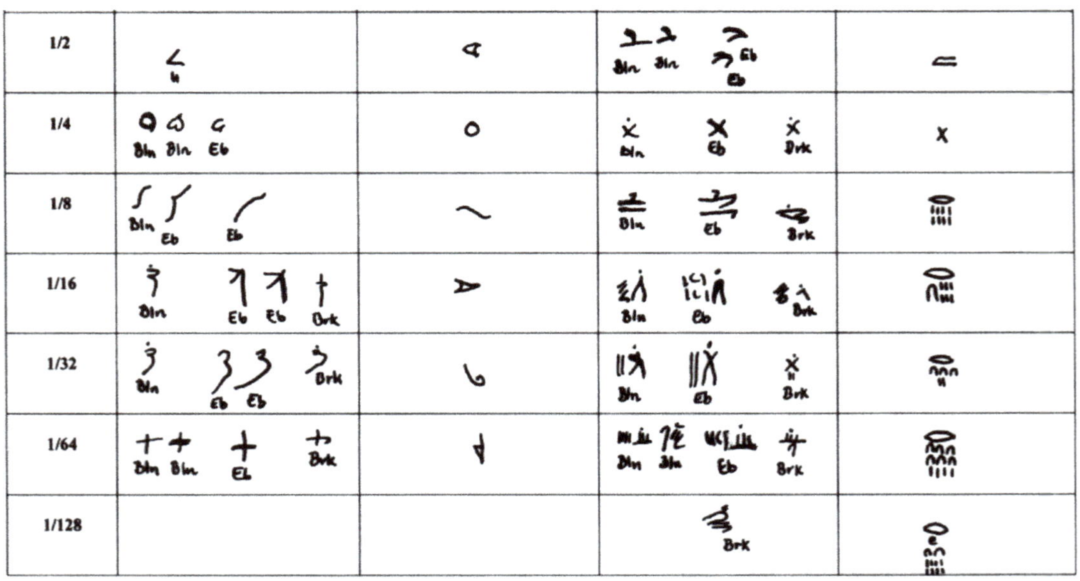

Figure 1: Horus Eye number series and normal fraction series hieratic / hieroglyphs

While the smallest number of the Horus Eye series is 1/64, the smallest number in the 'normal' fraction series is 1/128. Looking at the two systems a question arises: To which units of measurement do these fractions refer? Examination of numerous sources show the Horus Eye fractions to refer to the unit of volume called the hekat, its double, triple or quadruple – the latter later being called oipe (in Egyptian *jp.t*) – which conventionally are called grain-measures. The 'normal' fractions, on the other hand, are used to express the numerical value of any unit, even of length or weight. Besides, the normal notation can not only be used for dyadic fractions but exists for any unit fraction (like 1/5 or 1/7) and also for ⅔ and ¾. In the medicinal context, however, we do not find any fractions other than dyadic ones.

Let us take a closer look at the four interpretations suggested so far for the 'normal' fractions in a medicinal context, as exemplified by translations of pEbers 153 (32,15-17) (Fig. 3):

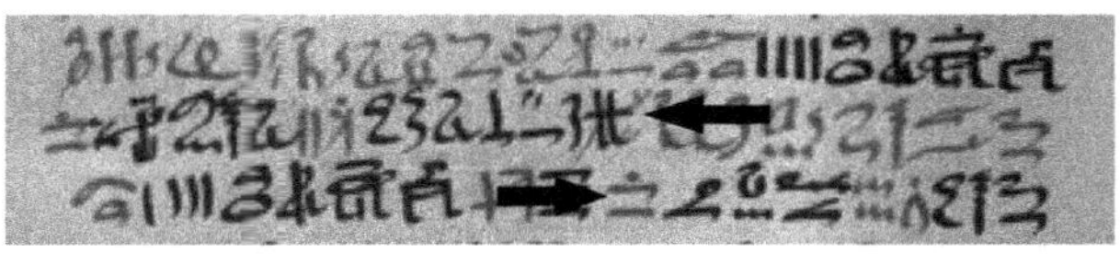

Figure 3: pEbers 153 (32,15-17) in Facsimile

Wolfhart Westendorf (1999, 572):
„...Inneres der Johannisbrotfrucht (*ḏ3r.t*) 1/32 ro;
frischer Brei (von Datteln ?) 1/8 ro;
Wachs 1/16 ro;
Fett der Gans 1/8 ro; ..."

Bendix Ebbell (1937, 44): [1 ro = 1/32 hin]
„...the interior of *ḏ3rt* 1 ro [= 1/32 hin],
fresh porridge 4 ro [= 1/8 hin],
wax 2 ro [= 1/16 hin],
goose-grease 4 ro [= 1/8 hin], ..."

Thierry Bardinet (1995, 271):
„...pulpe de plante-djaret: 1/32 [hekat];
pâte, fraîche: 1/8 [hekat];
cire: 1/16 [hekat];
graisse d'oie: 1/8 [hekat]; ..."

Hildegard von Deines et al. (1958, 142f.):
„...Inneres der Koloquinte (*ḏ3r.t*) 1/32 [5-ro];
frischer Brei (*3ḥ*) 1/8 [5-ro];
Wachs 1/16 [5-ro];
Fett (*ʿḏ*) der Gans 1/8 [5-ro]; ..."

Wolfhart Westendorf relates the numbers of the 'normal' fraction series to the unit ro, Bendix Ebbell to the unit hin. In Ebbell's translation the ro appears, because he converts the fractions assigned to the unit hin into ro units according to the equation 1 ro = 1/32 hin. However, he derives the measures 1 ro, 4 ro, 2 ro and 4 ro. Thierry Bardinet assigns the fractions to the unit hekat, Hildegard von Deines et al. assumes a so-called 5-ro-unit.

So far, the solutions proposed by modern philologists and medical historians have been confusing and contradictory. The translations of the metrological elements in the formulae differed according to the philological traditions of the translators. Only for the Horus Eye fractions behind the last ingredient water (1/16 + 1/64, cf. Fig. 5 column 1, line 5), are they in total agreement: All four authors relate them to the hekat measure, converting the hekat to ro via the formula 1/64 hekat = 5 ro.

The four units of measurement postulated until now for the 'normal' fraction series differ considerably in volume. It is difficult for the difference to be displayed graphically, since one hekat is 3200 times the size of one ro (Fig .4).

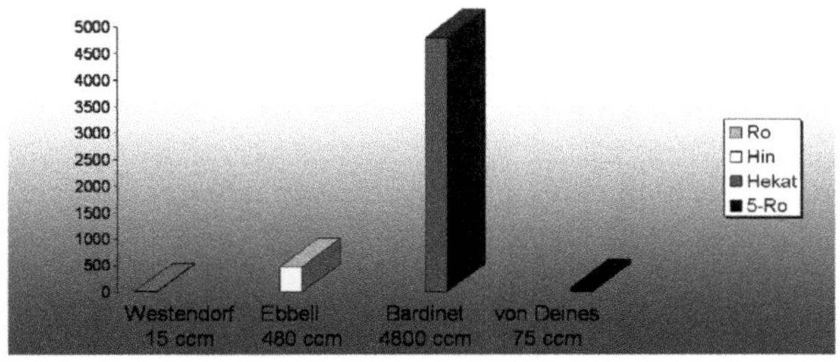

Figure 4: The approximate volumes of the suggested units

Figure 5 shows the volumes of each ingredient converted into millilitres according to the different interpretations of the fractional units. It is obvious that not only does the total volume of the four formulae range between 380 and 2025 millilitres, but the concentrations of the ingredients suspended in water also vary significantly. The effects of these interpretations of quantities on our understanding of ancient Egyptian medicines, including their manufacture and efficacy, are considerable.

	Westendorf 1-Ro-unit	Ebbell Hin-unit	Bardinet ¹Hekat-unit	v. Deines 5-Ro-unit
the interior of *ḏ3rt*	0,468 ml	15 ml	150 ml	2,34 ml
fresh porridge	1,875 ml	60 ml	600 ml	9,37 ml
wax	0,937 ml	30 ml	300 ml	4,68 ml
goose-grease	1,875 ml	60 ml	600 ml	9,37 ml
Water (¹Hekat-interpret.)	375,00 ml	375 ml	375 ml	375 ml
Σ	380,16 ml	540 ml	2025 ml	400,8 ml

Figure 5: Concrete volumes according to modern interpretations, pEbers 153

The aim of this paper is to summarize the most important results of my research which re-establishes the true units of volume – the dja and the oipe – used in these prescriptions. The results (Pommerening 2003a/b) have been corroborated by a complete and thorough examination of all relevant metrological data: reliefs, drawings, texts, and objects. All references are to be found *in extenso* in Pommerening (2005), except for the last proof in this paper, which is published in the present context for the first time.

The most instructive evidence is three measuring vessels inscribed with lines which subdivide the volume dyadically (Fig. 6). The two shown on the left bear hieroglyphic inscriptions above the lines indicating the name of the whole unit – dja – and numbers of the normal dyadic fractional sequence from 1/2 down to 1/128. The numbers display a remarkable correspondence to the 'normal' fractions found in medical texts. In addition to the dja-mark, a half and a whole hin-unit are recorded on the vessels, providing a strong argument for them being medicinal measuring cups, given that the hin-measure is the only unit of measurement appearing *expresso verbo* in the medical texts – even though it is used only in combination with whole numbers.

If we consider the vessel type, which would be suitable to measure all kinds of pharmaceutical ingredients (solid, liquid, molten, greasy), we have a second strong argument for assuming these objects were medicinal measuring cups and the dja a unit of medicinal measurement.

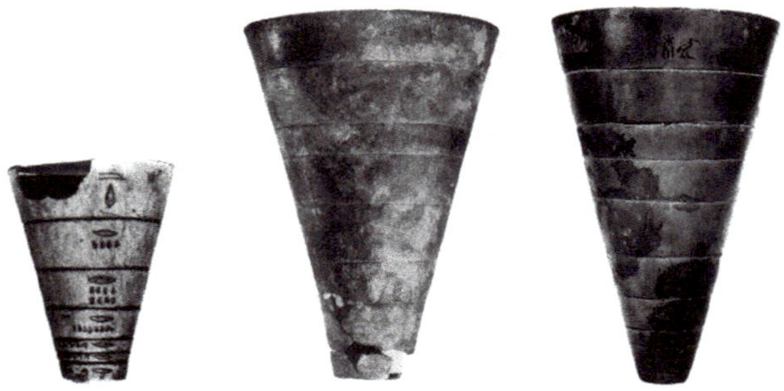

Figure 6: Conical cups with measurement details (Left – Bronze, Cairo Egyptian Museum JE28187 (CG3576); Centre – Silver, Cairo Egyptian Museum JE28493 (CG3577); Right – Bronze, Paris Louvre E2511-N891)

The oldest measuring cup (on the right in fig. 6) does not show metrological markings above the lines, but the volumes of the engraved segments leave no doubt that the units and their subdivisions are identical with those on the other cups. The only inscription is the name, Djehutjmes' = Thoth is born, which was very frequent in the 18th dynasty and from which we may infer that the cup dates back to the time when the innovation of exact measurements in medicine emerged.

The precise volume of each segment of the Louvre cup has been determined by Georges Daressy in 1897 (Daressy 1897), whilst Alfred Lucas and Alan Rowe determined the volumes of the Cairo cups in 1940 (Lucas/Rowe 1940). Both found a dja/hin proportion to be about 3 to 2, which fits very well with the Egyptian way of reckoning. On closer inspection however, the proportion is 8 to 5, which primarily would not appear to be an Egyptian system. From a different perspective however, it is precisely this proportion that permits us to reconstruct the foundations of ancient Egyptian metrology for medicinal units. Enlarging the relation 5 Hin = 8 Dja recovered from the measuring vessels (1) multiplying both – numerator and denominator – by 8 results in the equation where 40 hin is equal to 64 dja (2). From other texts it is evident that 40 hin equal 1 oipe (3); hence 1 oipe equals 64 dja (4).

(1) 5 hin = 8 dja

x 8

(2) 40 hin = 64 dja

(3) 40 hin = 1 oipe

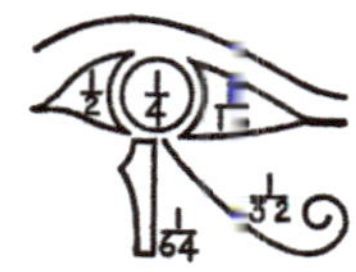

(4) 1 oipe = 64 dja

: 64

(5) 1/64 oipe = 1 dja!

As stated above, the fractional numbers used for the oipe, as well as those of the hekat and its multiples are represented hieroglyphically as the Horus Eye parts with 1/64 as the smallest fraction. The smallest fraction of the oipe, 1/64 oipe, therefore corresponds with one dja.

In the hieratic record, the smallest Horus Eye fraction is denoted by a shape similar to a modern plus-sign (Fig. 1) – hence, I will call it 'plus' from here on. In the medicinal texts we find multiples of this number expressed as several +-signs (eg.) or as one sign followed by strokes (eg.). Furthermore the combinations a–d are attested with 1/2 and 1/4 being fractions of the 'normal' fractional series.

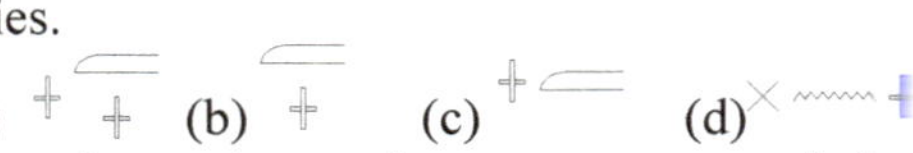

From these observations we may conclude that in the medicinal texts the smallest fraction in the Horus Eye series 1/64, written as +, is itself a base unit of measurement and a starting point for a new dyadic fraction series. This new series, to be found only in medico-magical and mythological contexts, subdivides progressively to the fraction 1/128, similar to the fractions marked on the measuring vessels. This smallest fractions volume given by the measuring cups is 2,34 millilitres and equals 1/8192 oipe (Fig. 7).

A hieratical text section in Papyrus Cairo, JdE 86637 also clearly shows the connection with the normal dyadic fractions to the Horus Eye numeral 1/64; it reads: "The Ennead is in adoration, when this eye is on its place, being revised in all its components. +, 1/2+, 1/4, 1/8, 1/16 [...] are in it every time it is counted." (numerals see below).

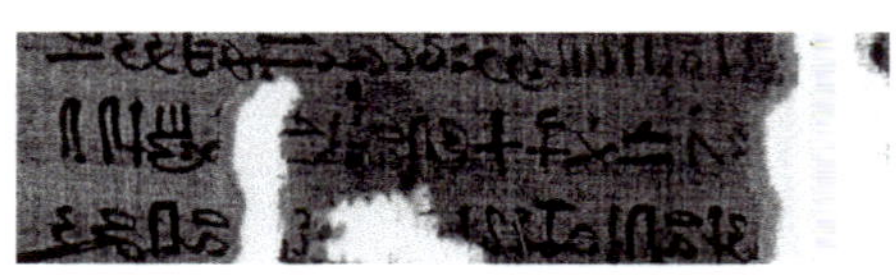

Starting with the + and 1/2+, a dyadic series of 'normal' fractional numbers follows, showing once more that the smallest fraction of the Horus Eye series (1/64), hieratically written as a +, is subdivided by 'normal' dyadic fractions. Once again the sequence of the numerals is identical with that on the measuring cups.

What is so remarkable about the Horus Eye fraction 1/64 is revealed by recalling the myth of the Horus Eye. According to this tradition, Seth robbed Horus of one Eye, and Thoth recovered it. In order to rebuild and heal the damaged eye, the latter counted its parts and made it whole. The restored eye was called Udjat, to be translated as 'that which is healthy, intact, complete'. Now if we add up the fractional parts of the grain measure, 1/2, 1/4, 1/8, 1/16, 1/32 and 1/64, we obtain 63/64, so it is 1/64 short of unity. This missing part of 1/64 or 1 dja is required to complete the Udjat and to heal it. 1 dja-measure is therefore the unit of measurement that heals the Udjat-eye

From the time of the New Kingdom onwards, Udjat could also be a designation for the cylindrical *jp.t*-measuring vessel and for the unit of measurement oipe.

Hence it should be noted that the hieroglyphic sign *ḏꜣ*, representing the unit dja on the measuring cups, is also a very common abbreviation for *wḏꜣ* = 'being whole'. Beyond that meaning, the word *(w)ḏꜣ*, written with the determinative of a scroll, stands for 'rest'.

The first traces of + being a unit relating to the hekat and double-hekat can be found in the MK. These MK-'+'-units had a maximum subdivision of 1/4. Later in the MK, when more precise results in reckoning were required, an arithmetic unit was invented which was called ro, with 5 ro = 1/64 hekat = 1 dja (of the basic hekat). The term ro does not constitute a specific unit of measurement but denotes a particular fraction of a whole, like the dja, both of which can depend on different base units, such as oipe, hekat, etc. Therefore, the absolute value of both, ro and dja, would be different depending on the respective base unit. pCarlsberg 182 + PSI 177, Fragment B, l. 25-29 mentions: 'The Udjat, which is intact, has been brought to 320 ro, corresponding to 40 hin'. We remember that 40 hin are equal to 1 oipe (= 1 quadruple-hekat). Here, 1 ro has a volume of 60 millilitres. The 'normal' fractions have often been misinterpreted by modern scholars as belonging to the unit ro.

How can we be sure that the dja units found in the medicinal recipes are based on oipe units rather than hekats or its multiples? The fundamental units in the MK had been the basic hekat and the double hekat, whilst in the NK it was the quadruple hekat, which came to be known as oipe. In medicinal texts from the period prior to the NK, no fractional units have been documented. The oldest surviving medicinal measuring cup dates back to the NK, its dja unit like that on the other two vessels being about 300 millilitres and therefore is based on the oipe. (The MK-dja is 75 millilitres). No vessels of this type have been found from the MK.

Therefore it is clear that the 'normal' fractions in the medicinal texts 1/2 to 1/128 have to be assigned to the dja measure based on the oipe and that the Horus Eye fractions 1/2 to 1/64 in the prescriptions must be assigned to the quadruple-hekat (i.e. the oipe) and not as previously recognised to the simple hekat (Fig. 7). Both series are linked to the fraction 1/64 oipe = 1 dja, so that there exists one single extended volume series with binary divisions. The fractions of the larger series, the Horus Eye fractions, may be measured in multiples of the dja-mark in the conical measuring cups as for instance 1/32 oipe equals 2 dja.

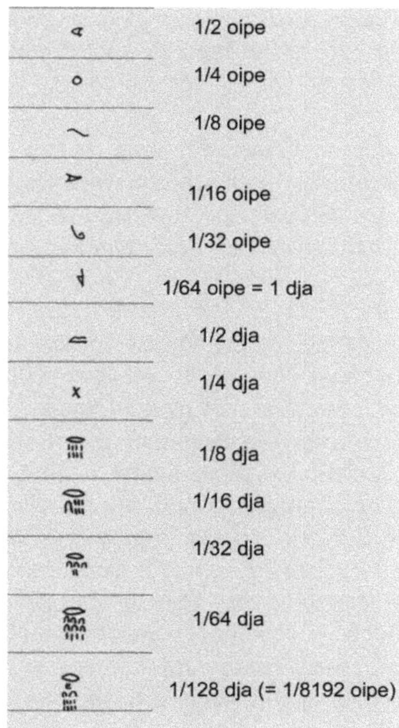

Figure 7: Relations between dja and oipe

The unit dja and the measuring cups move still deeper into a ritual and medicinal context when we consider the text and image of a temple relief in Kom Ombo (Kom Ombo II, 271, no. 950) (Fig. 8).

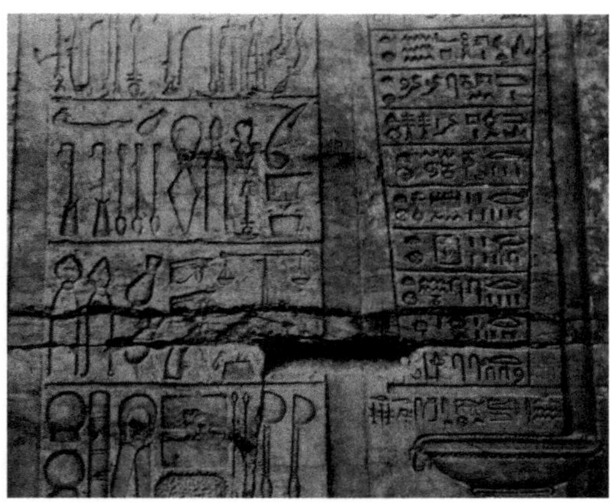

Figure 8: Kom Ombo, medical instruments and measuring cup

Next to the well-known depiction of a cupboard containing medical instruments, an image of one of these measuring cups is found, integrated into an offering ritual between the king and Haroeris. On the depicted cup, in addition to the inscriptions known from the actual objects preserved in the museums, place names are inscribed immediately after each measure. Starting from Elephantine, which marks the smallest fraction 1/128, these ancient Egyptian towns reproduce the course of the river Nile. Only in the Delta area do they deviate from the accurate south-north order. The inscribed units of measurement and their subdivisions on this cup are in every respect equal to those on the material cups analysed above. The measures carved are 1 and ½ hin, as well as 1 dja, which is subdivided dyadically down to 1/128 dja. An inscription inserted between the measuring cup and a water basin underneath reads: 'pleasant water coming from the interior to clean the Eye of Re and the Eye of Horus'.

The cup itself is integrated into a ritual in which medicinal instruments and healing water as well as two Udjat eyes are offered to Haroeris, a ritual closely connected with the myths of injured and healed eyes.

On the magical layer of reality any dja-fraction measurable with this archetypical measuring cup was considered to have an equal efficacy (Pommerening 2003a/b), which became part of the therapy. The healing effects were increased during the act of measuring as soon as the ancient Egyptian healer recited a particular incantation. For example: 'Spell for the *dbḥ*-measuring vessel when it is taken in order to measure a medicine. As far as this *dbḥ*-measuring-vessel is concerned in which I will measure this remedy: This is the *dbḥ*-measuring-vessel in which Horus has measured his eye, being corrected. Life, well-being and happiness were found. This remedy is being measured in this measure in order to drive away all diseases with it which are in this body' (pHearst 13,17-14,2).

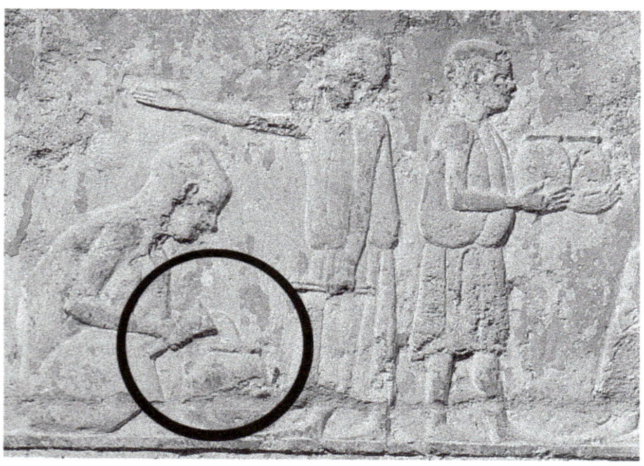

Figure 9: Unguentarius in the tomb of Petosiris

The measuring cup in use is shown in detail in a scene from the tomb of Petosiris (Cherpion et al. 2007; Lefebvre 1924) in which the preparation of ointments is depicted (Fig. 9). The two visual records – the only ones we have – therefore confirm the philological analysis, since the cup with its units dja and hin is used in a medicinal context.

The rediscovery of the dja and oipe measure as units of pharmaceutical measurement permits a more comprehensive understanding of the medicinal literature, materia medica, and the medical concepts of the ancient Egyptians. This is what I am investigating in my project, under the title 'Prescriptions of Ancient Egypt – Philology, cultural history, and pharmacology'.

Acknowledgements

I wish to express my sincere thanks to Rainer Broemer, Mainz, and to John Campbell, Manchester, for correcting my English and discussing this paper.

References

Bardinet, T. (1995) *Les papyrus médicaux de l'Égypte pharaonique: Traduction intégrale et commentaire.* Fayard, p. 271.

Cherpion, N. and J.-P. Corteggiani and J.-F. Gout (2007) *Le tombeau de Pétosiris à Touna el-Gebel. Relevé photographique*, Le Caire, p. 41.

Daressy, G. (1897) Deux vases gradués du Musée de Ghizeh. *Bulletin de l'Institut d'Égypte*, sér. 3, no. 8, pp. 149-152.

von Deines, H. and H. Grapow and W. Westendorf (1958) Übersetzung der medizinischen Texte. *Grundriss der Medizin der Alten Ägypter* IV/1, Berlin, pp. 142-143.

Ebbell, B. (1937) *The Papyrus Ebers: The Greatest Egyptian Medical Document.* Levin and Munksgaard, p. 44.

Grapow, H. (1958) Die medizinischen Texte in hieroglyphischer Umschrift autographiert. *Grundriss der Medizin der Alten Ägypter* V, Berlin, p. 249.

Kurth, D. (1996) Die Ritualszene mit den medizinischen Instrumenten im Tempel von Kom Ombo (Nr. 950). In Schade-Busch, M. (ed.) *Wege öffnen. Festschrift für Rolf Gundlach zum 65. Geburtstag*, ÄAT 35, Wiesbaden, pp. 153, 150.

Lefebvre, G. (1924) *Le tombeau de Pétosiris, Troisième Partie: Vocabulaire et Planches*, Le Caire, p. X.

Lucas A. and A. Rowe (1940) Ancient Egyptian Measures of Capacity. *Annales du service des antiquités de l'Égypte* 40, pp. 69-92.

Pommerening, T. (2003a) Neues zu den Hohlmaßen und zum Medizinalmaßsystem. In Loprieno, A. and Bickel, S. (eds.), *Basel Egyptology Prize 1. Junior Research in*

Egyptian History, Archaeology, and Philology, Aegyptiaca Helvetica 17, pp. 201-219

Pommerening, T. (2003b) Altägyptische Rezepturen metrologisch neu interpretiert. *Berichte zur Wissenschaftsgeschichte* 26, pp. 1-16.

Pommerening, T. (2005) Die altägyptischen Hohlmaße. *Studien zur altägyptischen Kultur* 10, pp. 239-261.

Pommerening, T. (2006) Überlegungen zur Wirksamkeit altägyptischer Arzneimittel aus heutiger Sicht. In Zibelius Chen, K. and Fischer-Elfert, H.-W. (eds.), *Von reichlich ägyptischem Verstande. Festschrift für Waltraud Guglielmi zum 65. Geburtstag*. Wiesbaden, pp. 103-112.

Westendorf, W. (1999) *Handbuch der altägyptischen Medizin, Handbuch der Orientalistik. Erste Abteilung. Der Nahe und Mittlere Osten* 36. Brill, pp. 6-79.

THE HISTORICAL TREATMENT OF MUMMIES AND THE IMPACT UPON MUSEUMS TODAY

G. Scott

University of York

Abstract: *The historical treatment of ancient Egyptian human mummies has been long, varied and in some cases, brutal. The unwrapped bodies that we see in museums today are the 'survivors' of these past deeds, but our desire to learn more about the people of ancient Egypt has left us in a quandary. How useful are these fragile unwrapped bodies for museum displays and scientific research considering their often vague histories? The following paper is a more detailed insight into the author's current PhD research following a poster presented at the Manchester conference. It aims to demonstrate how, by understanding what has gone before, museum staff and researchers can potentially avoid further damaging these ancient remains unnecessarily. The thesis also aims to aid the aforementioned groups with the creation of a detailed database documenting all known specimens within the UK. This thesis is now in its final stages and the results will be available in early 2011.*

Key words: mummification, unwrapping, 19th century, science, museums

Background

There is clear evidence within ancient Egyptian funerary texts that the mummified body was of crucial importance for the afterlife. In Ani's *Book of the Dead*, there are multiple passages which speak of horrors such as decay, mutilation and burning being inflicted upon the mummified body (Budge 1895; Faulkner 1985). However, if we investigate the long history of mummies and their treatment, we discover that many have been subjected to these very things.

Over the course of time, thousands of mummified bodies have been lost to us through medical enquiry, thievery, carelessness and even war. Written records from the 11th century onwards show us that Egypt was *the* place to find bitumen for medicinal use, as it was believed to coat the mummified bodies of the dead. However, as it is quite apparent that real bitumen was not employed by the ancient Egyptians in their funerary practices until much later on in their history, the likelihood of the blackened material covering the skin of mummies being pitch was often highly unlikely, but bodies were ground up in their thousands nonetheless!

Yet by the 1800s the mummies themselves, rather than their dark coating, had become the desirable commodities. The trade in bodies from Egypt boomed following the expulsion of Napoleon's army from Egypt in 1801. Wealthy Europeans took the *Grand Tour* of the country and brought back *antikas* to amuse family and friends at soirees. Not only were mummies now used by anatomists for public unwrapping demonstrations in hospitals, they were now being unrolled in private quarters for entertainment also. However, that is not to say that no scientific study of any value took place during this period, since individuals such as physicians John Davidson (1833) and Thomas 'Mummy' Pettigrew (1834) wrote detailed accounts of their findings from unwrapping mummies, both of which were pioneering works for their time.

At the turn of the 20th century, the focus appeared to have shifted towards scientific analysis and microscopic techniques in particular to reveal insights into the lives of the ancient Egyptians. Alfred Lucas also published a significant work in 1926, which was revised by Nicholson and Shaw (2000), and is still used as reference material for Egyptologists and scientists today. In the UK however, there was relatively little within the field of mummy studies and public autopsies until 1908 when Dr Margaret Murray, the first curator of Manchester Museum's Egyptology collections, unrolled 'The Two Brothers' (published 1910), whose remains are now housed in the Manchester Museum. Following this came two World Wars whose casualties include mummified bodies held in the Museum of Liverpool (El Mahdy 1989) and Ranefer, the Medum mummy destroyed by an air raid in London (Lucas, revised by Harris, 1962).

In total, the evidence destroyed and the amount of information lost is astonishing. This was the inspiration for the current study, whose purpose is to evaluate the way in which mummies were treated in the past and examine how this has impacted upon the modern conservation and display of unwrapped bodies. This, in turn, also delves into the scientific potential of these specimens. Despite the fact that science is now very much at the forefront of Egyptology, in some circumstances a lack of understanding of the subject's past can potentially hinder rather than help in our quest for knowledge.

Material and Methods

With this in mind, the author has devised a research methodology (for which there is not the space here to give a detailed breakdown of the specifics such as parameters) that aims to investigate all known unwrapped mummified remains within the UK. This project is a significant one, as there is no published work known which outlines all the known specimens, and assesses their historical treatment and how this has and will affect us in the future in terms of research and curation.

This process has been split into stages, comprising of the initial investigation into museum holdings around the

United Kingdom, followed by field visits (where possible), proceeded by the main body of analysis. This will then allow the author to compare and contrast the data in order to assess the different techniques and treatments employed historically through to the present day on these remains. It was necessary to devise a specialised field recording form ready for when the site visits commenced so that information was recorded in a consistent manner. Using examples from the Cairo Museum animal mummy recording form (2000), those used in the scientific investigations of mummies by Aufderheide (2003) and forensic crime scene documents, the author's form was developed and initially implemented in the case of two mummified bodies. Following this, suitable refinements and adaptations were made and the form was then used to give continuity for all case studies within the thesis. In addition to detailed written observations, photographs of each mummy were taken (where possible) for the purpose of reference and cross-analysis. For visits where photographs could not be taken, images were acquired through the generosity of the institution.

Running parallel with this process, a computerised recording database was devised using Microsoft Access. This system was initially designed to create a concise, easily accessible recording system, where different fields, such as provenance or date, could be cross-referenced and assist with the results' analysis of multiple specimens. All known subjects and reference images have been entered on to this system. Each record has been assigned a unique reference number that can be tracked and updated by the administrator (i.e. the author). More importantly, there is also the future potential for this to be a useful research tool for conservators, curators and Egyptologists who wish to find examples of particular treatments or methods of unwrapping that could potentially assist with their own projects. At the end of the thesis it is hoped that there will be the opportunity to expand this database to include known Egyptian mummies in European collections and eventually those from the rest of the world, with additional scope to incorporate mummified remains from many other ancient cultures.

Progress to Date

Currently, over 28 unrolled mummies have been examined for this PhD, which although a small sample size, is the number made available to the author and reasonable inferences can still be drawn. One of the biggest problems encountered has been access to collections. Many museums and similar institutions are currently undergoing gallery redevelopment, meaning that direct access to certain remains has not been possible. Some museums have not been able to facilitate a visit for other reasons, and so the author has had to draw conclusions based upon information given by the museum combined with any existing literature. Clearly this does not maintain the desired level of consistency, although the potential extension of this project beyond the duration of the thesis means it will be possible to add information to the database and any conclusions that are currently being drawn. The date for completion of this research is September 2010.

References

Animal Mummy Project in the Cairo Museum (2000) *Recording form*. Available from: http://www.animalmummies.com/projectfiles/datasheet.html [Accessed 14 January 2007].

Aufderheide, A.C. (2003) *The Scientific Study of Mummies*. Cambridge University Press.

Budge, E.A.W. (1895) *The Book of the Dead: The Hieroglyphic Transcript and Translation into English of the Ancient Egyptian Papyrus of Ani*. Random House Publishing (Reprint 1960).

David, R. and Archbold, R. (2000) *Conversations with Mummies: New Light on the Lives of Ancient Egyptians*. The Madison Press Ltd.

Davidson, J. (1833) *An Address on Embalming Generally*. London.

El Mahdy, C. (1989) *Mummies, Myth and Magic in Ancient Egypt*. Thames and Hudson.

Faulkner, R.O. (1985) *The Ancient Egyptian Book of the Dead*. British Museum Publications.

Lucas, A. (1926) *Ancient Egyptian Materials and Industries*. Longman, Green and Co.

Lucas, A. (1962) *Ancient Egyptian Materials and Industries*. (4th edn. revised J.R. Harris). Edward Arnold.

Murray, M.A. (1910) *The Tomb of Two Brothers*. Manchester Museum Handbook.

Nicholson, P.N. and I. Shaw (Eds.) (2000) *Ancient Egyptian Materials and Technology*. Cambridge University Press.

Pettigrew, T.J. (1834) *A History of Egyptian Mummies*. London.

STOMATOLOGICAL INVESTIGATION OF EGYPTIAN MUMMIES FROM THE PTOLEMAIC PERIOD IN HUNGARY

I. Szikossy[1], H. Győry[2], B. Tolnai[3] and I. Pap[1]

[1] Department of Anthropology, Hungarian Natural History Museum, Hungary
[2] The Egyptian Department, Museum of Fine Arts, Budapest, Hungary
[3] Semmelweis University, Budapest

Abstract: *The excavation of the Gamhud cemetery was initiated by Fülöp Back, a Hungarian merchant, in 1907. It was started by Taudeusz Smolenski, the Polish archaeologist, and finished by Ahmed Bey Kamal from the Cairo Museum. Almost half of the excavated objects were sent to the National Museum of Budapest, Hungary. The archaeological artefacts are now housed in the Museum of Fine Arts, and the human remains are located in the Hungarian Natural History Museum, Department of Anthropology.*

The purpose of this study is to present data on the oral health and nutrition of the people who lived at Gamhud, Egypt during the Ptolemaic Period. Oral pathological investigations were carried out on the mummified individuals. The frequency of caries, pre mortem loss of teeth and cysts/abscesses were studied.

Key words: Gamhud, mummy, palaeostomatology, oral pathology.

Introduction

The Excavation of the Gamhud Cemetery: The excavation of the Gamhud cemetery was initiated by Fülöp Back, a Hungarian merchant, in 1907. It was started by Taudeusz Smolenski, the Polish archaeologist (Smolenski 1907, 1908, 1910), a student of Maspero, and finished by Ahmed Bey Kamal from the Cairo Museum. Kamal had already published a general report and discussion of the finds during the mission; all the coffins he found himself were described in detail (Kamal 1908).

In Cairo, the finds were divided into two parts: the first remained in the Egyptian Museum and the second was put at the disposal of Fülöp Back. Five blocks from the temple in Sharuna and five coffins from Gamhud were given to the Court Museum in Vienna, three coffins were given to the Academy Collection in Krakow, now the Museum of Archaeology, and the majority of the other objects were sent to the National Museum of Budapest (Győry 1998a; 1998b). The archaeological artefacts are now housed in the Museum of Fine Arts, and the human remains are in the Hungarian Natural History Museum (HNHM), Department of Anthropology.

The Gamhud Cemetery: The Gamhud cemetery, measuring 480 meters by 120 meters, formed a semi-circular band in the desert. The tombs were dug into the flat ground on demand. Some of them were in underground chambers, which were hollowed out, with grave upon grave laid out alongside each other at random. These richer tombs usually surrounded the central area, whereas the more obviously poorer people were buried directly into the ground. Unfortunately, the burial site was disturbed by the activity of both ancient and modern grave robbers. By the time the Gamhud cemetery was used mummification had become widespread in Egypt, and developed into a social and commercial practice, which led to a decline in standards. The process concentrated more on the elaborate and permanent outer wrappings than on the preservation of the body (Győry 1998a; 1998b).

Material and Methods

Material: In the years of 1936 and 1937 almost 40 ancient Egyptian wooden coffins were opened in the Museum of Fine Arts in Budapest. The work was headed by a young Egyptologist, Aladár Dobrovits, who later organized the first Egyptian exhibition in the museum (Dobrovits 1939). The anthropological material was moved to the Department of Anthropology in 1938, where it is stored under the inventory numbers of 3823–3856. The mummies were unwrapped – as this was a common habit of that time – by Lajos Bartucz, a leading anthropologist (Győry 1998b). Unfortunately the authors have not found any documents of the unwrapping procedure. Later, the material was investigated by János Nemeskéri. He and his co-author published the case of the nose prosthesis from the Gamhud Collection (Mérei and Nemeskéri 1958; 1959).

Today, the material is in poor condition; a small number of body parts of the mummies are still in mummified condition, but most of them are skeletonised. During our research we found a lot of taphonomic changes, e.g. discolourations, post mortem fractures and other damage. Many skeletons were incomplete or mixed. These alterations might have happened during transportation from Egypt to the Austro-Hungarian Monarchy via camel and horse, as well as transport from one Hungarian institute to another. The unwrapping process also caused some serious impairment of the material.

The estimated number of specimens in the Gamhud Collection of the HNHM is approximately 34-41. The remains of the dried soft tissue are clearly visible on the bones. Resin, the material used during the mummification process, can still be found on the skulls, in some cases within the skull cavity and on the postcranial bones. The soft tissue and resin remains hindered the ageing, the sexing and the oral pathological investigations as well.

Methods: The age of adults was estimated from the ossification degrees of the endocranial surfaces of cranial sutures (Farkas 1972) and those of the ectocranial surfaces (Meindl and Lovejoy 1985). Ageing of the postcranial elements of adults was made from changes in the symphyseal face of the pubis (Nemeskéri et al. 1960). Age estimation based on the ribs was carried out on the basis of Işcan et al. (1984, 1985). The age of children was estimated by the sequence of the eruption of deciduous and permanent teeth and by the length of bones (Schour and Massler 1941; Stloukal and Hanákova 1978; Ferembach et al. 1979). Sexing was carried out on the basis of sexually dimorphic features of the cranium and the postcranial bones (Éry et al. 1963). The stomatological study was based on 21 adult and 6 child skulls of Egyptian mummies which were suitable for oral pathological examination.

The paleostomatological investigation was conducted using the Szikossy method (Szikossy 1999). The oral pathologies were scored by visual inspection under artificial light. Dental lesions were surveyed with a probe, an excavator and a magnifier. The skulls were individually recorded on examination sheets. Existing as well as pre-mortem and post-mortem lost teeth were recorded. The carious teeth were recorded; the location of caries on the carious teeth and the degree of the dental lesions were also indicated. Only the examples where the apex of the probe got caught in the enamel were considered as caries.

Radicular cavities caused by cysts or abscesses as the results of dental and alveolar diseases were recorded. These cavities evolve from the histolytic effect of pus (abscesses) or the pressure of a cyst. Their origin cannot be ascertained in archaeological terms because of the lack of filling material. Therefore, the term cysts/abscesses will be used further on. It should be noted that in some cases the cysts/abscesses could not always be recognised with certainty, due to the mummified skin remains on maxillae and/or mandibles. This fact may affect the results.

The degree of crown abrasion and dental calculus were determined. Remaining radices were also recorded with distinction of completely abraded teeth and those ones caused by caries. Wisdom-teeth (M3) were included in the survey and evaluation as well.

Results

No of skulls studied: 21 (Males: 9, Females: 12)
No of teeth studied: 294
No of post mortem lost teeth: 217
No of pre mortem lost teeth: 14
No of skulls with pre mortem lost teeth: 7
No of carious teeth: 9
No of skulls with caries: 5
No of cysts/abscesses: 4
No of skulls with cysts/abscesses: 3

The number of the post mortem lost teeth is high, although this is partly due to the taphonomic changes. The number of carious teeth is low, 3.1 %, but we have to be careful in the interpretation of the results, as we have few examinable teeth due to the high rate of post-mortem tooth loss. We found a high rate of abrasion at the interproximal surface of teeth. The degree of abrasion was very high among subadults, due to the effect of food containing sand particles. Cysts/abscesses were rare in the sample. We found one case of probable medical treatment; both mandibular second premolars are pre-mortem absent, and both first molars are in a leaning position. It is very probable that the second premolars were pulled out in her life (Inv. No. 3825, 40-50 year old female).

Conclusion

The newly recovered Gamhud Collection has a special history. Although a lot of potential information has been lost during the last hundred years, the anthropological material provided data on the oral health of the people who lived at Gamhud in Egypt during the Ptolemaic Period. The number of caries was very low in the sample. The teeth are strongly abraded, due to the effect of food containing sand particles. Further investigation is planned to identify the food remains in the dental calculi.

Acknowledgements

This research was partly supported by the Hungarian Scientific Research Fund (OTKA No 61155).

References

Dobrovits, A. (1939) Az Egyiptomi Gyűjtemény. *The Egyptological Collection*. Budapest, pp. 69.

Éry, K.K., Kralovánszky, A. and Nemeskéri, J. (1963) Történeti népességek rekonctrukciójának reprezentációja. (A representative reconstruction of the historic population.) *Anthrop. Közl.* 7, pp. 41-49.

Farkas, Gy. (1972) Antropológiai praktikum I. (Anthropological practice I). *Szeged,* pp. 233.

Ferembach, D., Schwidetzky, I. and Stloukal, M. (1979) Empfehlungen für die Alters- und Geschlechtsdiagnose am Skelett. *Homo* 30, pp. 1–32.

Győry, H. (1998a) Antiquities from Gamhud in Budapest. *KMT. A Modern Journal of Ancient Egypt* 9/1, Spring, pp. 27-30.

Győry, H. (1998b) *Az első magyar ásatás Egyiptomban, 1907 – Válogatás a gamhudi ásatás leleteiből, 1997.* (The first Hungarian excavation in Egypt, 1907 – Selection from the artefacts of the Gamhud excavation, 1997.) Szépművészeti Múzeum Budapest, pp. 39.

Işcan, M.Y., Loth, S.R. and Wright, R.K. (1984) Age estimation from the rib by phase analysis: white males. *Journal of Forensic Sciences* 29, pp. 1094–1104.

Işcan, M.Y., Loth, S.R. and Wright, R.K. (1985) Age estimation from the rib by phase analysis: white females. *Journal of Forensic Sciences* 30, pp. 853–863.

Kamal, A.B. (1908) Fouilles a Gamhoud. *Annales du service des antiquités de l'Égypte* 9, pp. 8-30.

Meindl, R. S. and Lovejoy, C. O. (1985) Ectocranial Suture Closure: A Revised Method for the Determination of Skeletal Age at Death Based on the Lateral-Anterior Sutures. *American Journal of Physical Anthropology* 68, pp. 57-66.

Mérei, Gy. and Nemeskéri, J. (1958) Paleopathológiai vizsgálatok ó-egyiptomi múmiákon. (Reserches paléopathologiques sur des momies Égyptiennes.) *Anthropológiai Közlemények* I/3-4, pp. 81-84.

Mérei, Gy. and Nemeskéri, J. (1959) Bericht über eine bei einer Mumie verwendete Nasenprothese. *Zeitschrift für ägyptische Sprache und Altertumskunde* 84, pp. 76–78.

Nemeskéri, I., Harsányi, L. and Acsádi, Gy. (1960) Methoden zur Diagnose des Lebensalters von Skeletfunden. *Anthrop. Anzeiger* 24, pp. 103-115.

Schour, J. and Massler, M. (1941) The development of the human dentition. *Journal of the American Dental Association* 28, pp. 1153-1160.

Smolenski, T. (1907) Le tombeau d'un prince de la VIe dynastie a Charouna. *Annales du service des antiquités de l'Égypte* 8, pp. 149-153.

Smolenski, T. (1908) Les vestiges d'un temple ptolémaique a Kom-el-Ahmar, pres de Charouna. *Annales du service des antiquités de l'Égypte* 9, pp. 3-6.

Smolenski, T. (1910) Nouveaux vestiges du temple de Kom-el-Ahmar pres de Charouna. *Annales du service des antiquités de l'Égypte* 10, pp. 26-27.

Stloukal, M. and Hanáková, H. (1978) Die Lange der Langsknochen altslawischer Bevölkerungen unter besonderer Berücksichtigung von Wachstumsfragen. *Homo* 29, pp. 53-69.

Szikossy, I. (1999) Studies on oral pathology in the cemetery of Vörs–Papkert B, Western Hungary. *Annls hist.-nat. Mus. natn. hung.* 91, pp. 219-230.

THE EBERS PAPYRUS' TREATISE ON TUMOURS 857-877 AND THE PHYTO-PHARMACOPOEIA PRESCRIBED

P.A. Veiga

KNH Centre for Biomedical Egyptology, The University of Manchester, UK

Abstract: *This paper focuses on part of my MSc dissertation: the plants prescribed as treatments for the illnesses described in the 21 paragraphs of the last section of the Ebers Papyrus. This is a treatise on tumours, which is now considered to relate to oncological concerns, bearing in mind the problem of the translations made so far, as some plants are still unidentified today.*

This paper will include a brief discussion of the Papyrus Ebers' description of pathogenic elements connected to the diseases referred to in this Treatise of Tumours and the phyto-pharmacopoeia prescribed will also be discussed.

Key words: Papyrus Ebers, Treatise, Tumours, pharmacopoeia

Papyrus Ebers: Description and Editions Published

This papyrus contains 877 prescriptions (Ebeid 1999, 23). As with other ancient Egyptian literature, it is considered likely to have been compiled from more ancient copies, with the knowledge contained within it being passed from generation to generation of doctors or *swnw* (Joachim 1997).

The Ebers Papyrus is a scroll measuring 0.30 x 18.63 m, dating to the reign of Amenhotep I, c.1553-1550 BC (Bryan 1930: 2). It is kept today in the University Library of Leipzig's special collections department. Unfortunately, some columns were damaged during the Second World War. It is written from right to left, in Hieratic, in black and red ink, and it is not accessible to the public for conservation reasons. The papyrus comprises 110 pages, and includes a last section on tumours (the so-called oncological concerns).

Several editions of this papyrus have been published – these are listed under *Appendix I: Editions of the Ebers Papyrus*. In 1987, Paul Ghalioungui, the head of the medical department at Ain Shams University in Egypt, provided a new English translation, based largely on the *Grundriss*, along with the support and encouragement of Wolfhart Westendorf; unfortunately the book, although printed and bound, was not on sale until 2004, 17 years after Ghalioungui's death (Farag 2005). Different translations of the Ebers Papyrus (EP) have produced different interpretations of words; therefore, the conclusions made by both Egyptologists and medical specialists can differ and influence the probable diagnosis.

The Ebers Papyrus and the Pathogenic Elements

The ancient Egyptians thought that the body contained *mtw*, and that these were both the carriers of bodily fluids, and were subject to obstructions that resulted in disease. They were not far from reality, as the human body is really a 'territory' served by highways and smaller roads, or more appropriately, by rivers and smaller affluents, that make its functioning dependent on the 'traffic': what we ingest; random exterior influences like infections and traumas: and, as the ancient Egyptians thought, untreatable conditions like cancer. Almost all of the authors studying ancient Egyptian medicine agree about the functions of the *mtw*.

The *metu*, *mtw*, can be interpreted as muscles and tendons, the vessels and ducts of the body together with the substances that flow through them such as blood, *senef*, (*snfw*) and urine *weseshet* (*wsš*) (Nunn 1996). Comparisons were drawn between these and the Nile, its tributaries, and its flow. As Ghalioungui states, quoting Marti-Ibañez, 'the physiology of ancient Egypt stated the existence of conduits in the human body to carry the blood and humours, where obstructions caused floods in some parts of the body and droughts in others (...). But the *mtw*, that conveyed health, could also carry disease' (Ghalioungui 1973, 57).

The *mtw* also converge in the anus (Majno 1975, 116; 129), and, if obstructed, gave rise to pathologies of all kinds. According to Ghalioungui, the *mtw* can contain air, water, faeces, blood, urine, sperm or mucus; disease appears when a certain matter is found in its improper place in the *mtw* (Ghalioungui 1987, 264). Sometimes, the described pathologies have recognisable symptoms such as obstructions, but also frequently untranslatable words such as *wekhedu (wḫdw)*. *Wekhedu* is written as a plural, but syntactically it is not a plural according to Grapow in the Grundriss (Majno 1975, 485, note 226). It is translated as purulence by Ebbell (1937, 130) or the word *aaa* (*ꜥꜣꜥ*) is used. These were considered to be malevolent substances which were the carriers of disease and transmitters of pain and pathology (Strouhal 1992, 245).

The *wḫdw* originated from a type of putrid process in the intestine and these substances circulated all over the body. Their removal was vital, and therefore ancient Egyptians carried out daily purges in order to make their bodies pure and cleanse them of disturbing substances and infections of all kinds. According to written sources like the medical papyri, these would be the provocative agents or circulating pathogens: the aforementioned ꜥ3ꜥ and *wḫdw*.

ꜥ3ꜥ is mentioned 28 times in the Ebers Papyrus, and, according to Ghalioungui, can be caused by a parasite (Ghalioungui 1973, 58-59); this would be consistent with an infection like schistosomiasis. However, this identification is doubtful because there are no references to hematuria in the fifty known prescriptions mentioning ꜥ3ꜥ and the ancient Egyptians were not able to identify microscopic parasites (Ghalioungui 1973, 60; Daglio 1998, 45). The only possible references to hematuria are in Ebers 49, referring to the word *wesesh* (urine) (Nunn and Tapp 2000). Although they were unable to identify microscopic parasites they often recognised the cause of a disease correctly as being a worm. However, if the determinative hieroglyph for ꜥ3ꜥ is a discharging phallus, this may be a possible visual aid for the schistosomiasis disease, an example of an infectious disease present in ancient Egyptian times.

Phyto-pharmacopoeia Prescribed by the Treatise of Tumours

From the German editions consulted the Ebers Papyrus paragraphs 857-877 (Westendorf 1961; 1999) translations made from the original writings including the use of plants as treatments and the number of applications, are described in the 21 paragraphs concerning tumours and the paragraphs concerning liver diseases (477-481) and these are given in Table 1 at the end of the manuscript. Other authors were consulted for more information on the plants' characteristics and meaning in ancient Egyptian thought (e.g. Manniche 1989; Loret 1887).

Some Italian forensic scientists (Lippi et al.) have already carried out research on ancient Egyptian medicine related to the Ebers Papyrus. They state that most of the anticancer agents available today in the oncology clinic are derived from plants (Lippi 2008). Contemporary plants used to treat liver infections include the native Egyptian glycyrrhizin (*Glycyrrhiza glabra*), which induces the production of natural interferon and protects and heals the liver cells from damage. It also acts as an anti-allergic, anti-inflammatory and detoxifying element. Olive (*Olea europaea*) leaf extract is another example; this interferes with the specific amino acid production processes vital for the life cycle of the virus and also interferes with viral invasion by inactivating the virus and prohibiting its shedding, budding or assembly at the cell membrane.

Strouhal claims that, although some authors state that malignant tumours are rare to find in ancient Egypt, literature favours the occurrence of these neoplasias, especially the EP that describes 21 cases. This is an indicator that, as well as the fact that this population may have been less exposed to these diseases, there is also a lack of material to study. This is not only because this type of disease is difficult to detect in ancient tissues (including bone tissue) but also because not everything has been excavated yet. The more cases that are studied, the more information we get about age, social rank, geographical location and gender of affected individuals, as well as about the specificity of the tumours.

Editions of the Ebers Papyrus

Ebers, G.M. and Stern, L. (1875) *Papyrus Ebers. Das hermetische Buch über die Arzneimittel der alten Aegypter in hieratischer Schrift, mit Inhaltsangabe und Einleitung versehen Mit hieroglyphisch-latei-nischem.* A facsimile with a partial translation, 2 volumes, Engelmann, Leipzig.

Joachim, H. (1890) *Papyros Ebers*, The first complete translation from the Egyptian. G. Reimer.

Wreszinski, W., (1913) *The papyrus Ebers, Transcription, translation and comment, I part: Transcription*, Leipzig.

Von Klein, C.H., (1905) *The Medical Features of the Papyrus Ebers*, English translation, publication announced and subject by 1000 subscriptions needed to undergo the endeavour; consisted of 650 pages, in red and black, similar to the original, with six plates in one volume, Chicago, USA: biology.bard.edu/ferguson/course/bio407/Carpenter_et_al_(1998).pdf;infoshare1.princeton.edu/rbsc2/pamphlets/Call_number_D810.P6.P356/185-%20contents%20listing.pdf)

Ebbell, B., (1937) *The papyrus Ebers, The greatest Egyptian Medical document*. Levin and Munksgaard.
Also available online at the University of Heidelberg Library:
http://www.ub.uniheidelberg.de/helios/fachinfo/www/aegypt/digilit/

References

Bardinet, T. (1995) *Les papyrus médicaux de l'Égypte pharaonique, traduction intégrale et commentaire.* Fayard.

Bryan, C.P. (1930) *Ancient Egyptian Medicine: The Papyrus Ebers*, translated from the German Version. Ares Publishers.

Carvalho, L.M. (2004) *The Gift of the Nile or the Use of Plants in Ancient Egypt*. Botanical Museum, Instituto Politécnico de Beja.

Creasy, W.A. (1969) Antitumoral Activity of the Fern Cibotium schiedei. *Nature* 222, pp. 1281-1282.

Daglio, C. (1998) *La medicina dei faraoni: malattie, ricette e superstizioni dalla farmacopea egizia*. Ananke.

Ebbell, B. (1937) *The Papyrus Ebers: the greatest Egyptian medical document*. Levin and Munksgaard.

Ebeid, N.I. (1999) *Egyptian medicine in the days of the pharaohs*. General Egyptian Book Organization.

Ebers, G. (1875) *Papyros Ebers. Das Hermetische Buch über die Arzneimittel der alten Ägypter in hieratischer Schrift* (Band 1): Einleitung und Text, Leipzig, 1875, http://digi.ub.uni-heidelberg.de/diglit/ebers1875bd1/ [accessed September, 1, 2008]

Farag, Talaat I. *The Unveiled Ebers Papyrus*, http://ambassadors.net/archives/issue17/selectedstudy4.htm

Faulkner, R.O. (1962) *A Concise Dictionary of Middle Egyptian*, Griffith Institute.

Ghalioungui, P. (1968) La notion de maladie dans les textes égyptiens et ses rapports avec la théorie humorale, *BIFAO* 66, IFAO, pp. 37-48.

Ghalioungui, P. (1973) *The House of Life: Per Ankh. Magic and Medical Science in Ancient Egypt* (2nd edition). B.M. Israel

Ghalioungui, P. (1987) *The Ebers papyrus: a new English translation, commentaries and glossaries*. Academy of Scientific Research and Technology.

Győry, H, (2006) *La Chirurgie dans l'Égypte ancienne*. presentation at the 40th International Congress of the History of Medicine, Budapest, August, 26-30, 2006, http://www.ishm2006.hu/scientific/abstract.php?ID=214 [accessed 30 August 2008]

Liber Herbarum, http://www.liberherbarum.com/Index.htm [accessed June 2, 2008]

Lippi, D. (1990). An aneurysm in the papyrus of Ebers (108, 3-9). *Medicina nei Secoli Arte e Scienza Journal of History of Medicine* 2, pp. 4.

Lippi, D., Bausi, L., Nobili, S., Mini, E. and Capaccioli, S. (2008) *Natural Compounds for Cancer Treatment and Prevention*. Florence (abstract): http://www.mdpi.org/ijms/specialissues/ncctp.htm [accessed 24 August 2008]

Loret, V. (1887) *La Flore Pharaonique d'après les documents hiéroglyphiques et les spécimens découverts dans les tombes*. Librairie J. B. Baillière and Fils.

Majno, G. (1975) *The Healing Hand, Man and Wound in the Ancient World*. Harvard University Press.

Manniche, L., (1989) *An Ancient Egyptian Herbal*. British Museum Press.

Montbriand, M.J. (2004) Herbs or Natural Products that protect against cancer growth, Part Three of a Four-Part Series, *Oncology Nursing Forum* 31 (6), pp. 127-146.

Nunn, J.F. (1996) *Ancient Egyptian Medicine*. British Museum Press.

Nunn, J.F. and Tapp, E. (2000) Tropical diseases in Ancient Egypt. *Transactions of the Royal Society of Tropical Medicine and Hygiene* 94, 147-153.

Osborn, D. (1968) Notes on Medicinal and other uses of plants in Egypt. *Economic Botany* 22, pp. 165-177.

Papyrus Ebers: http://www.medizinische-papyri.de/Papyrus_Ebers/ [accessed August, 20, 2008]

Strouhal, E. (1978) Ancient Egyptian case of carcinoma. *Bulletin New York Academy Medicine* 54, pp. 290-302.

Strouhal, E. (1991) Myeloma multiplex versus Osteolytic Metastic Carcinoma: Differential Diagnosis in Dry Bones. *International Journal of Osteoarchaeology* 1, pp. 219-224.

Strouhal, E. (1992) *Life of the Ancient Egyptians*. University of Oklahoma Press.

Strouhal, E. (2005a) *Evidence of Some Rare Pathologies from the New Kingdom Necropolis at Saqqara*. Wiesbaden.

Strouhal, E. (2005b) Examination of Mummies from the Tomb of Iufaa at Abusir (Egypt). In Massa, E.R. (ed). *V World Congress on Mummy Studies*. Compagnia di San Paolo.

Strouhal, E., A. N., Ecaron, Me, Ccaron and Ková, M. K. (2003) Palaeopathology of Iufaa and other persons found beside his shaft tomb at Abusir (Egypt). *International Journal of Osteoarchaeolog*, 13, pp. 331-338.

Strouhal, E. and Nemecková, A. (2004) Palaeopathological find of a sacral neurilemmoma from ancient Egypt. *American Journal of Physical Anthropology* 125, pp. 320-328.

Strouhal, E. and Jungwirth, J. (1980a) Paleopathology of the Late Roman-Early Byzantine Cemeteries at Sayala, Egyptian Nubia. *Journal of Human Evolution* 9, pp. 61-70.

Strouhal, E. and Vyhnanek, L. (1980b) *Egyptian mummies in the Czechoslovak collections*. Prague.

Strouhal, E. and Vyhnanek, L. (1981) New cases of malign tumours from Late Period cemeteries at Abusir and Saqqara (Egypt). *Ossa* 8, pp. 165-189.

Strouhal, E.A. (1999) Kissing osteochondroma: A case from Ancient Egypt. *International Journal of Osteoarchaeology* 9, pp. 361-368.

Temkin, O. (1938) Review of The Papyrus Ebers by B. Ebbell. *Isis 28*, pp. 126-131.

Terebinth:
http://www.violins.ca/varnish/violin_varnish_glossary.html
[accessed on July 17, 2008]

University of Leipzig, Papyrus Ebers, 2004:
http://www.uni-leipzig.de/ub/Wir_ueber_uns/sosa/scholl_4.htm
[accessed August, 20, 2008]

Wessely, C. (1931) Synopsis florae magicae. *BIFAO* 30, pp. 17-26.

Westendorf, W. (1999) *Handbuch der altägyptischen Medizin*. Brill.

Westendorf, W. and Von Deines, H. (1961) *Wörterbuch der medizinischen Texte*. Erste Hälfte; Akademie Verlag.

Yu, O. and Wong, S.L. (2004) *Secrets of Medicine in Ancient Egypt* In Whitelaw, W. A., (ed). *13th Annual History of Medicine Days*. Health Sciences Centre; Calgary, Canada.

Name of Plants	TT	L
Fruit *išd* from the persea tree The *ished* or persea tree existed in ancient Egypt and is recorded in literature from the pharaonic Period. The edible fruit is about 4 cm long and samples were found in Tutankhamun's tomb. Leaves were found in garlands like the one from Ramesses II. The fruit of the persea comes to maturity at the time of the Nile's rise so, it is associated with fecundity. The tree is shown in many tombs as surrounding the owner/king or not. The fruit resembled a heart and the leave a tongue, related in mythology to Thoth as he inscribed the king's name when ascending the throne. Spells 17 and 335 from The Book of the Dead show the *ished* tree and it is also mentioned in the Coffin Texts.		477 480
Bryony		477
pr.t-šny fruit (umbrella Pine of Byblos (Yu,2004))		478
Terebinth resin/frankincense Ebbell refers to this one as frankincense (Ghalioungui 1987: 237)	861	477 478 479 480
Acacia leave/thorn The thorn of an acacia seems to have been used for cutting up blisters; Ebers 504 says: "Another remedy for driving out the white spot of burn: *kšw* mineral 1, honey 1, fruit of the carob 1. It has to be pricked by the thorn of an acacia and ointed with them" (Győry 2006: 1). 'Kind of' acacia A tea made with dried flowers from acacia is used for treating gall bladder troubles in Kharga and Dakhleh Oases (Osborn 1968) gum	858 861 862 5 1	477
Sycamore figs (ripen fruit) The milky juice of the sycamore was used to heal wounds and abscesses		477 480 481
Figs		477 478 479 480 481
Peas	858 859 860 4	
Melon	858 (?)	
Barley grains Barley is one of the natural products to be considered potentially protective against cancer growth (Montbriand, 2004).		
Jujube bread/flour Jujube (wood powder, from bark?)		479 480 1
Long beans, (from lotus?)/ bean flour Leaves	857 (?) 858 859 877	
Juniper berries		479 481
Wine Raisins Grapes		477 479 478 480
Sweet beer		479 480
Onion bulbs	859	
Date syrup /wine/juice	859	
Cumin	859 861 862	
Fruit of *pyrethrum* (anti histaminic?)	2	
Honey	2	
Valerian ?	860	
Plant/fruit	2	
Incense (frankincense, myrrh)	861	

Table 1: Phyto-pharmacopeia prescribed by the Treatise on Tumours (TT) and liver (L) diseases' paragraphs

www.ingramcontent.com/pod-product-compliance
Lightning Source LLC
LaVergne TN
LVHW071217210926
848482LV00015B/830